D0004602

The
Psychiatry of Stroke

BY
D. Peter Birkett, M.D.

The
Psychiatry of Stroke

BY
D. Peter Birkett, M.D.

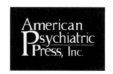

Washington, DC
London, England

Note: The author has worked to ensure that all information in this book concerning drug dosages, schedules, and routes of administration is accurate as of the time of publication and consistent with standards set by the U.S. Food and Drug Administration and the general medical community. As medical research and practice advance, however, therapeutic standards may change. For this reason and because human and mechanical errors sometimes occur, we recommend that readers follow the advice of a physician who is directly involved in their care or the care of a member of their family.

Books published by the American Psychiatric Press, Inc., represent the views and opinions of the individual authors and do not necessarily represent the policies and opinions of the Press or the American Psychiatric Association.

Copyright © 1996 American Psychiatric Press, Inc.
ALL RIGHTS RESERVED
Manufactured in the United States of America on acid-free paper
99 98 97 96   4 3 2 1
First Edition

American Psychiatric Press, Inc.
1400 K Street, N.W., Washington, DC   20005
Library of Congress Cataloging-in-Publication Data
Birkett, D. Peter.
    The psychiatry of stroke / D. Peter Birkett. — 1st ed.
        p.   cm.
    Includes bibliographical references and index.
    ISBN 0-88048-540-X
    1. Cerebrovascular disease—Psychological aspects. I. Title.
    [DNLM: 1. Cerebrovascular Disorders. 2. Cerebrovascular
Disorders—psychology.   WL 355 B619p 1996]
    RC388.5.B566   1996
    616.8'1—dc20
    DNLM/DLC   95-17692
    for Library of Congress   CIP
British Library Cataloguing in Publication Data
A CIP record is available from the British Library.

Contents

Part III. Outcome and Effects

Acknowledgments

In writing this book I have become deeply indebted to Roger Baretz and Latif Desouky for criticism and advice, to Mary Rafferty and Frank Appell for helpful and expert librarianship, to Hannelore Renud for secretarial and linguistic skills, and to Michael Hancock for computer expertise.

At American Psychiatric Press, Carol Nadelson, Claire Reinburg, Pamela Harley, and other editorial staff and reviewers contributed greatly. It has been a pleasure to work with Rebecca Richters, who has shown exemplary patience, attention to detail, and literary skill as project editor.

The illustrations were largely done by Ben Harris, using the CANVAS program. Several authors of first-person accounts have given generous permission to quote from their hard-won knowledge.

I owe more than I can say to my patients, and to Dylan, Rebecca, Susannah, and Isabella.

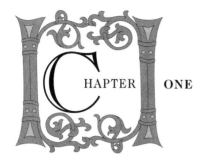

Introduction

This book is to meant to guide those who must deal with the behavioral and emotional disturbances that arise in stroke. Psychiatrists who treat stroke patients may find it of special interest, but the larger purpose of this work is to improve the treatment of stroke by increasing the attention paid to its emotional and intellectual aspects. Because those involved in treating stroke patients come from many and various disciplines, I have made an assumption of knowledge at a professional level, but have tried to write so that specialists in one field can understand contributions made to the subject from other fields. To make the book more widely understandable, technical terms are defined in the Glossary, and Appendix A explains the relevant basic neuro-anatomy in simple terms.

Several developments have led to this text being offered at this time. These include the advent of new brain-imaging techniques, greater precision in psychiatric diagnosis, new organic treatment methods, more recognition of the psychiatric needs of patients in nursing homes, increased psychiatric interest in dementia, and the development of the specialized field of geriatric psychiatry. There is increased medical interest in the treatment of chronically ill patients with multiple medical and psychiatric disabilities. With this heightened attention has come a realization that the limits to therapy and rehabilitation are largely set by mental impairment—and that because such impairment may be treatable, it must be evaluated.

Existing literature on the topic often emphasizes either neuropsychiatry or social psychiatry. Neuropsychiatrists and neuropsychologists are primarily concerned with the physical foundations of particular syndromes related to stroke. This is not a trivial preoccupation, because much of our knowledge of the relationships among brain, mind, and behavior comes from study of stroke, but often that knowledge seems remote from clinical psychiatry. Conversely, social psychiatrists are mostly concerned with the social and economic consequences of stroke, which are undeniably important; however, to alter these factors demands changes in the health care delivery system that are mostly outside the scope of the individual practitioner. Thus, a gap exists that needs to be filled. I attempt in this book to integrate the contributions of disparate fields to knowledge about stroke, emphasizing that of clinical psychiatry.

In deciding what material to include, I envisaged a health professional who is treating a stroke patient, encounters a psychiatric problem, and needs information about it. Because the advent of computerized literature searches has probably lessened the need for a comprehensive review of the literature on stroke, such a review is not attempted, although some classical papers, such as those that have given rise to eponyms, are discussed. In certain areas of controversy, fairness demands that the literature review be at a level of detail that may be tedious to those seeking a general overview of the subject. Such detailed reviews, and also summaries of papers containing single case reports, have been arranged so that they are preceded by more elementary outlines and can be skipped easily.

Part I of the book concerns the background and causative factors of stroke. Also covered is the basic science relevant to stroke. Part II describes the specific syndromes produced by stroke. Part III addresses the outcome and psychosocial consequences of stroke. Thus, Part I trespasses on neurology and Part III on social psychiatry.

Terminology dichotomizing the physical and the mental is used loosely. In many cases the terms *psychiatric* and *psychological* are used in antithesis to *organic* and *neurological*. Such loose terminology, or the existence of such a dichotomy, could be disputed, but the context should make clear what is meant. I use pronouns that reflect the sex incidence of the conditions discussed.

The broad intended audience of this book has inevitably resulted in inconsistencies in voice and level of sophistication, as well as variations in style. I hope that these stylistic errors are in the direction of oversimplification. Neurologists and internists may find Part I to be oversimplified, and psychiatrists may find Part II to be so. Simplification may be perceived as dogmatism by some readers, and their indulgence is requested. This especially applies to material that has been highly condensed and put in tabular form. Despite scientific advances, psychiatry continues to be a field in which opinions differ.

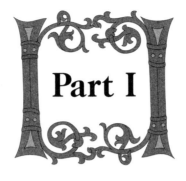

Part I

Background and Causation

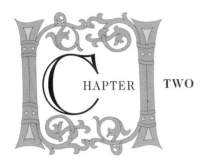

CHAPTER TWO

Diagnosis of Stroke

Defining Stroke

Someone who experiences a sudden attack of unconsciousness, then becomes paralyzed on one side and loses the power of speech probably has had a stroke, but ambiguities arise from any attempt to define more precisely what the word *stroke* means. Families often ask whether a patient's psychiatric illness could be due to a stroke. They may ask this because of the presence of physical symptoms at the onset of the illness, the suddenness of onset, the presence of stroke risk factors, or the finding of abnormalities on computed tomography (CT) scans or magnetic resonance imaging (MRI). The answer to the question "Was it a stroke?" may be needed to decide on an appropriate therapy, in which case the next questions probably will be about what is going on in the patient's brain: Is there an infarct? Is there an artery obstruction? Is there an embolism? Is there bleeding?

Official nomenclatures mostly ignore nonphysical symptoms (see Table 2–1). The World Health Organization (WHO) defines *stroke* as "rapidly developing clinical signs of focal (at times global) disturbance of cerebral function, lasting more than 24 hours or leading to death with no apparent cause other than that of vascular origin" (Hatono 1976, p. 541). The major classifications used in the United States are those of the Stroke Data Bank (Gross et al. 1986; Kunitz et al. 1984; Mohr et al. 1978) and the National Institute of Neurological Diseases and Stroke (NINDS; 1990).

The official definitions and classifications of stroke are largely neuropathological. Because they assume the ability to do a full physical examination and the availability of radiology facilities or autopsy follow-up, these definitions have only limited diagnostic usefulness in situations in which such opportunities and resources are not available—for instance, in research surveys of nonhospitalized populations (Bamford 1992; Gurland et al. 1977). However, less stringent diagnostic criteria can yield biased results; for example, a survey instrument that depends on self-reported symptoms rather than objectively observed signs can lead to overestimation of the association of stroke with depression and anxiety, because depressed and anxious respondents may be more likely than others to say that they have experienced strokelike symptoms (see also Chapter 3).

Silent and Inobvious Strokes

It is possible that some people with brain cavities produced by vascular disease have no symptoms at all. Such asymptomatic vascular events

Table 2–1.   Nomenclatures and instruments used in stroke diagnosis

World Health Organization definition of stroke	Rapidly developing clinical signs of focal (at times global) disturbance of cerebral function, lasting more than 24 hours or leading to death with no apparent cause other than that of vascular origin
Stroke Data Bank classification	Seven entities: 1) brain infarction due to atherosclerosis and distal insufficiency; 2) infarction of unproved etiology; 3) infarction due to embolism; 4) lacunar stroke; 5) parenchymal hemorrhage; 6) subarachnoid hemorrhage; and 7) TIA
National Institute of Neurological Diseases and Stroke classification	Four categories of cerebrovascular disease: 1) asymptomatic; 2) focal brain dysfunction; 3) vascular dementia; and 4) hypertensive encephalopathy. The focal brain dysfunction category contains two divisions: 1) TIA and 2) stroke.
Community survey instruments	Questionnaire (Gurland et al. 1977); recorded medical diagnosis (Bamford 1992)

Note.   TIA = transient ischemic attack.

have been referred to as *silent strokes* (Kempster et al. 1988). It is not always certain how silent these silent strokes really are. A stroke may produce neurological signs other than obvious hemiplegia. Although some of these signs may be quite subtle, they can be revealed in a full and careful examination by a skilled clinician, especially if the patient is alert and cooperative. Further uncertainty is added by the fact that published studies of this phenomenon often do not consider psychiatric symptoms. No difference in terminology has been formalized, but the term *silent* is more commonly used for strokes that produce no apparent nonpsychiatric clinical signs, and *inobvious* for those in which such signs were suspected and might have been found on full examination had one been carried out.

When a psychiatric patient is incidentally found to have an infarct on CT scan, he or she is not said to have had a stroke, as defined by NINDS, the Stroke Data Bank, and WHO. However, if a patient suddenly becomes mentally disturbed and is found to have a brain infarct that appears to have occurred at the same time as the onset of the disturbance, most physicians would probably say that patient had had a slight stroke.

Kase et al. (1989) found that among subjects with clinically diagnosed strokes in the Framingham study (a large, long-term study of the epidemiology of cardiovascular disease in a Massachusetts town), 10% showed CT evidence of previous strokes, which the authors referred to as "silent strokes." Retrospective examination of physicians' records showed no evidence of symptoms prior to the clinically diagnosed stroke, although the subjects might have had slight dementia that the records did not indicate as a symptom. Ricci et al. (1993) found CT evidence of a previous infarct in about one-third of a community sample of stroke patients. At 12-month follow-up of the entire sample, those patients with previous infarcts had no more dementia or disability than the rest.

Feinberg et al. (1990) carried out CT examination of the head on 141 asymptomatic patients with atrial fibrillation (a condition known to be a strong risk factor for stroke). Dementia patients and patients who had had strokes or transient ischemic attacks (TIAs) were excluded from the study. One-quarter of the asymptomatic patients were found to have probable infarcts on CT scan. Although most of the infarcts were small and deep, 13 patients had cortical or large, deep infarcts, and 12 had more than one infarct. The mean age of the patients with infarcts was 72 years; that of those without them was 67. Dunne et al. (1986) used the term *inobvious stroke* to describe patients who present with behavioral disturbance without accompanying physical symptoms. These authors found that, of patients who were hospitalized with a diagnosis of stroke, confirmed by CT scan or autopsy, excluding those with previous psychiatric or dementia histories, 3% presented with behavioral disturbance alone.

Transient Ischemic Attacks

In TIAs it is assumed that no brain tissue dies, and CT scans reveal no abnormalities. A reversible ischemic neurological defect (RIND) is a TIA that is less transient. Agreement among clinicians on the diagnosis of TIA is often far from unanimous (Landi 1992).

There is likewise disagreement about the use of the terms *minor stroke* and *little stroke*. These descriptors are sometimes applied to TIAs, sometimes to RINDS, and sometimes to small infarcts that give rise to strokes with limited symptoms.

Infarction Versus Hemorrhage

It used to be thought that parenchymal brain hemorrhage—bleeding into the substance of the brain—was an invariably fatal event with no impaired survivors. With the advent of the new imaging methods, however, small areas of hemorrhage have been recognized more frequently, and these often cannot be distinguished clinically from infarcts (Steinke et al. 1992). Subarachnoid hemorrhage differs considerably from infarction when a patient first presents for clinical examination, although survivors of such events have much in common with other stroke patients and often have mental impairment (Hütter 1993).

The New Brain-Imaging Techniques

The introduction of new brain-imaging techniques has added to our knowledge but generated new questions. Infarcts may be found in psychiatric patients who have no focal neurological signs or symptoms. Decisions must be made about which psychiatric patients should be subjected to scanning procedures, which can be frightening and may require patient cooperation and informed consent.

The two major imaging methods in clinical use are CT and MRI. Methods in research use are positron-emission tomography (PET), functional magnetic resonance imaging (fMRI, also called "fast MRI"), regional cerebral blood flow (rCBF), and a kind of rCBF called single photon emission computed tomography (SPECT). rCBF should be distinguished from methods—such as angiography—of determining whether arteries are obstructed. Regional blood flow may be reduced because a part of the brain is using less blood, even if there is no obstruction of the arteries.

Computed Tomography

An old infarct that has liquefied shows up clearly on a CT scan of the brain as a dark area. Before softening occurs, the picture is less clear, and immediately after the stroke, the CT is normal in 50% of cases (Bamford 1992).

Magnetic Resonance Imaging

MRI depends not on the radiopacity of objects but rather on the concentration of hydrogen ions or protons (in effect, how much water) they contain. Because nerve cell bodies contain more water than nerve fibers, the gray and white matter can be seen separately. There are two kinds of MRI pictures: T_1 and T_2.

Although MRI is very sensitive, cases have been described in which a patient with all of the signs and symptoms of a stroke—including hemiplegia and aphasia—had a negative MRI (Alberts et al. 1992; Besson et al. 1993).

MRI sometimes reveals areas of *rarefaction* that are not visible on CT scans. These areas are in the white matter, typically around the ventricles, and show up as high-intensity signals. (It can be confusing to hear the terms *high intensity* or *hyperintensity* used for an area that is [histologically speaking] an area of rarefaction. Such regions appear bright and white on the T_2 MRI because they are more watery.)

Functional MRI (fast MRI, or fMRI), which is still only in experimental use, can show the rate of oxygen use in different brain areas and has been used to indicate the localization of mental functions (David et al. 1994).

Positron-Emission Tomography

Available only on an experimental basis at present, PET scans reveal where the brain is working most actively by showing where the most glucose is being metabolized. In the most common PET method, a substance that goes through the same metabolic pathways as glucose is injected. This substance contains a positron-emitting isotope (which must be freshly produced in a cyclotron). The areas of the brain in which this is concentrated can be detected; these are areas of increased brain activity. The results of PET scans in patients with psychiatric disorders have suggested localizations of disturbed brain function that were not apparent from studies of brain injury and cerebral infarction. For example, decreased metabolism has been found in frontal areas in schizophrenic patients and in parietal areas in dementia patients. In patients with vascular dementia, the decreased brain activity may be in the parietal areas even if the infarct is not situated in these (see Chapter 16).

Regional Cerebral Blood Flow and Single Photon Emission Computed Tomography

rCBF estimation is an experimental procedure distinct from cerebral blood supply estimation, which is frequently performed in clinical practice. Cerebral blood supply measurement techniques (e.g., angiography) examine the patency of the artery; rCBF methods, on the other hand, determine how much blood the brain is using, and thus have more in common with PET than with angiography. Because rCBF techniques—unlike PET—do not demand a fresh supply of cyclotron-produced isotope, they are a little more widely available and less expensive than PET. An isomer of the inert gas xenon is mixed with the air the subject breathes for a few minutes. In the subsequent 10 minutes, the amount of the gas found in each part of the brain is measured. When CT is used for this measurement, the procedure is called SPECT.

Artery Investigations and Angiography

There are several ways of studying the blood supply to the brain. An old method, which still has advantages, was to inject a radiopaque dye into the carotid artery in the neck and take an X-ray picture (film/screen direct intra-arterial angiography). The decline of intra-arterial angiography may be responsible for the recent reduction in frequency of the diagnosis of obstruction of individual intracranial cerebral arteries.

Venous digital subtraction angiography replaced direct intra-arterial angiography for a while. Its advantage was that the dye could be injected into a vein rather than an artery; however, the images it produced were less clear than those from angiography and there was a risk of kidney damage from the dye.

Several examination techniques employing sound waves are in use. These include B-mode ultrasonography, which gives a picture of any bumps in the artery wall, and Doppler sonography, which measures the velocity of arterial flow. B-mode ultrasonography and Doppler sonography are combined in the technique called *duplex ultrasonography*. Although these commonly used techniques provide good information about the carotid arteries in the neck, they cannot detect artery disease inside the skull or in the vertebral arteries. Transcranial Doppler (TCD) can detect blockages of the basilar artery but is available in only a few centers. Magnetic resonance angiograms can provide pictures of intracranial arteries up to the circle of Willis, including the posterior, middle, and anterior cerebral arteries, but are still experimental.

Determining Which Patients Should Receive Further Tests

Deciding how extensively to investigate a psychiatric patient's physical state involves consideration of the extent to which the patient will cooperate with the investigation and benefit from it. It is reasonable to require a complete physical examination before resorting to more sophisticated technology. When stroke is suspected, several medical conditions must be ruled out, especially disorders of the heart and circulation such as hypertension, atrial fibrillation, and carotid stenosis. A detailed neurological examination includes inspection of the cranial nerves, optic fundi, visual fields, muscle power and tone, reflexes, and sensation. In addition to requiring patience and skill on the part of the examiner, such examinations necessitate a degree of patient cooperation of which mentally impaired persons may not be capable.

Several other medical tests are also needed, and the patient's reaction to these may be a useful guide as to whether brain imaging will be tolerated. If there is not enough cooperation to do a good physical examination and to get a readable chest X ray and electrocardiogram (ECG), then CT is not likely to be feasible.

MRI and CT both involve large and frightening machines. The CT scan is more informative if it is done with intravenously injected contrast. This usually means that the patient must sign a consent form, which can be problematic with some psychiatric patients. The newest CT machines can obtain an image with patients who are able to remain still for only a minute, so that it is often possible to obtain a usable image in a quiet patient with dementia who can follow simple commands, but it is impossible in the completely uncooperative violent patient.

For an MRI, the patient must lie recumbent for about 20 minutes in a small, confined space—a situation that can precipitate a panic attack even in individuals who have never had one before. Sedation with diazepam

(Valium) or lorazepam (Ativan) can be considered, but because stroke patients are often elderly and have heart problems, sedation must be carefully monitored and should be discussed by the primary care physician with the radiologist.

Personal contact by the referring physician will prepare the radiologist and X-ray technicians for the nervous or demented patient. Preliminary tours of the X-ray area and explanations can be helpful, as can be the presence of a family member or the patient's primary physician.

In practice, socioeconomic factors and family wishes often affect decisions about which investigations should be undertaken. The United States government is also involved because of the Omnibus Budget Reconciliation Act of 1987 (OBRA '87) rules, which mandate documentation of investigations for dementia in candidates for nursing-home placement who have psychiatric symptoms. In very elderly patients, the ethics and the risk-benefit ratio of elaborate tests may be questioned, but cases of dementia in young patients are usually fully investigated.

CT and MRI scans are often ordered for those with psychiatric conditions other than dementia. The implications of finding an infarct on CT in patients with such conditions will be considered in Part II of this volume.

Lacunes, Leukoareiosis, and Binswanger's Disease

The terminology used to describe abnormal spaces and areas of softening in the brain has become confusing. Because mental health professionals are often called upon to assess the clinical significance of radiology findings in psychiatric patients, they need to be aware of some fundamental brain-damage principles.

The basic concept remains that of the *infarct*. This is an area of the brain where tissue death has occurred because the blood supply has been cut off. Such areas soften and then liquefy to become fluid-filled cavities. Large fluid-filled cavities are readily identifiable on CT scan or at autopsy as infarcts; however, the confusion arises regarding what to call small cavities and areas of rarefaction without definite liquefaction.

Although the terms discussed in this section are often used descriptively by radiologists and neuropathologists today, in the original and classical descriptions these terms denoted actual disease entities, and some recent authors have also associated these names with specific clinical symptoms. Further compounding the issue is the fact that the original descriptions were based on autopsy examinations, whereas the more recent ones are based on CT and MRI findings. Thus, it is uncertain whether the terms as originally described and as used today actually represent the same entities.

Lacunes

Lacune[1] is sometimes used to denote any small hole or soft area in the brain, but there is confusion about the word's exact definition. Millikan and Futrell (1993) proposed that a small infarct should be called a small infarct, and that the term *lacune* should be used more generally for any small hole or soft area in the brain, regardless of whether it is caused by an infarct.

The first definition of lacunes was that of Marie (1901), who considered that they were distinct from infarcts, consisting rather of small holes in the brain and representing a discrete clinical entity that he termed *état lacunaire*.

Fisher (1969) described small infarcts due to specific types of artery lesions. These were more common in the area supplied by the lenticulostriate arteries of Charcot, and their sites of predilection were the lenticular nucleus, base of pons, caudate nucleus, thalamus, internal capsule, subcortical central white matter of the hemispheres, and cerebellar white matter.

A third definition of lacune is any small hole in the brain found at autopsy, regardless of its location or etiology (i.e., the type of artery disease responsible for it). Some such lacunes are not infarcts but just empty spaces around blood vessels (i.e., perivascular spaces of Virchow-Robin).

The term *lacune* is also applied to rarefied areas seen on CT and MRI scans. Although many areas of rarefaction are being revealed through these imaging techniques, it is not clear how these areas are related to behavioral or cognitive changes and to brain changes found at autopsy. In the words of Bogousslavsky (1992), "radiologists report lacunes on CT or MRI to describe any kind of small voids in the brain, whatever their aspects, potential causes, or clinical correlates" (p. 629).

Some authors (Huang et al. 1987; Norrving and Staaf 1991) recognize *lacunar stroke* as a distinct condition with a specific set of symptoms.

---

[1] Although *lacuna* is the more correct form of the noun, *lacune* is by far the more widely used and recognized term in the neurological literature, probably because the original work on the concept was in French.

They say that the damage caused by this event is concentrated in the area of the basal ganglia and internal capsule and is the result of obstruction of the branches of the lenticulostriate arteries of Charcot (see Figure 2–1) and other small basal perforating arteries that arise from the carotid and middle cerebral arteries. These authors describe precise clinical syndromes: pure motor stroke, pure sensory stroke, sensorimotor stroke, ataxic hemiparesis, and acute focal movement disorders.

These syndromes are those that might be expected from damage to localized areas of the internal capsule and basal ganglia (see Figure 2–2). Fisher (1969, 1982) has claimed as manifestations of lacunar strokes every syndrome that can arise from a small cerebral infarction not affecting the cortex. There are thus more than 20 lacunar syndromes. He stated that the presence of aphasia, isolated severe memory impairment, stupor, coma, loss of consciousness, or seizures almost always excludes a lacunar diagnosis (Fisher 1982). However, when Huang et al. (1987) used the absence of such symptoms to delimit a group of stroke patients, they found only a minority of the patients to have CT evidence of lacunes as defined by Fisher.

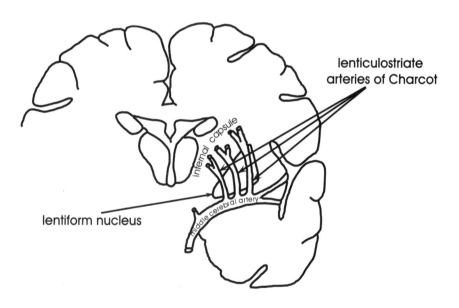

Figure 2–1.   Coronal section, showing middle cerebral artery with lenticulostriate arteries of Charcot.

On the other hand, authors who define lacunes in purely histological terms go further than Fisher and include dementia as a possible manifestation. Among these authors are Ishii et al. (1986), who defined *lacunes* in histological terms (with autopsy follow-up) rather than according to anatomical location. The patients studied by Ishii and co-workers had lacunes predominantly in the frontal lobe, with clinical manifestations including dementia, lack of volition, emotional lability, and akinetic mutism.

Some texts describe an entity of *lacunar dementia* in which "epileptiform attacks may occur, and various forms of aphasia, agnosia, and apraxia are met with. Corticospinal tract lesions are common and the grasp reflex may be encountered. In walking there is a tendency to take short shuffling steps. Arteriosclerotic parkinsonism also occurs" (Brain 1985, p. 293). This definition is somewhat supported by the work of Loeb et al. (1992), who defined lacunes as small low-density lesions, seen on

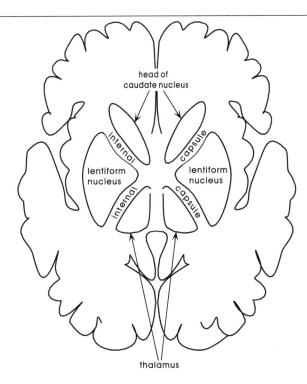

Figure 2–2. Transverse section, showing the internal capsule, the lentiform nucleus, and the head of the caudate nucleus.

CT, that are situated within the basal ganglia, thalamus, or internal capsule and are associated with neurological symptoms. Loeb and colleagues found that about one-quarter of their patients who had such lesions had dementia. However, Scheinberg (1988) concluded from a review of the literature that there was no solid experimental evidence to support the existence of lacunar dementia as a distinct entity.

Leukoareiosis

Some of the abnormalities revealed by the newer imaging techniques have yet to be classified as diseases. Small areas of rarefaction in the white matter are especially common in MRI scans. Neurologists have christened these *leukoareiosis* but have not been able to find a disease associated with them. Although such areas are more frequently found in elderly patients, they are also quite common in healthy young people (Brown et al. 1992). Elderly individuals with extensive white-matter changes revealed on MRI have been found to retain normal cognitive function when followed up for more than 7 years (Fein et al. 1990).

The significance of leukoareiosis differs depending on whether the areas of rarefaction are seen on CT or only on MRI, where they are located, and whether stroke risk factors are also present. The three most widely agreed-on conclusions are that 1) rarefaction seen on CT is more likely to be associated with dementia and to be caused by infarction than is rarefaction seen only on MRI; 2) periventricular rarefaction is associated with dementia; and 3) areas of rarefaction in the presence of stroke risk factors are associated with dementia. Such findings are not yet useful in clinical psychiatric practice, but there are indications that vascular disease that causes cognitive impairment without definite infarcts can be recognized, and this diagnostic ability may be useful in the future.

It is probable, as Brown et al. (1992) suggested based on their own work and on a review of the literature, that "white-matter hyperintensity signals represent subtle anatomical changes that occur as a result of vascular insults, producing an expression of psychiatric symptoms that is determined by location of the vascular insult. Many late-onset psychiatric disorders may in fact be a direct result of such injury" (p. 623).

CT-diagnosed leukoareiosis is more common in dementia patients than in control subjects (Kobari et al. 1990). MRI-diagnosed leukoareiosis in general is no more frequent in dementia patients than in control subjects, but periventricular rarefaction on MRI is more frequent in dementia patients (Matsubayashi et al. 1992; Mirsen et al. 1991). Kumar et al.

(1992) suggested that areas of rarefaction may be associated with vascular dementia even though they do not constitute definite infarcts. These authors found that such areas were just as common in control subjects without dementia as in dementia patients in general. However, among subjects with stroke risk factors, areas of rarefaction were more frequently seen in those with dementia. In other words, these areas are characteristic of a group of dementia patients who do not have definite infarcts but who do have stroke risk factors.

The work of Kawamura and Meyer (1993) points in a similar direction. They found that CT-diagnosed leukoareiosis was more common in patients with vascular dementia than in those with Alzheimer's disease.

Binswanger's Disease

Binswanger's disease, as Binswanger originally described it in 1894, was a dementing illness unrelated to stroke. It was considered a rarity until the advent of CT and MRI (Olszewski 1962). Although Binswanger's patients did not have the areas of softening that characterize a fully developed infarct, gross examination revealed atrophy of the white matter of the brain. The cortex was spared.

Binswanger called his disease *encephalitis subcorticalis chronic progressiva*. (In the 1963 edition of *Greenfield's Neuropathology*, it was called "chronic progressive subcortical encephalitis of Binswanger" [Blackwood et al. 1963, p. 126].) Binswanger neither provided histological descriptions nor measured his patients' blood pressure. Alzheimer (1902) thought that the condition was caused by artery disease, specifically disease of the arteries within the white matter.

With today's brain-imaging methods, many cases of thinning of the white matter without definite infarcts have been found, and there has been a tendency to widen the definition of Binswanger's disease to include such cases. Suggested criteria for a Binswanger's diagnosis are long-standing hypertension and a history of frequent minor strokes, in combination with MRI findings of diffuse white-matter lesions (Kuwabara 1992). However, if patients with large areas of white-matter rarefaction revealed on MRI or CT are followed to autopsy, they seldom have the white-matter atrophy and other changes of classical Binswanger's disease (Alston et al. 1990; Janota et al. 1989).

The case described by Mahler et al. (1987) and followed to autopsy appeared to meet all criteria for Binswanger's disease. Noted in this 57-year-old patient were excessive somnolence and gait disturbance. When examined at age 65, he was alert, had dysarthric speech, and would cry when trying to talk. Although the patient could follow simple commands and repeat long sentences, he was disoriented and could not calculate. A spastic left-sided weakness with a positive left Babinski was present. The patient died at the age of 68.

Working Definition of *Stroke*

This book covers all vascular disease affecting the brain. *Neurologically evident stroke* will be used to refer to strokes that have caused manifestations that are not exclusively behavioral, cognitive, or emotional. *Paralytic stroke* will be used to refer to strokes that have caused paralysis to distinguish them from brain infarcts that have not caused paralysis. When discussing the work of other authors, I will accept their use of the generic term *stroke,* with additional comment if they have used an unusual definition.

Summary

The World Health Organization defines stroke as a vascular lesion of the brain, resulting either in a neurological deficit persisting for more than 24 hours or in death. Several other definitions and classifications exist, none of which emphasize psychiatric symptoms.

Brain infarcts in patients who have no physical symptoms may be referred to as "silent" or "inobvious" strokes. In transient ischemic attacks (TIAs) or reversible ischemic neurological defects (RINDs), no brain infarcts are present.

The terms *minor stroke* and *little stroke* are sometimes applied to TIAs or RINDS and sometimes to strokes caused by small infarcts that give rise to limited symptoms.

There are limitations on which diagnostic tests can be performed in stroke patients, who are often elderly individuals with heart problems and/or mental impairments.

The two major imaging techniques in clinical use are computed tomography (CT) and magnetic resonance imaging (MRI). Positron-emission tomography (PET), fast MRI (fMRI), regional cerebral blood flow (rCBF), and single photon emission computed tomography (SPECT) are methods in research use.

Doppler and sonographic techniques yield information about the patency of the carotid arteries in the neck. Transcranial Doppler (TCD) can detect blockages of the vertebral and basilar arteries.

Although the word *lacune* is sometimes used to mean any small hole or soft area in the brain, there is disagreement about its exact definition. Areas of rarefaction in the white matter are termed *leukoareiosis* and are most common in elderly patients. MRI sometimes reveals areas of rarefaction that are not visible on CT. Rarefaction seen on CT is more likely to be associated with dementia and to be caused by infarction than is rarefaction seen only on MRI. Periventricular rarefaction and areas of rarefaction in the presence of stroke risk factors are associated with dementia.

As originally defined, Binswanger's disease was a dementing illness characterized by atrophy of the white matter. The definition of Binswanger's disease is sometimes widened to include some cases of leukoareiosis.

References

Alberts MJ, Faulstich ME, Gray M: Stroke with negative brain magnetic resonance imaging. Stroke 23:663–667, 1992

Alston SR, Boyko OB, Clark CM, et al: The utility of post-mortem magnetic resonance in distinguishing Alzheimer's disease from vascular dementia (abstract). J Neuropathol Exp Neurol 49:269, 1990

Alzheimer A: Die Seelenstörungen auf arteriosklerotisher Grundlage: Jahresversammlung des Vereins der deutschen Irrenärzte. Allgemeine Zeitschrift für Psychiatrie 59:695–711, 1902

Bamford J: Clinical examination in diagnosis and subclassification of stroke. Lancet 339:400–402, 1992

Besson G, Hammel M, Clavier I, et al: Failure of magnetic resonance imaging in the detection of a pontine lacune (letter). Stroke 23:1535, 1993

Binswanger O: Die Abgrenzung der allgemeinen progressiven Paralysie. Berliner Klinische Wochenschrift 31:1103–1105, 1137–1139, 1180–1186, 1894

Blackwood W, McMenemy WH, Meyer A, et al: Greenfield's Neuropathology. London, Edward Arnold, 1963, p 126

Bogousslavsky J: The plurality of subcortical infarction. Stroke 23:629–631, 1992

Brain WR: Disorders of the cerebral circulation, in Brain's Clinical Neurology, 6th Edition. Revised by Bannister R. London, Oxford University Press, 1985, pp 285–327

Brown FW, Lewine RJ, Hudgins PA, et al: White matter hyperintensity signals in psychiatric and non-psychiatric subjects. Am J Psychiatry 149:620–625, 1992

David A, Blamire D, Breiter H: Functional magnetic resonance imaging. Br J Psychiatry 164:2–7, 1994

Dunne JW, Leedman PJ, Edis RH: Inobvious stroke: a cause of delirium and dementia. Aust N Z J Med 16:771–778, 1986

Fein G, Van Dyke C, Davenport L, et al: Preservation of normal cognitive function in elderly subjects with extensive white matter lesions of long duration. Arch Gen Psychiatry 47:220–223, 1990

Feinberg WM, Seeger JF, Carmody RF, et al: Epidemiologic features of asymptomatic cerebral infarction in patients with nonvalvular atrial fibrillation. Arch Intern Med 150:2340–2344, 1990

Fisher CM: The arterial lesions underlying lacunes. Acta Neuropathol (Berl) 12:1–15, 1969

Fisher CM: Lacunar strokes and infarcts: a review. Neurology 32:871–876, 1982

Gross CR, Shinar D, Mohr JP, et al: Interobserver agreement in the diagnosis of stroke type. Arch Neurol 43:893–898, 1986

Gurland B, Kuriansky J, Sharpe L, et al: The comprehensive assessment and referral evaluation (CARE): rationale, development, and reliability. Int J Aging Hum Dev 8:9–41, 1977

Hatono S: Experience from a multicenter stroke register: a preliminary report. Bulletin of WHO 54:541–553, 1976

Huang CY, Woo E, Yu YL, et al: When is sensorimotor stroke a lacunar syndrome? J Neurol Neurosurg Psychiatry 50:720–726, 1987

Hütter BO: Which neuropsychological defects are hidden behind a good outcome after aneurysmal subarachnoid hemorrhage? Neurosurgery 33:999–1006, 1993

Ishii N, Nishihara Y, Imamura T: Why do frontal lobe symptoms predominate in vascular dementia with lacunes? Neurology 36:340–345, 1986

Janota I, Mirsen TR, Hachinski VC, et al: Neuropathologic correlates of leukoareiosis. Arch Neurol 46:1124–1128, 1989

Kase CS, Wolf PA, Chodosh EH, et al: Prevalence of silent stroke in patients presenting with initial stroke: the Framingham study. Stroke 20:850–852, 1989

Kawamura J, Meyer JS: Correlations of leukoareiosis with cerebral atrophy and perfusion in elderly normal subjects and demented patients. J Neurol Neurosurg Psychiatry 56:182–187, 1993

Kempster PA, Gerraty RP, Gates PC: Asymptomatic cerebral infarction in patients with chronic atrial fibrillation. Stroke 19:955–957, 1988

Kobari M, Meyer JS, Ichigo M: Leuko-areiosis, cerebral atrophy, and cerebral perfusion in normal aging. Arch Neurol 47:161–165, 1990

Kumar A, Yousem D, Souder E, et al: High intensity signals in Alzheimer's disease without cerebrovascular risk factors: a magnetic resonance imaging evaluation. Am J Psychiatry 149:248–250, 1992

Kunitz SC, Gross CR, Heyman A, et al: The pilot stroke data bank: definition design and data. Stroke 15:740–746, 1984

Kuwabara Y: Cerebrovascular responsiveness to hypercapnia in Alzheimer's dementia and vascular dementia of the Binswanger type (response to Birkett). Stroke 23:1534–1535, 1992

Landi G: Clinical diagnosis of transient ischemic attacks. Lancet 339:402–405, 1992

Loeb C, Gandolfo C, Croce R, et al: Dementia associated with lacunar infarction. Stroke 23:1225–1229, 1992

Mahler ME, Cummings JL, Tomiyasu U: Atypical dementia syndrome in an elderly man. J Am Geriatr Soc 35:1116–1126, 1987

Marie P: Des foyers lacunaires de desintegration et de différents autres états cavitaires du cerveau. Revue Médicale 21:281–298, 1901

Matsubayashi K, Shimada K, Kawamoto A, et al: Incidental brain lesions on magnetic resonance imaging and neurobehavioral functions in the apparently healthy elderly. Stroke 23:175–180, 1992

Millikan C, Futrell N: Response to Mendez and Estanol (letter). Stroke 24:328, 1993

Mirsen TR, Lee DH, Wong CJ, et al: Clinical correlates of white-matter changes on magnetic resonance imaging scans of the brain. Arch Neurol 48:1015–1021, 1991

Mohr JP, Caplan LR, Melski JW, et al: The Harvard Cooperative Stroke Registry: a prospective registry. Neurology 28:754–762, 1978

National Institute of Neurological Diseases and Stroke: Classification of cerebrovascular diseases, III. Stroke 21:637–676, 1990

Norrving B, Staaf G: Pure motor stroke from presumed lacunar infarct. Cerebrovasc Dis 1:203–209, 1991

Omnibus Budget Reconciliation Act of 1987 (OBRA), Public Law 100-203

Olszewski J: Subcortical arteriosclerotic encephalopathy: review of the literature on the so-called Binswanger's disease and presentation of two cases. World Neurology 3:359–375, 1962

Ricci S, Celani MG, La Rosa F, et al: Silent brain infarctions in patients with first-ever stroke. Stroke 24:647–653, 1993

Scheinberg P: Dementia due to vascular disease: a multifactorial disorder. Stroke 19:1291–1299, 1988

Steinke W, Sacco RL, Mohr JP, et al: Thalamic stroke: presentation and prognosis. Arch Neurol 49:703–710, 1992

CHAPTER THREE

Stroke Risk Factors

Stroke risk factors involve mental health professionals in several ways. Some stroke risk factors (e.g., drugs, alcohol) present practical and immediate psychiatric management problems because they cause behavioral disturbances. Other factors raise broader issues of public policy and preventive medicine that nonetheless impinge on clinical practice: because the prognosis for a stroke survivor largely depends on the likelihood of a second stroke, prevention of another stroke is an important part of clinical treatment. When this prevention depends on reducing behaviors that increase stroke risk, mental health professionals are still further involved.

What follows is a survey of the stroke risk factors that are amenable to psychiatric treatment, of psychiatric disorders arising from conditions that are also stroke risk factors, and of behavioral problems in stroke management related to stroke risk factors. Some of the stroke factors have an independent main effect in causing stroke; that is to say, it can be statistically shown that their effect is not a result of some other factor. In other cases, we must discuss a tangled interaction between the behavioral and biochemical factors.

Common Risk Factors in Heart Attack and Stroke

The major risk factors for stroke are old age, a previous stroke or transient ischemic attack (TIA), high blood pressure, heart disease with atrial fibrillation, and carotid artery narrowing. There are many other possible risk factors, some of which are behavioral.

Although there is considerable overlap among stroke risk factors and heart attack risk factors, the overlap is not complete. Hypertension, for example, is more specific to stroke, but obesity, smoking, and lack of exercise are more associated with heart attacks. Strokes generally occur at older ages than heart attacks. A worksheet of risk factors based on the Framingham study is available from the American Heart Association (address in Appendix B); the contents of this worksheet are summarized in Table 3–1.

A man is more likely to suffer a stroke than is a woman of the same age (except for subarachnoid hemorrhage, which is more common in women). The prevalence and overall incidence of stroke is higher in women because women live longer, and elderly people get more strokes (Kelly-Hayes 1992). Incidence rises in women after menopause and is lower among postmenopausal women who take estrogens, who tend to be better educated and wealthier than those not receiving estrogen (Finucane et al. 1993). The typical female stroke patient is more likely to be socially isolated (because widowhood is more common than widower-

Table 3–1.   Heart attack and stroke risk factors

Risk factors		
Heart attack	**Heart attack and stroke**	**Stroke**
• Elevated total cholesterol • Low levels of high-density lipoprotein (HDL)	• Older age • Male sex • Hypertension • Cigarette smoking • Diabetes • Electrocardiogram-diagnosed left-ventricular hypertrophy	• Atrial fibrillation • Myocardial infarction • Angina pectoris • Coronary insufficiency • Intermittent claudication • Congestive heart failure

Source.   Adapted from American Heart Association: Risk Factor Prediction Kit (#64–9590). Dallas, TX, American Heart Association, 1990.

hood) and institutionalized. Disabled male patients are more likely to remain in their own homes, looked after by their wives.

Some factors associated with stroke can be shown statistically not to be independent risk factors. Frequent church attendance, for example, is associated with lower incidence of stroke, but this is because of the generally better health of churchgoers (Colantonio et al. 1992). Obesity can be associated with diabetes and high blood pressure, and thus with stroke, but does not in and of itself cause stroke (Aronow 1990). Some factors, such as drug use, are important in certain populations, but surveys done on other populations may fail to detect them. Ellekjaer et al. (1992), in northern Norway, were not able to confirm that smoking, drinking, salt intake, obesity, or lack of exercise was related to stroke.

Personality and Temperament

The possibility that, in addition to contributing to other stroke risk factors, having a certain personality type predisposes a person to stroke is not entirely settled (Johnston 1989). The following personality factors have been found to be linked to stroke risk.

Anger and hostility.   Several of the earliest accounts of stroke suggest an association with anger, and phrases such as "apoplectic with rage" have passed into the language. Studies have also suggested that hostility is important in the development of cerebrovascular disease (Adler 1993; Ecker 1954; Gianturco et al. 1974; Williams 1992). Matsumoto et al. (1993) found a correlation between questionnaire responses indicating anger and the severity of carotid atherosclerosis.

Most of this anger research has been done with men. Linden (1993) found that venting rather than restraining hostility tended to produce a prolonged rise in blood pressure in women. He linked this effect to the social disapproval women risk when they display anger. Goetz et al. (1992) found what they described as a "pressured" pattern, which included difficulties in handling anger, significantly more often in women with ischemic stroke than in women in a control group.

Type A behavior.   Type A behavior is less well-accepted as an entity than it used to be, and some studies have failed to confirm its link with cardiovascular disease (Bass and Wade 1982). As originally described by Rosenman et al. (1975), this behavioral pattern consisted of excessive competitiveness, a sense of being under pressure, and easily provoked hostility and was said to be an independent risk factor for coronary artery disease (stroke was not under study). Other characteristics of the Type A individual that have been listed are an excessive sense of time urgency and extremes of ambition, aggressiveness, punctuality, and impatience.

Stevens et al. (1984) found that the Type A pattern correlated with carotid artery atherosclerosis. Eaker and Feinleib (1983) studied data from the Framingham study and found that Type A behavior predicted an increased stroke risk for women in general, and for men who were experiencing work overload.

Anxiety.   Weissman et al. (1990) found, in a community survey, that respondents with panic disorder were more likely than those without anxiety symptoms to report having suffered a stroke. These authors suggested that the two disorders may be linked via the condition of mitral valve prolapse. In some surveys, mitral valve prolapse has been associated with panic attacks, and in others it has been linked with stroke (Jackson 1984), although both of these associations have been queried, and the condition may also be asymptomatic.

The relationship between anxiety and hypertension is discussed in Chapter 15.

Ethnicity

Americans of African ancestry have one of the highest stroke rates in the world. Mortality from stroke in the 35- to 74-year age group is twice as high among blacks as among whites in the United States. In general, stroke in African Americans is likely to be more severe, and to be followed by a slower recovery and worse outcome, than stroke in members of other racial groups in the United States. This poorer prognosis is partly attributable to the presence of more severe stroke risk factors in the African-American population, the most prominent being high blood pressure. Although high blood pressure increases with age in blacks and whites of both sexes, it begins to appear at a younger age in black men and to be more extreme. The type of high blood pressure that is particularly common in young black men is essential hypertension with low plasma renin, a condition that is affected by salt intake.

Although efforts have been made to determine whether social stress is a cause of hypertension in Americans of African ancestry, findings have been inconclusive. In Africa itself, increased incidence of stroke has been associated with increased urbanization, but there are considerable—and as yet incompletely studied—variations among African groups (Lisk 1993). Rural Zulu who migrate to South African cities have more psycho-

logical distress and higher blood pressure than those who remain in traditional villages, but a study of the Sere of West Africa found that mental
health and blood pressure among villagers who moved to a city were no
worse than among those who stayed at home (Beiser 1990).

Age

Advancing age is a strong risk factor for stroke. Of the 500,000 new
strokes in the United States each year, about 5% occur in young adults
between the ages of 15 and 45 years (Love and Biller 1991). Among
adults over 45 years of age, the incidence rises steadily with age, subject
to the sex differences previously mentioned. Thus, there is a considerable overlap between geriatric psychiatry and stroke. Practitioners often
must attempt to determine whether conditions such as memory loss,
delusions, failure to rehabilitate, or social isolation are attributable to
the stroke itself or to advancing age. They must also face the medical,
ethical, and economic dilemmas that arise in dealing with multiple
medical illnesses, retirement, nursing-home legislation, and Medicare.
The recently developed specialty of geriatric psychiatry has brought precision to the diagnosis and treatment of such symptoms as apathy and
agitation, which might previously have been attributed to irreversible
dementia or "senility."

Despite its strong association with old age, stroke is so common that
many cases occur in the young. The study of these can be informative in
revealing how much of the psychiatric and rehabilitative difficulties in
stroke are intrinsic to the illness itself and how much are due to old age.

Stroke in the Young

Injury to the developing nervous system in early childhood gives rise to
a complex interaction of neurophysiological and psychological factors
that is further discussed in Chapter 17. Heart disease accounts for half
of the cases of stroke in children. Child abuse may also cause some cases
of stroke. Buchanan and Oliver (1977) found that child abuse was the
cause of brain damage leading to mental retardation in at least 4 of
140 children in an institution. Focal cerebral infarction was present on
the computed tomography (CT) scans of 2 of 712 physically abused children reviewed by Merten et al. (1984). Trauma is the most frequent cause
of cerebral hemorrhage in childhood (Wehrmacher and Gonzalzles 1990).

Aside from cocaine (discussed later in this section) and hypertension, there are a large number of rare conditions that are listed as causing stroke in the young. Often, no particular cause can be found. Rare diseases present special challenges to a clinician's psychiatric and diagnostic skills. When stroke is due to a rare disease or condition, diagnosis may be delayed, resulting in frustration and resentment in the patient and difficulty in dealing with the family. Their feelings of isolation and bewilderment can often be helped by contact with support groups dedicated to the particular illness.

Although in the older literature, syphilis was mentioned as a stroke risk factor, these days a positive reagin test for syphilis (e.g., the rapid plasma reagin [RPR] and the venereal disease research laboratory [VDRL] tests) in a stroke patient is more suggestive of antiphospholipid antibody syndrome (APLAS). More specific tests for syphilis, such as the fluorescent treponemal antibody (FTA), are negative in APLAS.

Systemic lupus erythematosus.   Systemic lupus erythematosus (SLE) has many psychiatric manifestations, including psychosis (Iverson 1993). Much of the psychiatric disturbance in lupus is thought to be due to the emotional effects of the illness rather than having a direct organic basis (Lim et al. 1991).

Delirium, impaired consciousness, and memory loss can occur with lupus and may be associated with cerebrovascular lesions (Abel et al. 1980). Stroke is reported in 5%–20% of SLE patients, and those who have had one stroke are likely to have another (Olsen 1992). Most neuropsychiatric manifestations of SLE clear completely with resolution of the lupus flare, but focal neurological deficits from stroke persist.

Terao et al. (1994) described two cases of depression in corticosteroid-treated patients with SLE-related stroke, both of which responded well to lithium.

Medications and Other Drugs and Substances

Contraceptive pills.   Birth control pills have been implicated as a risk factor for ischemic stroke and, less consistently, for subarachnoid hemorrhage, especially among smokers (Stern et al. 1991). Evidence concerning the connection between stroke and these medications has recently been questioned (Norris and Bladin 1993).

Many female psychiatric patients of childbearing age already have behavioral risk factors for stroke, such as heavy cigarette smoking (common in chronic schizophrenia) and cocaine use. In assessing the risk-benefit ratio of prescribing contraceptives for such patients, the potential effect of pregnancy on the course of their illness must be considered along with their reproductive rights and the fact that pregnancy itself constitutes a risk factor for stroke (Allbert and Morrison 1992).

Tobacco. Tobacco use is an independent stroke risk predictor. The younger the patient, the stronger a predictor it is (Woo et al. 1992). Smoking may be a specific risk factor for subarachnoid hemorrhage in young women (Longstreth et al. 1992). Risk of stroke is significantly diminished 2 years after quitting smoking, and is the same as that of a nonsmoker 5 years after smoking cessation (Kawachi et al. 1993; Love 1990).

In the original Framingham study, cigarette smoking was found to be a strong risk factor for heart disease but a relatively weak risk factor for stroke. Some recent studies (Dempsey and Moore 1992; Homer et al. 1991; Jamrozik et al. 1994) have shown smoking to have a stronger correlation with stroke and a tendency for smoking to cause extracranial carotid artery atherosclerosis. Rogers et al. (1984) found that cigarette smoking reduces the responsiveness of intracranial blood vessels to changes in oxygen concentration, perhaps by making them more rigid and inelastic.

Alcohol. Drinking may cause strokes or prevent them. A number of studies have pointed to an association between alcohol and stroke, especially cerebral hemorrhage in young adults, with acute intoxication immediately preceding stroke in several instances (Matthew and Wilson 1991). There is also evidence of a reverse, protective, effect from moderate drinking. Epidemiologists call the graphic depiction of this effect, in which what is good in moderation is bad in excess, the J-shaped curve.

Because alcoholism and stroke are both common illnesses, their occurrence in combination may often be seen. A practical management issue is that a stroke may cause an alcoholic person who has been steadily drinking to be hospitalized and thus abruptly withdrawn from alcohol. Alcohol withdrawal seizures and delirium tremens may ensue. If the physician does not know about the alcohol history, these symptoms can produce a puzzling diagnostic picture, especially if the onset of delirium tremens occurs, as can sometimes happen, days after the alcohol consumption ceased.

Henrich and Horwitz (1989) found no evidence for an association between alcohol use and ischemic stroke risk. Using a case-control study design, they compared 89 hospitalized patients with ischemic stroke documented by CT scan with a control group of hospitalized nonstroke patients. These authors noted in their report that some of the previous case-control studies had used control groups that excluded subjects with alcohol-related illnesses.

The Honolulu Heart Program, a prospective study of cardiovascular disease in 8,000 men followed for 12 years, found no association between drinking and thromboembolic stroke, but did find a relationship between drinking and hemorrhagic stroke, especially subarachnoid hemorrhage (Donahue et al. 1986). Longstreth et al. (1992) also observed a specific association of alcohol use with subarachnoid hemorrhage.

Binge drinking may be particularly likely to cause stroke. Taylor (1982), in St. Louis, compared drinking habits in stroke patients with those in a control group of hospitalized patients. Of 14 patients under the age of 50 hospitalized for stroke, 3 admitted to having drunk, within the preceding 24 hours, "one fifth of whisky, three fifths of whisky, and 12 cans of beer," respectively.

Wilkins and Kendall (1985), under the admonitory heading "Lesson of the Week" in the *British Medical Journal,* described a 30-year-old and a 36-year-old who developed hemiplegia with cerebral infarction after "alcoholic binges," although these binges were mild by the St. Louis standards.

Moderate alcohol intake may benefit the cardiovascular system. In some studies, it has been found that consuming two or three drinks a day reduces the risk of stroke, at least in whites (Gorelick 1990). Gill et al. (1986) found that moderate drinking—up to 90 grams of alcohol (about nine drinks) a week—protected against stroke, but that above that level it was a contributory factor. Sophisticated epidemiological methods are needed in these studies to account for such potentially confounding factors as recovered alcoholic patients who have become teetotalers (Lazarus 1991; Rimm et al. 1991).

All population surveys must cope with the fact that respondents may not be truthful about their alcohol intake. Long-term prospective surveys, such as the Framingham study, also must allow for change in social customs regarding drugs and alcohol over time.

The mechanism by which alcohol causes (or prevents) strokes is not clear. Hillbom et al. (1983) found that alcohol increased the coagulability of the blood by decreasing fibrinolytic activity and increasing factor VIII. They suggested that this increased coagulability predisposed patients to thrombosis (although hemorrhage rather than thrombosis seems to be the specifically alcohol-related risk).

Cocaine.   In the older studies, cocaine did not emerge as a risk factor for stroke. This may simply reflect the fact that there was less cocaine around or that the studies were done in areas of low addiction prevalence. Since the first report relating cocaine to stroke (Brust and Richter 1977), the association between cocaine and stroke has become generally accepted, so that stroke in a young person from a drug-using background raises the possibility of illicit drugs as a precipitating factor. The typical infarct occurs within a few hours following cocaine abuse or in the morning after a party (Tuchman and Daras 1990).

The first epidemiological study of cocaine and stroke was done by Kaku and Lowenstein (1990). They examined the records of more than 200 young stroke patients admitted to San Francisco General Hospital between 1978 and 1988 and compared them with those of a control group of patients admitted with other diagnoses. The stroke patients were significantly more likely to have used drugs. Cocaine was used most frequently, followed by heroin, amphetamine, methylphenidate, and phencyclidine.

In a study of 116 Maryland stroke cases in 1988 and 1989, Sloan et al. (1991) found 11 associated with illicit drug use, mostly younger patients (mean age of 41). The associated drugs in order of frequency were cocaine (5), over-the-counter sympathomimetics (3), phencyclidine (2), and heroin (1). Some studies show differences in liability to cause stroke between cocaine hydrochloride and alkaloidal cocaine.

The mechanism by which cocaine produces stroke is not yet exactly known. Depletion in intracellular magnesium, followed by intracellular acidosis, has been found to be the primary event in rats that developed cerebral bleeding after cocaine administration (Altura and Gupta 1992). Cocaine is sympathomimetic and increases blood pressure. The increased blood pressure may be especially likely to be a cause of hemorrhagic stroke and rupture of intracranial aneurysms. This type of stroke is more common among those who sniff cocaine (cocaine hydrochloride users), whereas those who smoke "crack" (alkaloidal cocaine) are more likely to suffer an occlusive (ischemic) stroke (Brust 1993). In some studies, reduced cerebral blood flow has been shown, suggesting vasospasm, which might cause ischemic infarcts. In several kinds of drug abuse, vasculitis has been suspected (Citron et al. 1970), and in two cocaine users, this was confirmed by biopsy (Krendel et al. 1990). In one reported cocaine stroke, there was a left atrial thrombus, and embolism was suggested as a likely mechanism (Petty et al. 1990).

There is dispute as to whether cocaine is a long-term risk factor as well as an immediate precipitant of stroke. According to Tuchman and Daras (1990), any stroke occurring several months after the last cocaine use, in the presence of a negative drug screen, is a chance event. Others say that the risk may be persistent (Deringer et al. 1990). Levine et al. (1990) studied 28 stroke patients who had used crack within 72 hours before their attack and found that most of them had developed neurological symptoms within 1 hour of using crack, although for some patients 2 or 3 days intervened. Twenty-six had been regular crack users for 2 or 3 years before their stroke, one had smoked crack only occasionally, and one was a claimed first-time user.

Other drugs.   Several other drugs have been associated with stroke, but a cause-and-effect relationship has been difficult to establish in humans because of the small numbers reported and the possibility of multiple drug use. Many cocaine users also use alcohol intermittently as a "downer" when cocaine makes them too "jittery." Among the 28 crack users with stroke studied by Levine et al. (1990), 3 had used intravenous heroin and 5 had consumed alcohol in the preceding day.

Intravenous drug use can cause brain infarcts through arterial occlusion from vasculitis (Citron et al. 1970)) or from bacterial endocarditis (Kaku and Lowenstein 1990) with septic embolism. Caplan et al. (1982) found that nine patients had been reported in the literature whose strokes were directly attributable to the use of heroin, and in each case the stroke was due to cerebral infarction and had followed immediately or within 24 hours after intravenous use.

In some intravenous users, particles of foreign substances injected into veins along with the addictive drugs have reached the brain, especially if oral or rectal preparations were injected into a vein. This has happened with pentazocine (Talwin; also known as "T's" and "blues"), methylphenidate (Ritalin), and hydromorphone (Dilaudid). It is not clear how such particles pass into the left side of the heart in the absence of congenital septal defects. Bitar and Gomez (1993) postulate occult functional arteriovenous shunts. Possibly there can be inadvertent intracarotid injection when neck veins are used.

Three cases in young men have been reported of basal ganglia infarct that was thought to be associated with heavy marijuana smoking, but the association remains speculative (Zachariah 1992).

Amphetamine use has been linked to stroke, but the numbers have been too small to allow statistical conclusions. Harrington et al. (1983) described four patients in whom cerebral hemorrhages occurred while they were taking oral amphetamines or diethylpropion, and the authors reviewed literature suggesting an association between intravenous amphetamine use and cerebral hemorrhage. Two of their cases had characteristic small artery deformities seen on carotid angiography.

On the other hand, there has also been evidence for a therapeutic use of amphetamines after stroke; work on the use of amphetamines in stroke rehabilitation has been reviewed by Mcdowell (1991). Positive results have been reported, but the numbers treated have been small because of the need to exclude patients with cardiac risk factors when using amphetamines. Methylphenidate has been used for treatment of depression after stroke with no adverse effects (Lingam et al. 1988).

Caffeine is probably safe—in fact, there is even evidence that it protects against stroke. A possible mechanism suggested for this effect is that caffeine acts at receptor sites for adenosine, an excitatory neurotransmitter. As is discussed in Chapter 5, one of the mechanisms of brain damage in stroke is overstimulation at the nerve cell receptor sites for excitatory neurotransmitters. Frequent use of caffeine renders the receptor sites resistant to adenosine. The moral drawn by some authors is that people should drink plenty of coffee before having a stroke, but abstain afterward (Longstreth and Nelson 1992).

Several other drugs have been suggested as causing strokes on the basis of indirect evidence and reports of isolated cases. Mueller (1983) described seizures and headaches associated with use of phenylpropanolamine in humans. She subsequently demonstrated that hypertensive rats given a combination of phenylpropanolamine and caffeine (such as found in certain diet preparations and "look-alike" pills) at a high and prolonged dosage were liable to subarachnoid and cerebral hemorrhage (Mueller et al. 1984). Kokkinos and Levine (1993) reported two cases of stroke in young women taking phentermine, one of whom was also taking phendimetrazine. Ephedrine use was associated with stroke in three patients described by Bruno (1993).

Sobel et al. (1971) reported a case of a 14-year-old boy who had seizures after taking LSD, and then a few days later developed a left hemiplegia. A total obstruction of the carotid artery was found on arteriography.

The effect of drugs of abuse on cerebral blood flow varies. Cerebral blood flow is increased by small doses of alcohol, recent smoking of a cigarette, recent cocaine use, and sometimes recent marijuana use. It is reduced by caffeine, amphetamine, large doses of alcohol, and chronic use of alcohol and most addictive substances (Matthew and Wilson 1991).

Migraine

The role of migraine in stroke and of psychological factors in migraine are both uncertain. It has not been proved that true migraine can cause a true stroke. Migraine is so common that 15%–30% of stroke patients would be expected to have a history of migraine (Bartleson 1984). Although a causal relationship has not been established statistically, such a relationship seems likely in some patients who, following a migraine attack, develop a stroke with visual field defects. There are also cases in which a recurrent transient hemiplegia follows migraine, and an entity of *migrainous cerebral infarction* is recognized by the International Headache Society (Welch and Levine 1990).

A relationship exists between severe headache and the presence of antiphospholipid antibodies, which constitute a stroke risk factor, and it has been suggested that these antibodies may play a role in some cases of "migraine-related stroke" (Hess 1992). On the other hand, an absence of headache has sometimes characterized those cases of migraine that are followed by stroke (Rothrock et al. 1988).

In a group of patients with migraine, Rothrock et al. (1991) compared those who had had strokes with those who had not, and followed them for over 2 years. There was no difference between the two groups in age, contraceptive use, or prevalence of other stroke risk factors. Those with stroke were more likely to have had a history of migraine with aura, or so-called complicated migraine.

Management of Stroke Risk Factors

Diet

In theory, weight reduction is a method of reducing blood pressure and thus reducing stroke risk that is under mental control; however, the status of obesity as an independent stroke risk factor is in doubt. Some kinds of hypertension can be influenced by salt restriction and some types of hyperlipidemia, by special diets.

After a stroke that has led to hospitalization, a patient's food intake is initially limited by the need for assessment of swallowing ability. As solid food is reinstated, the dietitian will meet with the treatment team to discuss the nutrition plan. At such meetings, the patient's cooperation in a reducing diet can be enlisted.

In later stages, especially with the dementia patient in a nursing home, some caregivers may disagree with restricting pleasure in so deprived a life. Although the medical and dietary staff should ensure that the case for diet restriction is adequately presented, the ultimate decision must meet with the agreement of the primary caregivers.

Drugs for Hypertension

The management of hypertension after a stroke offers special challenges because of the psychiatric effects of antihypertensive drugs, some of which are listed in Table 3–2. In the alert office patient taking a single drug, the adverse effects of antihypertensive drugs are easy to detect. In fact, efforts often must be made to prevent patients from attributing all of their symptoms to the medication and using this as a reason to stop taking it. In the demented or poorly communicating patient who has had a stroke, more care is needed to detect adverse drug effects.

Drowsiness and postural hypotension can present severe and unrecognized obstacles to rehabilitation and may be mistaken for signs of poor motivation. A careful and knowledgeable review of the drugs a patient is taking, and has recently been taking, should form part of the psychiatric assessment of any stroke patient. The mental effects of drugs such as propranolol and reserpine are so marked that these drugs have a separate use as psychotropic agents.

Psychiatric symptoms are so common that a cause-and-effect relationship between them and antihypertensive drugs must not be too readily assumed. In one large trial of treatment of hypertension in the elderly, where the drugs used were chlorthalidone and reserpine or atenolol, no differences in dementia or depression were found between the treated and the untreated groups (Systolic Hypertension in the Elderly Program [SHEP] Cooperative Research Group 1991).

Some patients on beta-adrenergic–blocking drugs report vivid dreams and nightmares. It has been suggested that such symptoms occur because some of these drugs are lipophilic and therefore able to cross the blood-brain barrier. Dimsdale and Newton (1989) reviewed the literature on the neuropsychological effects of beta-blockers and found no general support for the proposition that drugs that were more lipophilic were especially likely to have such effects. They found that cognitive functions and memory were as likely to improve as to diminish with use of beta-blockers, but they also noted that many patients report not feeling well on these drugs, with vague complaints that may reflect sedation, such as sluggishness or fatigue.

Sometimes a psychotic patient is found by coincidence, on routine medical examination, to have hypertension. There is little literature on the management of such patients. The antipsychotics are generally not useful for the treatment of high blood pressure, because their hypotensive

Table 3–2. Psychiatric effects of antihypertensive medications

Drug class	Medications	Effects
Diuretics	Hydrochlorothiazide (Hydrodiuril, Esidrix), chlorthalidone (Hygroton), indapamide (Lozol), metolazone (Zaroxolyn), bumetanide (Bumex), furosemide (Lasix), spironolactone (Aldactone), triamterene (Dyrenium), and many combinations, the trade names of which include Aldactazide, Dyazide, and Moduretic	Interact with lithium to raise blood level Depression and impotence have been reported
Angiotensin-converting enzyme (ACE) inhibitors	Captopril (Capoten), enalapril (Vasotec), lisinopril (Prinivil), benazepril (Lotensin)	Enalapril is more likely than captopril to produce mild depression (Testa et al. 1993) Loss of taste sensation (ageusia)
Calcium channel blockers	Diltiazem (Cardizem), nifedipine (Procardia), verapamil (Calan)	Dizziness, headache, constipation, joint pain
Peripheral sympatholytic action	Beta-adrenergic blockers: propranolol (Inderal), atenolol (Tenormin), labetalol (Normodyne), metoprolol (Lopressor), timolol (Blocadren)	Vivid dreams, nightmares sedation, sluggishness or fatigue
	Peripheral adrenergic neuron antagonist: reserpine (Ser-Ap-Es)	Sedation and depression
	Alpha-adrenergic blocker: prazosin (Minipress)	Dizziness, vertigo, palpitations, headache, drowsiness, weakness, priapism, urinary incontinence
Central sympatholytic action	Clonidine (Catapres)	Sedation or insomnia Sympathetic overactivity on sudden withdrawal, with nervousness and palpitations

effect is largely a postural hypotension that tends to wear off after a week or so at a constant dose. Postural hypotension can be a hindrance to treatment when antipsychotic and antihypertensive drugs are started together. However, if antipsychotic drugs are withheld and the patient remains psychotic, management of the hypertension may become impossible. Clinical experience suggests that it is best to first stabilize the patient on an antipsychotic medication, unless there is malignant hypertension or the presence of end-organ damage requiring urgent hypotensive treatment.

Smoking

The patient who has had a single TIA is usually amenable to simple education about the danger of cigarettes. Material can be obtained from the American Cancer Society (see Appendix B for address) and reinforced by attendance at one of the smoking prevention meetings the society organizes in many areas. Nicotine can be prescribed as a gum (Nicorette) or as a skin patch (Nicoderm, Habitrol). Taking pure nicotine in these forms instead of smoking cigarettes provides no great advantage from the stroke-prevention point of view, because nicotine, although not carcinogenic, is probably the ingredient of the cigarette that causes cardiovascular disease. In practice, however, it is rare to find persistent use of medicinal nicotine. Some give it up and stop smoking; some give it up to return to smoking.

In acute-care general hospitals in the United States, smoking is now usually forbidden. Many patients circumvent this by surreptitiously breaking the rules, but the limited mobility of stroke patients forces them to be law-abiding.

For the hemiplegic patient at home, the risk of fire is almost as great as the vascular disease risk, and the fear of fire will usually prompt caregivers to restrict the patient's smoking. Patients with severe dementia almost always stop smoking.

Cocaine

Although no special withdrawal treatment is necessary in the acute phase, it is worthwhile to test for cocaine in young stroke patients. Upon recovery of consciousness, there may be a paranoid psychosis in chronic users. A classical symptom is *formication,* or *signe de Magnan,* the delusion of insects running over the skin. Panic attacks are also associated with cocaine use.

Most behavioral management problems in cocaine-induced stroke arise from preexisting personality factors rather than from any pharmacologically specific drug effect. Many of these problems are the same as those of young stroke patients in general. Sometimes cocaine use will continue, even in the institution, so that precautions such as urine testing for cocaine may be advisable.

In the hospital, the treatment team should institute early discussions with the discharge planner. Good rapport and communication are needed to prevent patients from absconding and signing out against medical advice. Getting the cocaine-addicted individual into a drug rehabilitation center can be helpful to the family and the community. The effectiveness of treatment of cocaine addiction has been reviewed by Hubbard et al. (1989).

Alcohol

Regardless of alcohol's standing as a stroke risk factor, the presence of alcohol problems strongly affects stroke management. Clues to alcohol use can be obtained from by reviewing the patient's history, by smelling his or her breath, by observing clinical signs of other alcohol-related illness, or by measuring blood alcohol levels. Thiamine should be given if there is any suspicion of Wernicke's encephalopathy, and this may forestall the subsequent development of a Korsakoff-type amnesia. If the blood alcohol level is high, a detoxification regimen should be initiated as soon as the patient is conscious and the alcohol level is falling. Sometimes delirium tremens can begin several days after alcohol withdrawal, with an interval of clear consciousness between. Indeed, this condition should be one of the first to be suspected when a patient begins experiencing delusions and hallucinations and demonstrates confusion after a lucid interval in the 2 weeks after a stroke.

Summary

Prevention of another stroke is an important part of stroke treatment. Some stroke risk factors produce behavioral problems, and others require behavioral management. Personality factors leading to stroke have not been well established.

Cocaine is emerging as a common cause of stroke in the young. Other addictive drugs may also cause stroke. Alcohol withdrawal must be considered as a possible cause of psychiatric complications in stroke management.

Compliance with treatment for hypertension is often poor. Several antihypertensive drugs can cause psychiatric side effects. Diuretics may interact with lithium. Antipsychotic drugs may cause orthostatic hypotension.

References

Abel T, Gladman DD, Urowitz MB: Neuropsychiatric lupus. J Rheumatol 7:325–333, 1980

Adler RH: Do anger and aggression affect carotid atherosclerosis? (letter). Stroke 24:1761, 1993

Allbert JR, Morrison JC: Neurologic diseases in pregnancy. Obstet Gynecol Clin North Am 19:765–781, 1992

Altura BM, Gupta RJ: Cocaine induces intracellular free Mg deficits, ischemia and stroke as observed by in vivo ^{31}P-NMR of the brain. Biochim Biophys Acta 1111:271–274, 1992

American Heart Association: Risk Factor Prediction Kit (#64–9590). Dallas, TX, American Heart Association, 1990

Aronow WS: Risk factors for geriatric stroke. Geriatrics 45:37–44, 1990

Bartleson JD: Transient and persistent neurological manifestations of migraine. Stroke 15:383–386, 1984

Bass C, Wade C: Type A behavior not specifically pathogenic? Lancet 2:1147–1151, 1982

Beiser M: Migration: opportunity or mental health risk? Triangle 29:83–90, 1990

Bitar S, Gomez CR: Stroke following injection of a melted suppository. Stroke 24:741–743, 1993

Bruno A: Stroke associated with ephedrine. Neurology 43:1313–1316, 1993

Brust JCM: Clinical, radiological, and pathological aspects of cerebrovascular disease associated with drug use. Stroke 24 (suppl 1):129–133, 1993

Brust JCM, Richter RW: Stroke associated with cocaine abuse. N Y State J Med 77:1473–1475, 1977

Buchanan A, Oliver JF: Abuse and neglect as causes of mental retardation. Br J Psychiatry 131:458–467, 1977

Caplan LR, Hier DB, Banks G: Current concepts of cerebrovascular disease–stroke: stroke and drug abuse. Stroke 13:869–872, 1982

Citron BP, Halpern N, Mccarron M, et al: Necrotizing angiitis associated with drug abuse. N Engl J Med 283:1003–1011, 1970

Colantonio A, Kasi SV, Ostfeld AM: Depressive symptoms and other psychosocial factors as predictors of stroke in the elderly. Am J Epidemiol 136:884–894, 1992

Dempsey RJ, Moore RW: Amount of smoking independently predicts carotid artery atherosclerosis severity. Stroke 23:693–696, 1992

Deringer PM, Hamilton LL, Whelan MA: Strokes associated with cocaine use (reply to Tuchman and Daras). Arch Neurol 47:1170, 1990

Dimsdale JE, Newton RP: Neuropsychological side effects of beta-blockers. Arch Intern Med 149:514–525, 1989

Donahue RP, Aboot RD, Reed DM, et al: Alcohol and hemorrhagic stroke: the Honolulu program. JAMA 255:2311–2314, 1986

Eaker ED, Feinleib M: Psychological factors and the 10-year incidence of cerebrovascular disease in the Framingham Heart Study (abstract). Psychosom Med 45:84, 1983

Ecker A: Emotional stress before strokes: a preliminary report of 20 cases. Ann Intern Med 40:49–56, 1954

Ellekjaer EF, Wyller TB, Sverre JM, et al: Life-style factors and risk of cerebral infarction. Stroke 23:829–834, 1992

Finucane FF, Madans JH, Bush TL, et al: Decreased risk of stroke among postmenopausal hormone users. Arch Intern Med 153:73–79, 1993

Gianturco DT, Brestin MS, Heyman A, et al: Personality patterns and life stress in ischemic cerebrovascular disease, I: psychiatric findings. Stroke 5:453–460, 1974

Gill JS, Zezulka AV, Shipley MJ, et al: Stroke and alcohol consumption. N Engl J Med 315:1041–1046, 1986

Goetz S, Adler RH, Weber R, et al: "High need for control" as a psychological risk in women suffering from stroke: a controlled retrospective exploratory study. Int J Psychiatry Med 22:119–129, 1992

Gorelick PB: Stroke from alcohol and drug abuse. Postgrad Med 88:171–178, 1990

Harrington H, Heller A, Dawson D, et al: Intracranial hemorrhage and oral amphetamine. Arch Neurol 40:503–507, 1983

Henrich JB, Horwitz RI: Evidence against the association between alcohol use and ischemic stroke risk. Arch Intern Med 149:1413–1416, 1989

Hess DC: Stroke associated with antiphospholipid antibodies. Stroke 23 (suppl I):I-23–I-28, 1992

Hillbom M, Kaste M, Rasi V: Can ethanol intoxication affect hemocoagulation to increase the risk of brain infarction in young adults? Neurology 33:381–400, 1983

Homer D, Ingall TJ, Baker HI, et al: Serum lipids and lipoproteins are less powerful predictors of extracranial carotid arteriosclerosis than are cigarette smoking and hypertension. Mayo Clin Proc 66:259–267, 1991

Hubbard RL, Marsden ME, Rachal JV, et al: Drug abuse and treatment: a national survey of effectiveness. Chapel Hill, NC, University of North Carolina Press, 1989

Iverson GL: Psychopathology associated with systemic lupus erythematosus: a methodological review. Semin Arthritis Rheum 22:242–251, 1993

Jackson AC, Boughner DR, Barnett JM: Mitral valve prolapse and cerebral ischemic events in young patients. Neurology 34:784–787, 1984

Jamrozik K, Broadhurst RJ, Anderson CS, et al: The role of lifestyle factors in the etiology of stroke. Stroke 25:51–59, 1994

Johnston DW: Prevention of cardiovascular disease by psychological methods. Br J Psychiatry 154:183–194, 1989

Kaku DA, Lowenstein DH: Emergence of recreational drug abuse as a major risk factor for stroke in young adults. Ann Intern Med 113:821–827, 1990

Kawachi I, Colditz GA, Stampfer MJ, et al: Smoking cessation and decreased risk of stroke in women. JAMA 269:232–236, 1993

Kelly-Hayes M: Framingham data: Stormy Monday linked to high risk of stroke (news report of presentation at American Academy of Neurology 44th Annual Meeting). Geriatrics 47:21, 1992

Kokkinos J, Levine SR: Possible association of ischemic stroke with phendimetrazine. Stroke 24:310–313, 1993

Krendel DA, Ditter SM, Frankel MR, et al: Biopsy-proven cerebral vasculitis associated with cocaine abuse. Neurology 40:1092–1094, 1990

Lazarus NB, Kaplan GA, Cohen RD, et al: Change in alcohol consumption and risk of death from all causes and from ischemic heart disease. BMJ 303:553–556, 1991

Levine SR, Brust JCM, Futrell N, et al: Cerebrovascular complications of the use of the "crack" form of alkaloidal cocaine. N Engl J Med 323:699–704, 1990

Lim LC, Lee T, Boey M: Psychiatric manifestations of systemic lupus erythematosus in Singapore: a cross-cultural comparison. Br J Psychiatry 159:520–523, 1991

Linden W: Sex differences in social content of anger expression. Paper presented at the meeting of the American Psychological Association, Toronto, Ontario, Canada, August 1993

Lingam VR, Lazarus LW, Groves L, et al: Methylphenidate in treating poststroke complications. J Clin Psychiatry 49:151–153, 1988

Lisk DR: Stroke risk factors in an African population: a report from Sierra Leone (letter). Stroke 24:139–140, 1993

Longstreth WT, Nelson LM: Caffeine and stroke (letter). Stroke 23:117, 1992

Longstreth WT, Nelson LM, Koepsell TD, et al: Cigarette smoking, alcohol use, and subarachnoid hemorrhage. Stroke 23:1242–1249, 1992

Love BB: Cigarette smoking: an important risk factor for stroke in young adults. Be Stroke Smart 7:9, 1990

Love BB, Biller J: Stroke in the young—cardiac cause. Stroke Clinical Updates 1:13–16, 1991

Matsumoto Y, Uyama O, Souichiro S, et al: Do anger and aggression affect carotid atherosclerosis? Stroke 24:983–986, 1993

Matthew RJ, Wilson WH: Substance abuse and cerebral blood flow. Am J Psychiatry 148:292–305, 1991

Mcdowell FH: Activation of rehabilitation. Arzneimittel-Forschung/Drug Research 41:355–359, 1991

Merten DF, Osborne DRF, Radkowski MA, et al: Craniocerebral trauma in the child abuse syndrome. Pediatric Radiology 14:272–277, 1984

Mueller SM: Neurological complications of phenylpropanolamine use. Neurology 33:623–628, 1983

Mueller SM, Muller J, Asdell SM: Cerebral hemorrhage associated with phenylpropanolamine in combination with caffeine. Stroke 15:119–123, 1984

Norris JW, Bladin CF: Stroke in the young (letter). Stroke 24:1417, 1993

Olsen ML: Autoimmune disease and stroke. Stroke Clinical Updates 3:13–16, 1992

Petty GW, Brust JCM, Tatemichi TK, et al: Embolic stroke after smoking "crack" cocaine. Stroke 21:1632–1635, 1990

Rimm EB, Giovannucci EL, Willett WC, et al: Prospective study of alcohol consumption and risk of coronary artery disease in men (letter). Lancet 338:464, 1991

Rogers RL, Meyer JS, Shaw TG, et al: The effects of chronic cigarette smoking on cerebrovascular responsiveness to 5% CO_2 and 100% O_2 inhalation. J Am Geriatr Soc 32:415–420, 1984

Rosenman RH, Brand RJ, Jenkins CD: Coronary heart disease in the Western Collaborative Group study. JAMA 233:872–877, 1975

Rothrock J, Walicke P, Swenson MR, et al: Migrainous stroke. Arch Neurol 45:63–67,1988

Rothrock J, Murray J, Madden K, et al: Migraine and migraine-associated stroke: risk factors and long term prognosis (abstract). Cephalgia 11 (suppl 2):185, 1991

Sloan MA, Kittner SJ, Rigaminti D, et al: Occurrence of stroke associated with use/misuse of drugs. Neurology 41:1358–1364, 1991

Sobel RJ, Espinas OE, Friedman SA: Carotid artery obstruction following LSD capsule ingestion. Arch Intern Med 127:290–291, 1971

Stern BJ, Kittner S, Sloan M, et al: Stroke in the young. Md Med J 40:453–462, 565–571, 1991

Stevens JH, Turner CW, Rhodewalt F, et al: The type A behavior pattern and carotid artery atherosclerosis. Psychosom Med 46:105–113, 1984

Systolic Hypertension in the Elderly Program (SHEP) Cooperative Research Group: Prevention of stroke by antihypertensive drug treatment in older persons with isolated systolic hypertension. JAMA 265:3255–3264, 1991

Taylor JR: Alcohol and strokes (letter). N Engl J Med 306:1111, 1982

Terao T, Mizuki T, Ohji T, et al: Anti-depressant effect of lithium in patients with systemic lupus erythematosus and cerebral infarction, treated with corticosteroid. Br J Psychiatry 164:109–111, 1994

Testa MA, Anderson RB, Nackley JF, et al: Quality of life and antihypertensive therapy in men: a comparison of captropril with enalapril. N Engl J Med 328:907–913, 1993

Tuchman AJ, Daras M: Strokes associated with cocaine use (letter). Arch Neurol 47:1170, 1990

Wehrmacher WH, Gonzalzles A: Stroke in the young. Internal Medicine for the Specialist 11:88–93, 1990

Weissman MM, Markowitz JS, Ouellette R, et al: Panic disorder and cardiovascular problems. Am J Psychiatry 147:1504–1508, 1990

Welch RM, Levine SR: Migraine related stroke in the context of the International Headache Society classification of head pain. Arch Neurol 47:458–462, 1990

Wilkins MR, Kendall MJ: Stroke affecting young men after alcoholic binges (letter). BMJ 291:1342, 1985

Williams RB: Cynical hostility pinpointed as type A behavior conducive to coronary heart disease (news report of paper presented at 1992 American Psychiatric Association annual meeting). Psychiatric News 27(13):8, July 3, 1992

Woo J, Lau E, Kay R: Elderly subjects aged 70 years and above have different risk factors for ischemic and hemorrhagic strokes compared with younger subjects. J Am Geriatr Soc 40:124–129, 1992

Zachariah SB: Stroke following marijuana smoking: response to Barnes, Palace and O'Brien (letter). Stroke 22:1381, 1992

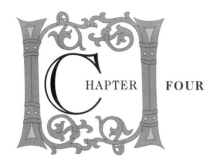

CHAPTER FOUR

Stroke and Localization of Brain Function

Evidence and Usefulness of Localization

The traditional methods of localizing functional areas of the brain were clinical observation and autopsy follow-up. The original numbers examined were small, but the findings have been confirmed over time. Many of the early anecdotal accounts compensated for their lack of statistical rigor by giving full descriptions of individual patients. The advent of brain imaging has enabled greater numbers to be studied, and larger study populations may, in turn, yield better statistical evidence, such as interrater reliability of descriptions of syndromes. However, brain-imaging techniques are in many ways less precise than brain examinations at autopsy. Table 4–1 shows the effects of localized brain lesions on selected mental functions.

Most possible sources of error lead to falsely describing a set of symptoms as specific to a particular localization. Misinterpretations of this kind are especially applicable to mental symptoms; indeed, such errors have been termed fallacies of overspecific conclusions that follow from the "bull in a Royal Worcester china shop" strategy (American Psycho-

Table 4–1.   Functional effects of localized brain lesions

Effect of lesion	Location of lesion	Evidence from infarct or hemorrhage cases	Consensus of agreement or quality of evidence	Chapter or other reference
Inability to produce speech	Broca's area	+	****	Chapter 6
Inability to understand speech	Wernicke's area	+	***	Chapter 6
Apathy	Frontal lobes	+	*	Chapter 10
Disinhibition	Frontal lobes	+	**	Chapter 12
Depression	Left frontal	+	**	Chapter 14
Hemineglect	Parietal lobes	+	***	Chapter 8
Visual hallucinations	Occipital lobes	+	***	Chapter 7
Inability to recognize faces or written words	Connections between parietal and occipital lobes	+	**	Chapter 7
Aggression and seizures	Temporal lobe		**	Chapter 11
Inability to register recently acquired information	Hippocampus	+	**	Chapter 16
Dementia	Lower part of genu of internal capsule	+	*	Chapter 16
Hypersexuality	Amygdala		*	Chapter 9
Subcortical dementia with bradyphrenia	Basal ganglia and thalamus	+	**	Chapter 16
Inability to learn skills as opposed to facts	Head of left caudate nucleus and surrounding white matter		*	Damasio 1992

(continued)

Table 4–1.   Functional effects of localized brain lesions *(continued)*

Effect of lesion	Location of lesion	Evidence from infarct or hemor- rhage cases	Consensus of agreement or quality of evidence	Chapter or other reference
Apathy	Caudate nucleus	+	*	Chapter 10
Repetitive behavior	Head of both caudate nuclei	+	*	Croisile et al. 1989
Apathy and lack of motivation	Both lentiform nuclei	+	*	Strub 1989
Spontaneous unilateral pain	Thalamus	+	**	Chapter 8
Mania	Right thalamus	+	*	Chapter 12
"Utilization behavior"	Bilateral thalamus		*	Chapter 12
Episodes of apathy and of hyper- activity	Thalamus	+	*	Chapter 12
Visual hallucinations	Midbrain	+	**	Chapter 7
Coma	Brain stem	+	****	Chapter 17
Acute confusion with rapid recovery	Brain stem	+	**	Chapter 16

Note.   + = Evidence from infarct or hemorrhage cases. Consensus of agreement or quality of evidence: * = Supported by a single published article or author; ** = Both supported and contradicted by several published articles and authors; *** = Contradicted by a single published article or author; **** = Not contradicted by any published article or author.

logical Association 1974, p. 22). If, for example, a psychotic patient happens to have an infarct, and also has a particular kind of delusion, then failure to do a complete psychiatric assessment may lead to regarding the delusion as caused by the infarct, when it is really part of a larger picture of psychosis.

In everyday psychiatric practice, the usefulness for management purposes of linking a mental disability to a brain location may be doubted. Some brain localizations are of only theoretical significance. What is useful to the patient is often an exact delineation of his or her disability rather than information about its anatomical basis. If, however, an abnormal speech pattern is found to be part of a certain type of aphasia rather than a manifestation of an emotional illness, this finding can be helpful in its management. In some such cases, localization of the lesion is made by neurological and radiological examination. This localization is then useful in explaining the mental symptoms, rather than the mental symptoms being useful in determining the location of the lesion.

Stroke and Other Keys to Localization

Stroke has played a large part in increasing our knowledge about the effects of localized brain damage because it is the most common cause of such damage. However, stroke-caused lesions do not provide clear information about cerebral localization because such lesions are often multiple and accompanied by other conditions that obscure the clinical picture. A strictly localized experimental lesion is ideal, but this can only be attained in animals, and animal experiments are of limited use in investigating mental effects and aphasia.

Head injuries are a better source of information about the mental effects of localized brain damage in humans, but even here the patient does not always get a circumscribed lesion without complications.

It is possible that the effects of destruction of an area of the brain vary according to what has caused the destruction. Strokes cause more severe effects than tumors, relative to the area destroyed. Anderson et al. (1990) compared stroke patients with brain tumor patients. Despite close matching of the location of lesions, they found that subjects with stroke in the left hemisphere had more severe language deficits than subjects with left-hemisphere tumors, and some of the tumor subjects performed normally on all neuropsychological tests.

Gerstmann's Syndrome and Localization

Gerstmann's syndrome is worth considering in detail as an example of the process of designating a new syndrome and associating it with a particular brain area.

Gerstmann (1927) described a syndrome consisting of disorientation for right and left, inability to name the fingers correctly, and inability to write or to calculate. Obviously, many dementia patients have all four of these defects. Gerstmann contended that this syndrome was due a lesion of the left angular gyrus (see Figure 4–1). Gerstmann's syndrome was subsequently described in texts and cited as evidence of the remarkable localization of certain language skills to certain areas of the cortex.

Investigators who reexamined the topic pointed out that Gerstmann's original data were scanty, and included subjects with widespread brain lesions and generalized mental confusion. The alleged syndrome could not be substantiated, and one paper about it—called "The Fiction of the Gerstmann Syndrome"—pointed out that

> a patient with parieto-occipital disease may show one or more of a relatively large number of diverse behavioral deficits. When he presents with two, three, or more of these symptoms, the latter may be viewed by the clinical observer as forming a naturally occurring combination of deficits and given the status of a syndrome, this status implying that the concurrence of deficits is not a chance one, that there is an underlying factor responsible for it, and that it possesses a distinctive neuropathological significance. Once such a special combination or syndrome is established, not only is it used in the observation and description of subsequent cases but it may also determine what aspects of a patient's behavior are selected for study and which are not. (Benton 1961, p. 176)

Gerstmann seemed to be vindicated by the case of a patient who showed all four Gerstmann deficits in the absence of dementia, 1 week

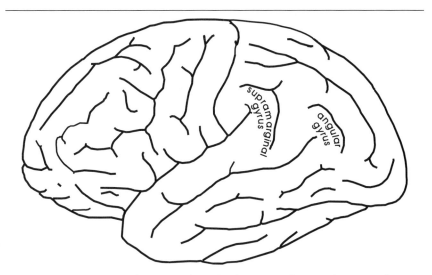

Figure 4–1.   Lateral surface view of cerebral cortex indicating location of angular and supramarginal gyri.

after an ischemic cerebral infarction (Roeltgen et al. 1983). A computed tomography (CT) scan showed a cortical lesion involving the upper part of the left angular and supramarginal gyri. However, whether a single case can be considered enough evidence for localization is debatable (Benton 1992). A further complication has been the description of a case in a patient with a right parietal infarct (Moore et al. 1991).

Brain Pathways and Projection Systems

Traditional studies of the localization of mental functions in the brain were mainly concerned with ascribing functions to single areas, especially of the cerebral cortex. Function may also be identified as being performed by a single system with widespread connections. An analogy might be the various systems in an automobile. If a car overheats, the reason could be damage to the water pump, the thermostat, the radiator, the fan belt, or any of the connections between these. Tracking down such connections in the brain is done primarily in three ways.

The first is the old-fashioned method of dissection of the formalinized brain. This remains a basic source of information. An example of a pathway that can be traced out by dissection is the *limbic system,* or *Papez circuit* (Figure 4–2). The fornix, the stria terminalis, the mammillothalamic tract, the habenula, the cingulum, and the medial forebrain bundle can all be demonstrated to the naked eye by scalpel and forceps.

A second classical way to determine the connections between parts of the brain is to track down the effects of damage to one part histologically. Myelin stains will show the complete course of axons that have been damaged in one part of their length. A nerve cell may degenerate because of damage either to its own axon or to that of a cell that makes a synaptic connection with it. Cells in the lateral geniculate bodies, for example, degenerate after the loss of an eye or infarction of the occipital lobe (Figures 4–3 and 4–4). Nerve cells in the dorsomedial thalamic nucleus (Figure 4–3) degenerate after infarction of the frontal lobe.

A third method is now displacing the older ones. Projection systems are mapped by following the tracks of neurotransmitter substances. The site of neurotransmitter production is identified, and the receptor sites can be localized by using neurotransmitters labeled with isotopes.

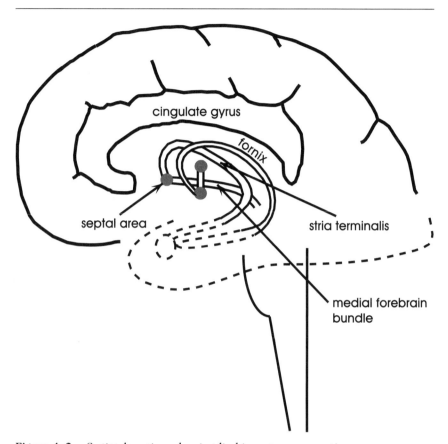

Figure 4–2.   Sagittal section, showing limbic system connections.

Psychological Testing

Several psychological tests were originally devised to provide evidence of the existence of a brain lesion in a particular area. Because of the advent of imaging techniques, such tests now are more often used to provide evidence of the severity, rather than the brain location, of a disability. Sometimes a test originally designed to diagnose damage to a particular brain area constitutes a useful measure of a specific disability without actually providing valid evidence of a localized lesion. Although it may be inaccurate to designate such a test as an assessment of parietal or frontal function, that does not diminish its practical utility. The statistical qualities of a test may prove that it measures a real entity,

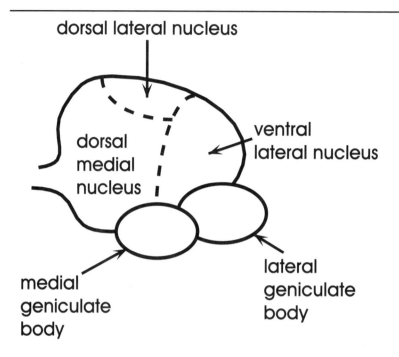

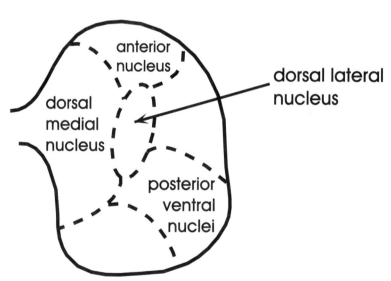

Figure 4–3. Thalamus seen from behind *(top)*, showing the lateral and medial geniculate bodies, and from above *(bottom)*, showing the location of some of the nuclei.

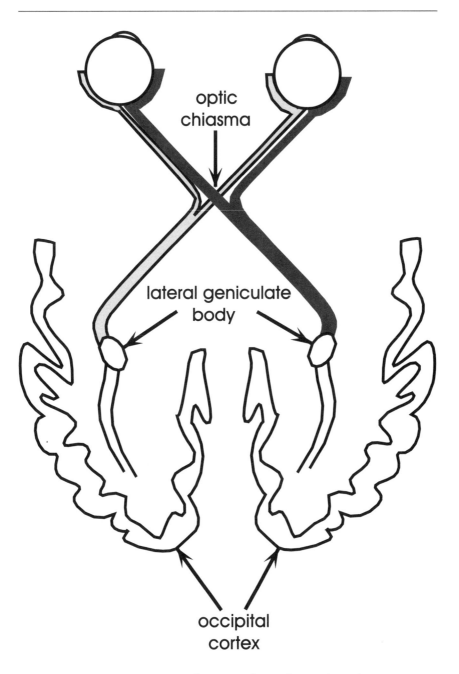

Figure 4–4. Transverse section, showing pathway of vision from the retina to the occipital cortex.

even if that entity is not a particular localized type of brain damage.

Examples of tests commonly mentioned in the stroke literature are listed in Table 4–2. The annually updated volumes of the *Mental Measurements Yearbook* (Buros 1938–) provide full listings. Often used in neuropsychological practice are batteries of tests, the most popular in the United States being that of Halstead-Reitan (Reitan and Wolfson 1985).

In the Wisconsin Card Sorting Test (Heaton 1985), subjects are instructed to sort cards with various colors and shapes according to certain rules, but are not told the rules. In the Stroop Test (Stroop 1935), the task of naming colors is made more difficult by supplying the wrong color names. Other possible tests of frontal lobe function are the Radial Arm Maze Test and the Computerized Tower of London Test (Orrell et al. 1989).

Several tests of parietal lobe function are in use, but any patient with dementia will find some of them difficult (Stone et al. 1991). In the Kew Parietal Test (McDonald 1969), the patient is asked to touch the left ear with the right hand, show the left hand, identify a coin placed in the right hand, construct a square with matches, and distinguish between being touched in two places. The frequent failure of elderly patients without focal brain lesions to complete items in such tests was been addressed by O'Carroll et al. (1991), who used age-matched control subjects in developing the Behavioral Inattention Test for hemineglect.

Various tests of memory have been used as measures of temporal lobe function, including the Visual Reproduction subtest of the Wechsler Memory Scale (Wechsler 1987) and the Block-Tapping Test of Corsi (Milner 1971).

Table 4–2. Psychological tests of localized cortical function

Brain location	Functional assessment tests
Parietal lobe	Kew Parietal Test (McDonald 1969) Behavioral Inattention Test for hemineglect (O'Carroll et al. 1991)
Frontal lobe	Wisconsin Card Sorting Test (Heaton 1985) Stroop Test (Stroop 1935) Radial Arm Maze Test (Orrell et al. 1989) Computerized Tower of London Test (Orrell et al. 1989)
Temporal lobe	Visual Reproduction subtest of Wechsler Memory Scale (Wechsler 1987) Block-Tapping Test of Corsi (Milner 1971)

Left Brain Versus Right Brain

The fact that patients with infarcts on the left side of the brain lose their power of speech has inspired a search for some kind of mental power unique to the right side of the brain. Much has been written about this phenomenon, mostly suggesting that a nonverbal type of mental ability resides in the right side of the brain. According to one reviewer of the literature on this topic, "The left brain–right brain story, while giving rise to much creative scientific enquiry, has also spawned some rather dubious psychophantasy" (David 1989, p. 422).

Among the defects suggested to be caused by right cerebral hemisphere damage have been loss of understanding of the metaphoric or humorous use of language, inability to understand motivations of characters and logical interrelationships among events in a narrative passage, deficiency in verbal problem solving (Benowitz et al. 1990), disorders of spatial manipulation (right parietal), schizophrenia-like psychosis (right temporal), loss of creativity, loss of willpower, loss of ego boundaries with "response to next-patient-stimulation," Capgras' syndrome, incorrect proverb interpretation, impaired ability to estimate the cost of common objects, tendency to overcategorize objects, and incoherent and tangential speech (Cutting 1992).

Ross (1981; Ross and Rush 1981) has coined the term *aprosodia* to describe a specific set of disturbances of the ability to express or understand the emotional component of speech. He believes that aprosodia is due to lesions of the right side of the brain, in the area of the Sylvian fissure, and that these lesions are an exact mirror of the lesions of the left side of the brain that are known to cause aphasia. The Ross theory is of great interest but is based on small numbers of cases without statistical analysis.

Many of the experimental studies of right-brain function have been done with subjects with split brains, capitalizing on the fact that the right side of the brain sees objects in the left side of the visual field. When blindfolded, split-brain subjects cannot correctly name objects placed in their left hands, but can pick them out from an array of objects later—a finding that has been taken to mean that although the brain receives the information and can use it, the object never gets named by the brain.

Splitting the brain means effectively severing the corpus callosum (see Figure A–1 in Appendix A), which is supplied by the anterior cerebral artery. Such severance is unlikely to occur as a result of a stroke unless there is very extensive damage.

Comparing Left-Sided and Right-Sided Strokes

The consensus is that mental disturbance is a more prominent and con-
spicuous feature of stroke damage to the right hemisphere than of damage to the left. However, this may not necessarily mean that mental
disturbance is truly more common in right-hemisphere damage than in
left-hemisphere damage, because a problem of comparability of groups
arises whenever the mental effects of the site of the brain infarct are
considered.

The fact that damage to the left side of the brain causes right-sided
paralysis and loss of speech makes it difficult to detect mental deficits in
individuals who have sustained left-hemisphere infarcts. Patients who cannot speak or otherwise express themselves will not be able to perform
well on tests requiring communication, and paralysis of the dominant
hand may impede tasks such as copying drawings in tests of visuospatial
ability (Kirk and Kertesz 1989). This means that the tester faces the task
of deciding how the patient's deficits affect the test results.

Another reason that individuals with left-sided lesions cannot always
be used as matched control subjects for those with right-sided lesions in
studies of hospitalized patients is that left-side and right-side stroke patients may be hospitalized for different reasons. For example, infarcts on
the left side of the brain cause right-sided hemiplegia and aphasia; such
infarcts might therefore be expected to cause more disability than those
on the right side of the brain. These differences in disability might be
reflected in differences in hospitalization rates. More hospital patients
have left-hemisphere infarcts than have right-hemisphere infarcts, but
even in the United States, 40% of people who have a stroke are not hospitalized (Alberts et al. 1992).

Almost any population we study is skewed. The direction of this bias
must be taken into account when using patients with left-brain infarcts
as control subjects to study patients with right-brain infarcts.

The right-handed person who has lost both the use of the right hand
and the power of speech is obviously severely handicapped. The impairments of the left hemiplegia patient are less obvious but may also be
severe. Left hemianopsia and hemineglect may be present. Because these
deficits are more subtle, the effect of therapy may be to point them out
and to make them more evident, and the patient may resent this. In
obvious right hemiplegia, the therapist does not have to begin with the
task of showing patients that they are more disabled than they had
thought.

In practice, behavioral problems are more obvious in left-hemiplegia patients, for reasons that are still speculative. It may be simply that the *physical* handicaps are less obvious. Compared with right-hemiplegia patients, those with left hemiplegia are more mobile and more able to talk, and thus more capable of expressing or acting on negative feelings. Such patients are sometimes described as quick and impulsive (Vance 1993). Their tendency to deny their disabilities *(anosognosia)* is discussed in Chapter 18. A publication these patients and their families may find helpful is "How Stroke Affects Behavior" (American Heart Association 1991), which explains the impairments of left hemiplegia in lay terms.

Summary

Aphasia is the best-established impairment predicting the location of a brain lesion. Prefrontal lesions are generally supposed to cause personality and emotional disorders, of which the most distinctive is the disinhibited type. Parietal lesions can cause apraxia and subtle sensory disturbances. Several temporal lobe syndromes have been described, but these are not well documented for stroke patients. Certain types of memory deficits may be localized to the hippocampus. The occipital lobes are concerned with vision, but evidence for the location of specific types of psychovisual disturbance is often conflicting. Dementia in which there is slowing of thought processes rather than memory loss is considered to be subcortical. Brain stem lesions characteristically produce deep coma and localizing neurological signs rather than mental symptoms, but may give rise to confusional states. Psychological tests are useful in determining the severity and type of impairment, even if they are not diagnostic of lesion location. Patients with left hemiplegia are generally more likely to have behavioral disturbances than are those with right hemiplegia.

References

Alberts MJ, Perry A, Dawson DV, et al: Effects of public and professional education on reducing the delay in presentation and referral of stroke. Stroke 23:352–356, 1992

American Heart Association: How Stroke Affects Behavior. Dallas, TX, American Heart Association, 1991

American Psychological Association: Publication Manual of the American Psychological Association. Washington, DC, American Psychological Association, 1974

Anderson SW, Damasio H, Tranel D: Neuropsychological impairments associated with lesions caused by tumor or stroke. Arch Neurol 47:397–405, 1990

Benowitz LI, Moya KL, Levine DL: Impaired verbal reasoning and constructional apraxia in subjects with right hemisphere damage. Neuropsychologia 28:231–241, 1990

Benton AL: The fiction of the Gerstmann syndrome. J Neurol Neurosurg Psychiatry 24:176–181, 1961

Benton AL: Gerstmann's syndrome. Arch Neurol 49:445–447, 1992

Buros OK (ed): Mental Measurements Yearbook. New Brunswick, NJ, Rutgers University Press, 1938 (annual updates)

Croisile B, Tourniaire D, Confavreux C, et al: Bilateral damage to the head of the caudate nucleus. Ann Neurol 25:313–314, 1989

Cutting J: The role of right hemisphere dysfunction in psychiatric disorders. Br J Psychiatry 160:583–588, 1992

Damasio AR: Aphasia. N Engl J Med 326:531–539, 1992

David AS: Reading about the split-brain syndrome. Br J Psychiatry 154:422–425, 1989

Gerstmann J: Fingeragnosie und isolierte Agraphie, ein neues Syndrom. Zeitschrift für die gesamte Neurologie und Psychiatrie 108:152–177, 1927

Heaton R: Wisconsin Card Sorting Test. Odessa, FL, Psychological Assessment Resources, 1985

Kirk A, Kertesz A: Hemispheric contributions to drawing. Neuropsychologia 27:881–886, 1989

McDonald C: Clinical heterogeneity in senile dementia. Br J Psychiatry 115:267–273, 1969

Milner B: Interhemispheric differences in the localization of psychological processes in man. British Medical Bulletin 27:272–277, 1971

Moore MR, Saver JL, Johnson KA, et al: Right parietal stroke with Gerstmann's syndrome: appearance on computed tomography, magnetic resonance imaging, and single photon emission computed tomography. Arch Neurol 48:432–435, 1991

O'Carroll RO, Whittick J, Baikie E: Parietal signs and sinister prognosis in dementia. Br J Psychiatry 158:358–361, 1991

Orrell MW, Sahakian BJ, Bergmann K: Self-neglect and frontal lobe dysfunction. Br J Psychiatry 155:101–105, 1989

Reitan RM, Wolfson D: The Halstead-Reitan Neuropsychological Test Battery: Theory and Clinical Interpretation. Tucson, AZ, Neuropsychology Press, 1985

Roeltgen DP, Sevush S, Heilman KM: Pure Gerstmann's syndrome from a focal lesion. Arch Neurol 40:46–47, 1983

Ross ED: The aprosodias: functional-anatomical organization of the affective components of language in the right hemisphere. Arch Neurol 38:561–569, 1981

Ross ED, Rush JA: Diagnosis and neuroanatomical correlates of depression in brain-damaged patients. Arch Gen Psychiatry 38:1344–1354, 1981

Stone SP, Halligan PW, Wilson B, et al: Performance of age matched controls on a battery of visuo-spatial neglect tests. J Neurol Neurosurg Psychiatry 54:341–344, 1991

Stroop JR: Studies of interference in serial verbal reactions. J Exp Psychol 18:643–662, 1935

Strub RL: Frontal lobe syndrome in a patient with bilateral globus pallidus lesions. Arch Neurol 48:1024–1027, 1989

Vance B: An open letter to family, relatives and friends of stroke survivors. Be Stroke Smart 10:15–16, 1993

Wechsler D: Wechsler Memory Scale—Revised. San Antonio, TX, Psychological Corporation, 1987

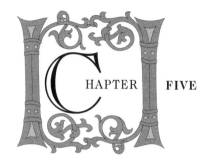

CHAPTER FIVE

Neuropsychopharmacology of Stroke

Neurotransmitters

Among the neurotransmitters especially relevant to the psychiatric aspects of stroke are glutamate (an excitatory amino acid), gamma-aminobutyric acid (GABA, an inhibitory amino acid), acetylcholine, the catecholamines (norepinephrine, epinephrine, and dopamine), and serotonin (5-hydroxytryptamine, or 5-HT).

To transmit messages from one nerve cell to another, neurotransmitters must act at precisely one spot and at one time. This precision is accomplished in five main ways: by the arrangement of the nerve cell synapses; by the packaging of the neurotransmitter substance in discrete vesicles within the cell; by the presence in the fluid around nerve cell endings of enzymes that can destroy surplus neurotransmitters; by a process whereby nerve cell endings snatch back any spare neurotransmitter as soon as they have used it to pass a message (reuptake); and by the presence on the surface membrane of the receiving cell of localized and specific receptors and channels. The arrival of the neurotransmitter at these receptors results in changes in the interior of the receiving nerve cell.

The action of a psychotropic drug is often to reduce the reuptake of a particular neurotransmitter, thereby enhancing the latter's action. Several antidepressants work in this way. Many sedatives and anticonvulsants act on inhibitory receptors. Lithium acts within the receiving nerve cell on the "second messenger."

Some receptors are doughnut-shaped proteins in the walls of the receiving cell that can allow chloride to flow in or out of the cell through the hole in the doughnut. Such receptors are called *ligand-gated*. The glutamate receptor and the GABA$_A$ receptor are of this type. Others, such as the dopamine receptor, are called G protein–linked. These do not themselves have holes, but act by transduction, causing production of a second-messenger substance inside the cell, which then causes the opening of other gates (voltage-gated ion channels) in the cell wall.

Infarct Location and Neurotransmitters

The neurotransmitter-producing areas, other than those for glutamic acid and GABA, tend to be localized: norepinephrine in the locus coeruleus, acetylcholine in the nucleus of Meynert, serotonin in raphe nuclei in the pons and medulla, and dopamine in the substantia nigra. Usually the receptor sites are more diffusely distributed, but some of these can also be mapped, as can the pathways (also called *projection systems*) the neurotransmitters follow to them (Figures 5–1, 5–2, 5–3, and 5–4).

Our knowledge of the anatomical status of these pathways varies. In some cases, the pathways conform to the bundles of axons mapped out by traditional anatomical dissection and are given conventional names, usually including the word *tract*. In other cases, their direction and general location can be deduced from neurochemical studies but their precise structure is not known.

The discovery of these specialized neurotransmitter-producing areas and distribution pathways suggests that a strategically situated infarct might produce a specific deficiency of a particular neurotransmitter. For example, the finding of acetylcholine deficiency in Alzheimer's disease and the recognition that acetylcholine's principal origin in the brain is the nucleus basalis of Meynert have led to the suggestion that infarcts of this area might specifically cause dementia—a hypothesis that has not been confirmed empirically. The relationships between specific emotional disorders in stroke and serotonin and catecholamine deficiencies are discussed further in Chapters 11, 12, and 14.

Poisonous Messengers

In brain injury of any kind, including stroke, the damaged nerve cells send out a surge of uncoordinated messages, so that there is a flood of neurotransmitters, which become "poisonous" to the receptor cells at high doses. Glutamic acid is primarily involved (Baethmann et al. 1989; Longstreth and Nelson 1992), but catecholamines, adenosine, and other neurotransmitters may also act in this way (Napier and Friedman 1989). This excitotoxic effect takes place at the kind of glutamic acid receptors called N-methyl-D-aspartate (NMDA) receptors. It results in an excessive flow of calcium into the receptor nerve cell and a sequence of chemical changes that kills the cell.

One approach to treating acute stroke has therefore been to use drugs that counteract glutamic acid (Marangos 1990) and that block the NMDA receptors. A limitation has been that these NMDA-receptor–blocking

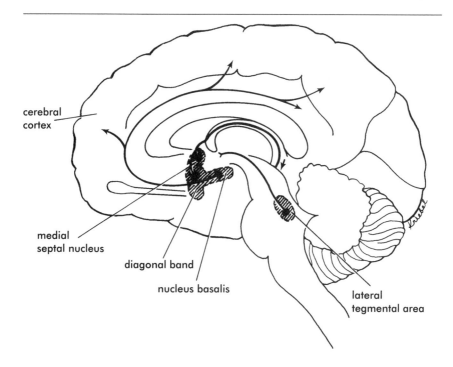

Figure 5–1.   Cholinergic projection systems in the brain.
Source.   Adapted from Hyman SE, Nestler EJ: *The Molecular Foundations of Psychiatry.* Washington, DC, American Psychiatric Press, 1993, p. 88. Copyright 1993, American Psychiatric Press, Inc. Used with permission.

drugs (such as the synthetic opioids) may cause mental disturbance (Albers et al. 1992; Buchan 1992; Scheinberg 1991).

Interaction of Drug Effects and Stroke Effects

Antianxiety Drugs

Drugs that reduce anxiety have many side effects in common. Among those effects particularly relevant to stroke are drowsiness, liability to falls, and impairment of memory. The effects of antianxiety drugs can include a slight immediate deleterious effect on memory, a long-term damaging effect on the brain at high dosages, and acute confusion if the drug is stopped abruptly after being used for an extended period. Seizures and mental disturbance can occur during withdrawal. As with alcohol, the withdrawal and its effects may occur upon hospitalization of a

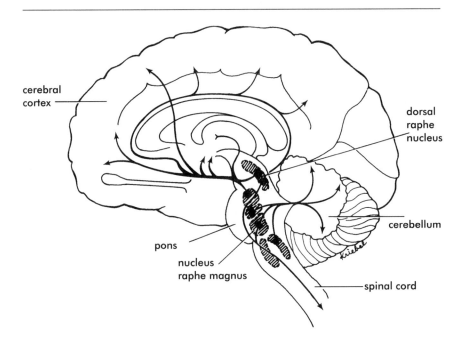

Figure 5–2.   Serotonergic projection systems in the brain.
Source.   Adapted from Hyman SE, Nestler EJ: *The Molecular Foundations of Psychiatry.* Washington, DC, American Psychiatric Press, 1993, p. 86. Copyright 1993, American Psychiatric Press, Inc. Used with permission.

patient about whose prior intake nothing is known, thus causing diagnostic errors if superimposed on a stroke.

These similarities in effect are probably due to the fact that all of these substances act on the doughnut-shaped GABA receptor. GABA encourages chloride ions to go into the cell through the hole in the doughnut. Chloride ions are negatively charged, so that more chloride in the cell makes it more negatively charged inside, thus inhibiting it.

Benzodiazepines.   The benzodiazepines are the most commonly used drugs for anxiety (see Chapter 15). Benzodiazepines bind to a part of the GABA receptor called the benzodiazepine site and make the receptor more attractive to GABA.

These drugs are used in stroke patients to treat insomnia or anxiety, to reduce muscle spasticity, as anticonvulsants, and for emergency seda-

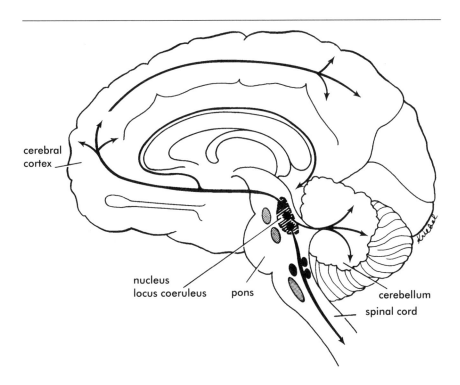

Figure 5–3.   Noradrenergic projection systems in the brain.
Source.   Adapted from Hyman SE, Nestler EJ: *The Molecular Foundations of Psychiatry.* Washington, DC, American Psychiatric Press, 1993, p. 78. Copyright 1993, American Psychiatric Press, Inc. Used with permission.

tion. A disadvantage of benzodiazepines for seizure control is that tolerance develops and they stop working (Rall and Schleifer 1985). Some controversy surrounds the long-term use of benzodiazepines for insomnia and anxiety (Elliot-Baker and Tiller 1990; Rickels et al. 1991). Potential problems with such use in stroke patients include confusion, unsteady gait, and tolerance that renders these agents ineffective for insomnia. Health Care Financing Administration (HCFA) guidelines mandate careful monitoring of benzodiazepine use in nursing homes (HCFA 1992; Zito 1989).

Anticonvulsants.   About 15%–20% of stroke patients develop seizures (Larkin 1991), and anticonvulsant drugs are used to treat or forestall

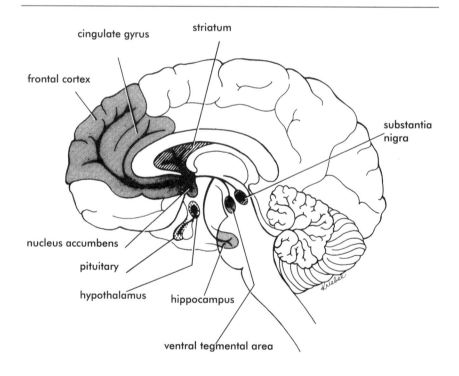

Figure 5–4.   Dopaminergic projection systems in the brain.
Source.   Adapted from Hyman SE, Nestler EJ: *The Molecular Foundations of Psychiatry.* Washington, DC, American Psychiatric Press, 1993, p. 77. Copyright 1993, American Psychiatric Press, Inc. Used with permission.

these. Some anticonvulsant drugs act on the inhibitory $GABA_A$ receptor and can cause cognitive impairment, drowsiness, or motor impairment. Phenobarbital is more likely to cause these side effects than is phenytoin (Dilantin), but Dilantin can cause cognitive and motor impairment if too high a dose is given, possibly even one within the therapeutic range (Trimble and Reynolds 1976).

Some drugs originally developed as anticonvulsants are also used to treat behavioral or mood disturbances. Carbamazepine (Tegretol) and valproic acid (Depakote) are frequently used for this purpose. Both of these drugs are atypical in that they do not have the sedative and antianxiety properties of most anticonvulsant drugs, such as benzodiazepines and barbiturates that act on the $GABA_A$ receptor. Their probable action is not on the $GABA_A$ receptor (which controls chloride channels) but rather directly on the channels for transmission of ions other than chloride across the nerve cell membrane. The ion channels involved are the voltage-gated sodium channels in the case of carbamazepine, and the voltage-gated calcium channels in the case of valproic acid (MacDonald and Kelly 1993).

Carbamazepine.   Carbamazepine is used for a variety of psychiatric and neurological conditions. It has been suggested that its usefulness is related to a specific effect on the limbic system (Sugarman 1992). In addition to being the drug of choice for complex partial seizures, carbamazepine is used to treat mania, especially rapid-cycling bipolar disorder (Ballenger 1988; Chou 1991) and various psychiatric conditions accompanied by behavioral dyscontrol (Keck et al. 1992). It is widely used for treating antisocial behavior in patients with brain damage, although its empirical use for this purpose has been criticized (Bridgman 1993).

Based on a review of the literature, Richardson (1992) suggested that there are two groups of patients who develop a psychosis after a right-hemisphere stroke. One group is relatively young and free of other chronic physical or mental illness. People in this group develop psychotic symptoms a month to several years after a stroke and "tend to have [electroencephalograms] demonstrating epileptiform activity" (Richardson 1992, p. 382). These individuals are helped by anticonvulsant medication. A second group is older and develops abnormal behavior soon after the stroke. This group is sometimes helped by antipsychotic medication.

Successful use of carbamazepine in combination with phenelzine to treat poststroke depression has been described (Yatham et al. 1990). Carbamazepine showed no significant advantage over placebo in a trial of drug treatments for central poststroke pain (Liejon and Boivie 1989). Although dizziness, drowsiness, and ataxia have been the most frequently reported side effects relevant to carbamazepine's use in stroke patients, hematological and other adverse effects also occur.

Valproic acid.   Valproic acid is especially effective in preventing *absence seizures* (a type of seizure in which the patient is briefly unaware of the surroundings but does not have convulsions). Its use in psychiatry has been primarily for recurrent affective disorder (Lovett et al. 1986), but there are several reports of its utility in panic disorder and behavioral dyscontrol syndromes (Keck et al. 1992). The psychiatric indications for valproic acid closely parallel those for carbamazepine but are less well-established by controlled trials (Chou et al. 1993). It is probably less likely than carbamazepine to cause cognitive impairment, blurring of vision, or ataxia.

The risk-benefit ratio must be considered in seizure control. If a patient is to return to work and to driving a car, attempts to control seizures must be vigorous. If those activities are not realistic goals, the untoward effects of the drugs must be balanced against the risks from seizures. These risks include an element of danger to life from status epilepticus.

Fully alert epileptic patients seen in office practice sometimes refuse to take anticonvulsant medications, mostly because of adverse effects on alertness and general psychological well-being. Because stroke patients who have communication problems may not be able to describe adverse symptoms they may be experiencing, clinicians must carefully monitor for such effects.

Antipsychotic Drugs

Antipsychotics are often used following stroke as nonspecific sedatives for agitation. These drugs include thioridazine (Mellaril), chlorpromazine (Thorazine), trifluoperazine (Stelazine), perphenazine (Trilafon), and fluphenazine (Prolixin), which are phenothiazines, and haloperidol (Haldol) and thiothixene (Navane). Their equivalent effectiveness in psychosis, as well as their similar neurological side effects, is probably related to their blockage of dopamine effects. Most antipsychotics block all types of dopamine receptors. The primary sites of dopamine production are the substantia nigra and the adjacent areas of the midbrain. Dopamine receptors are mainly in the corpus striatum and the frontal cortex. The blockage of dopamine receptors causes movement disorders, partly as the result of increased action of acetylcholine in the corpus striatum. These disorders can be counteracted with anticholinergic drugs. The more recently introduced antipsychotics block only specific types of dopamine receptors and are not as likely to cause movement disorders.

The neurological side effects of antipsychotic drugs can exacerbate or mimic the effects of stroke. These effects include drowsiness, parkinsonism, dystonia, akathisia, and tardive dyskinesia. Drowsiness usually begins about 2 hours after the drug is taken and lasts for about 12 hours. Parkinsonism and dystonia are dose related. Tardive dyskinesia is related to the length of time the drug has been taken, and is more common in elderly and brain-damaged patients, which means that stroke patients are at high risk. Akathisia can take the form of pacing or restlessness, which may lead to a mistaken decision to increase the dose of the causative drug.

Single doses of dopamine-blocking drugs given to animals with experimentally produced stroke delay recovery of mobility. On the other hand, the properties of phenothiazines include an antioxidant effect, which might protect against the acute effects of ischemia. The dopamine blockers currently used in psychiatry are not potent in this regard, but a phenothiazine with strong antioxidant capacity has been found to reduce rat brain damage after focal ischemia (Yu et al. 1992).

Since dopamine-blocking drugs reduce psychosis, a hypothetical danger exists that dopamine-stimulating drugs may aggravate psychosis. Nonetheless, dopamine-stimulating drugs such as levodopa have been used experimentally in stroke patients to treat aphasia (Albert and Helm-Estabrooks 1988), hemineglect (Fleet et al. 1987), and emotional incontinence (Wolf et al. 1979). None of these uses is well established.

Anticholinergic Drugs

There are two types of acetylcholine receptor: the nicotinic receptor is the ligand-gated type, and the muscarinic receptor is G protein–linked. Mental effects are mostly mediated by the muscarinic receptors.

Several drugs have the capability to block the action of acetylcholine. These drugs are likely to be encountered in the management of stroke patients because individuals in this population often take multiple medications. Anticholinergic drugs such as benztropine (Cogentin) are used to treat the neurological side effects of the dopamine-blocking antipsychotic drugs, although some of the latter have an intrinsic anticholinergic action. Antihistamines and tricyclic antidepressants are also potent in this regard. The *anticholinergic intoxication syndrome* can present as an acute mental disorder, with delirium, dry mouth, and dilated pupils. Elderly patients are especially vulnerable to cognitive impairment from this cause (Molloy 1987).

The Stroke Patient on Psychotropic Drugs

Because so many individuals take psychotropic drugs, clinicians often encounter patients who were taking such medications before they had a stroke. Complications may arise from either continuing or stopping these drugs. Such complications can be divided into three categories: direct effects of drug withdrawal, relapse of the patient's mental condition due to drug withdrawal, and adverse effects of the psychotropic drug on the patient's physical illness.

Withdrawal Effects

Delirium and seizures can result from sudden withdrawal of benzodiazepines, barbiturates, or anticonvulsants (see Chapter 15). No life-threatening effects are produced by abrupt withdrawal of phenothiazines or antidepressants. Charney et al. (1982) described anxiety and increased noradrenergic activity, but no changes in blood pressure or heart rate, following antidepressant withdrawal.

The pharmacokinetics of dopamine-blocking antipsychotic drugs are such that the effects of stopping their administration are slow and unlikely to become clinically evident during the acute stage of stroke treatment. If benztropine, being used to counteract drug side effects, is stopped at the same time as a dopamine-blocking antipsychotic drug, an acute dystonia may be precipitated because antipsychotics have a longer half-life (i.e., stay in the system longer).

Several psychiatric conditions require long-term drug maintenance medication to prevent recurrence. Relapse may be delayed for weeks or months after withdrawal. Psychosis that occurs in a stroke patient in a rehabilitation or nursing-home setting sometimes represents a relapse of an illness that was being treated with antipsychotic medications that were withdrawn during the course of acute medical treatment.

Adverse Drug Effects

Orthostatic hypotension can be produced by several psychotropic drugs. This condition can be quite debilitating. Its detrimental effects may become more marked after a stroke. The possible role of hypotension in vascular dementia is discussed in Chapter 16. The frequent co-occurrence of cardiovascular disease and stroke enhances the hazards of cardiotoxic effects such as the quinidine-like actions of tricyclic antidepressants.

One of the risks of continuing psychotropic medications when a psychiatric patient suffers a stroke is the possibility of drug interactions. Stroke may lead to the patient's receiving several additional drugs that interact with the psychotropic drug. For example, phenytoin (Dilantin) blood levels are increased by phenothiazines or diazepam (Valium), and the action of warfarin (Coumadin) is prolonged by haloperidol (Haldol) or chlordiazepoxide (Librium). The interaction of lithium and diuretics can result in lithium toxicity.

Summary

Neurotransmitters include glutamate (an excitatory amino acid), gamma-aminobutyric acid (GABA, an inhibitory amino acid), acetylcholine, the catecholamines (norepinephrine, epinephrine, and dopamine), and serotonin (5-hydroxytryptamine, or 5-HT).

The main neurotransmitter-producing areas are in the locus coeruleus for the catecholamines, in the nucleus of Meynert for acetylcholine, in the gray matter in the pons and medulla for serotonin, and in the substantia nigra for dopamine. It is possible that some strokes can cause specific deficiencies in certain neurotransmitters. This mechanism may be one by which stroke causes depression.

The NMDA (N-methyl-D-aspartate) glutamate receptor and the GABA$_A$ receptor are ligand-gated. The dopamine receptors and the muscarinic acetylcholine receptor are G protein–linked.

The excitotoxic effect in brain injury takes place at the NMDA receptor. The result is an excessive inflow of calcium into the receptor nerve cell, which kills the cell. Drugs used to prevent the neurotoxic effects of excitatory neurotransmitters in stroke may cause psychiatric symptoms.

Drugs that reduce anxiety and those that prevent seizures have many clinical effects in common, probably because both types of drugs act on the GABA$_A$ receptor. Benzodiazepines bind to a part of the GABA$_A$ receptor called the benzodiazepine site and make the receptor more attractive to GABA.

Approximately 15%–20% of stroke patients develop seizures. Carbamazepine and valproic acid were originally developed as anticonvulsants but are also used to treat behavioral or mood disturbances.

Antipsychotic drugs block dopamine effects. The blockage of dopamine receptors causes movement disorders, some of which are produced by increased action of acetylcholine in the corpus striatum and can be counteracted by anticholinergic drugs. The anticholinergic intoxication syndrome can present as an acute mental disorder.

Withdrawal from previously used psychotropic drugs may complicate stroke management.

References

Albers GW, Goldberg MP, Choi DW: Do NMDA antagonists prevent neuronal injury? Yes. Arch Neurol 49:418–420, 1992

Albert ML, Helm-Estabrooks N: Diagnosis and treatment of aphasia, II. JAMA 259:1205–1210, 1988

Baethmann A, Maier-Hauff K, Schurer L, et al: Release of glutamate and of free fatty acids in vasogenic brain edema. J Neurol Neurosurg Psychiatry 70:578–571, 1989

Ballenger JC: The clinical use of carbamazepine in affective disorders. J Clin Psychiatry 49 (suppl):13–19, 1988

Bridgman P: Terminology raises concern (letter). Headlines 4:30, 1993

Buchan AM: Do NMDA antagonists prevent neuronal injury? No. Arch Neurol 49:420–421, 1992

Charney DS, Heninger GR, Sternberg G, et al: Abrupt discontinuation of tricyclic antidepressant drugs: evidence for noradrenergic activity. Br J Psychiatry 141:377–386, 1982

Chou JCY: Recent advances in treatment of acute mania. J Clin Psychopharmacol 11:3–21,1991

Chou JCY, Tuma I, Sweeney EA: Treatment approaches for acute mania. Psychiatr Q 64:331–344, 1993

Elliot-Baker SJ, Tiller JW: The damnation of benzodiazepines (letter). Br J Psychiatry 156:278, 1990

Fleet WS, Valenstein E, Watson RT, et al: Dopamine agonist therapy for neglect in humans. Neurology 37:855–857, 1987

Health Care Financing Administration: Appendix P: Guidance to Surveyors. State Operations Manual for Provider Certification, Transmittal 250. Washington, DC, Department of Health and Human Services, 1992

Keck PE, McElroy SL, Friedman LM: Valproate and carbamazepine in the treatment of panic and posttraumatic stress disorders, withdrawal states, and behavioral dyscontrol syndromes. J Clin Psychopharmacol 12 (suppl 1):368–418, 1992

Larkin M: Risk of seizures associated with neurologic injuries and conditions: review of the literature. Headlines 2:6–7, 1991

Liejon G, Boivie J: Central post-stroke pain in a trial of amitriptyline and carbamazepine. Pain 36:27–36, 1989

Longstreth WT, Nelson LM: Caffeine and stroke (letter). Stroke 23:117, 1992

Lovett L, Watkins SE, Shaw DM: The use of alternative drug therapy in nine patients with recurrent affective disorder resistant to conventional prophylaxis. Biol Psychiatry 21:1344–1347, 1986

MacDonald RL, Kelly KM: Antiepileptic drug mechanisms of action. Epilepsia 34 (suppl 5):51–58, 1993

Marangos PJ: Adenosinergic approaches to stroke therapeutics. Med Hypotheses 32:45–49, 1990

Molloy DW: Memory loss confusion and disorientation in an elderly woman taking meclizine. J Am Geriatr Soc 35:454–456, 1987

Napier TC, Friedman AH: Stroke, II: neurotransmitters and the pathophysiology of stroke. Internal Medicine for the Specialist 10:113–117, 1989

Rall TW, Schleifer LS: Drugs effective in the therapy of the epilepsies, in The Pharmacological Basis of Therapeutics. Edited by Gilman AG, Goodman LS, Rall TW, et al. New York, Macmillan, 1985, pp 446–472

Richardson JK: Psychotic behavior after right hemispheric accident: a case report. Arch Phys Med Rehabil 73:381–384, 1992

Rickels K, Case WG, Schweizer E, et al: Long-term benzodiazepine users 3 years after participation in a discontinuation program. Am J Psychiatry 148:757–761, 1991

Scheinberg P: The biologic basis for the treatment of acute stroke. Neurology 41:1867–1874, 1991

Sugarman P: Carbamazepine and episodic dyscontrol (letter). Br J Psychiatry 161:721, 1992

Trimble MR, Reynolds EH: Anti-convulsant drugs and mental symptoms: a review. Psychol Med 6:169–178, 1976

Wolf JK, Santana HB, Thorpy M: Treatment of "emotional incontinence" with levodopa (letter). Neurology 29:1435–1438, 1979

Yatham LN, Barry S, Mobayed M, et al: Is the carbamazepine-phenelzine combination safe? (letter). Am J Psychiatry 147:367, 1990

Yu MJ, McCowan JR, Smalstig EH, et al: A phenothiazine derivative reduces rat brain damage after global or focal ischemia. Stroke 23:1287–1291, 1992

Zito JM: Psychotherapeutic Drug Manual for Use in New York State Mental Health Facilities. Albany, NY, New York State Office of Mental Health, 1989, pp 5–10

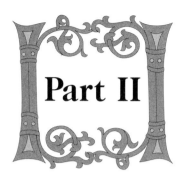

Part II

Psychiatric Syndromes

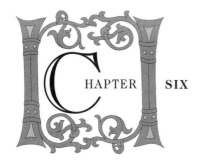

CHAPTER SIX

Speaking and Understanding

T he separation of speech disorders from psychiatric disorders
is not always complete or easy. Psychiatric disorders can
affect speech, and speech disorders can mimic or produce
psychiatric disorders.

Stupor and *mutism* are conditions in which the level of consciousness
or the motivation to talk is questionable (Segarra 1970). They are more
commonly due to general medical conditions, or to psychiatric conditions
such as catatonia or depression, than to cerebral infarction.

Damasio (1992) ascribed akinetic mutism to lesions on the internal
(mesial) surface of the left cerebral hemisphere. Segarra (1970) attributed somnolent cases of mutism to infarcts in the upper part of the midbrain that prevented impulses from the reticular formation (Figure 6–1)
from going down to the thalamus. More severe damage to this area can
produce the "locked-in" syndrome, in which there is complete immobility,
although consciousness is preserved (Mauss-Clum et al. 1993).

Disorders of articulation such as *aphonia* and *dysarthria,* which do
not affect reading and writing or the understanding of speech, are usually
assumed to be due to disturbance of the mechanical production of speech,
but even these may have a psychological component. These conditions
may occur in stroke because of damage to the lower part of the pathway

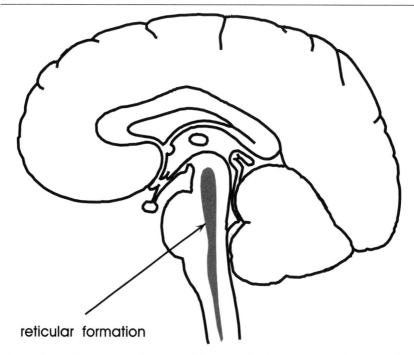

reticular formation

Figure 6–1. Approximate location of the reticular formation in relation to the sagittally cut brain.

through the centrum ovale and internal capsule to the cranial nerve nuclei controlling the mouth and vocal cords. *Aphasia,* on the other hand, is a disturbance of the ability to formulate or to understand speech. Reading and writing as well as vocal speech are affected, and the causative lesion is likely to be at a higher cerebral level.

The distinctions are not complete. Most right-handed right-sided hemiplegia patients, for example, will have a disturbance of the motor functions of the tongue and palate in addition to aphasia, so that there is dysarthria as well as aphasia. Several of the first-person accounts of stroke in the literature describe concerns about speech in terms such as "I had no volume to my voice" (Mason 1992). This subjective sense of loss of volume may not match what listeners of the voice hear, but in some cases of subcortical aphasia with lesions in the thalamus or basal nuclei, the volume of speech is specifically affected.

Bruyn (1989) reviewed 20 case reports of patients with lesions confined to the left thalamus, including 4 of his own cases. The characteristic speech disorder was reduced spontaneous speech and reduced volume of speech,

with retention of the ability to repeat; most patients had memory disturbance, nominal aphasia, and perseveration. Bruyn was unable to localize
speech disturbance to any particular part of the thalamus. The picture
he describes is rather similar to that seen in Parkinson's disease with
dementia.

Lazzarino et al. (1991) described two patients in whom there was a
pure reduction in the loudness of speech without aphasia, with paramedian thalamic-subthalamic infarcts in the territory supplied by the tha-
lamomesencephalic branches of the posterior cerebral arteries. In one
patient, the infarct was on the left side, and in the other it was bilateral.
Both recovered completely within a few months and showed no aphasia
or dementia. This syndrome seems to be what was described by earlier
authors as "pure word dumbness," "aphemia," "apraxic anarthria," or
"subcortical motor dysphasia" (Benson 1973).

Classifications of Aphasia

There are several classifications of aphasia, some of which may reflect
philosophical theories about speech rather than experimental evidence.
Reformers often announce a new and simplified classification, and thus
complicate matters by adding new terminology. The list of aphasias in
Table 6–1 is meant to be simple and eclectic. It is based on multiple
sources, ultimately deriving from the 19th-century writings of Lichtheim and Wernicke (as summarized in Eggert 1977).

Anterior Aphasias

Some authors use the term *anterior aphasia* for *any* difficulty in speech
production, because they say such a problem must be due to damage to
the front of the brain (that is, anterior to the central sulcus). There are
exceptions to this localization, and the nomenclature is not universally
accepted. In general, however, anterior aphasias are easier to distinguish clinically from psychiatric illness than are the posterior aphasias,
which affect the understanding rather than the production of speech.

Expressive (Broca's) Aphasia

Expressive aphasia—described by Broca, and sometimes named after
him—is the best-evidenced of all the aphasias. Despite the small number

of cases observed by Broca, his work has withstood the test of time and the advent of new imaging methods, so that *Broca's area* (Figure 6–2) remains the best example of localization of a mental function in the brain. In a "pure" case of expressive aphasia, the power of uttering speech is lost, but the ability to understand it is retained. Sometimes islands of speech are preserved, such as the ability to shout obscenities when angry or to repeat single words. Broca's aphasia is associated strongly with right hemiplegia and with damage to the left side of the brain. Users of American Sign Language who acquire expressive aphasia lose their ability to communicate with signs (Corina et al. 1992). Other kinds of aphasia are not as well defined and are more difficult to distinguish from dementia.

Transcortical Motor Aphasia

In transcortical motor aphasia, the ability to repeat is retained but spontaneous speech is lost. This condition is traditionally held to be due to damage above and in front of Broca's area. Some patients with transcortical motor aphasia cannot talk at all but can sing the entire words of a song (usually a well-known song, such as the national anthem) if someone sings along with them.

Nominal Aphasia

Nominal aphasia (also sometimes called *anomic aphasia, anomia,* or *amnestic aphasia*) is the inability to name things. The patient with this

Table 6–1.   Types of aphasia

Type	Functional effects
Broca's aphasia	Can understand. Cannot repeat. Cannot talk.
Transcortical motor aphasia	Can understand. Can repeat. Can name objects. Cannot talk.
Nominal aphasia	Can understand. Cannot name objects. Can talk.
Wernicke's aphasia	Cannot understand or repeat. Can talk.
Transcortical sensory aphasia	Cannot understand. Can repeat. Can talk.
Conduction aphasia	Can understand. Cannot repeat. Can talk.
Global aphasia	Cannot understand. Cannot talk.

Source.   Based on reports of Lichtheim and Wernicke (as summarized in Eggert 1977).

condition cannot name common objects put in his or her hand or provide the names of family members. Nominal aphasia is traditionally held to result from damage above and behind Wernicke's area (see Figure 6–2).

Mental disorder can impede testing for this disability, and the more severe a patient's dementia is (as measured by behavioral rating scales), the more difficulty he or she will have in naming objects (Skelton-Robinson and Jones 1984). Some criteria therefore specify that for the diagnosis of nominal aphasia to be made, dementia must be absent.

Margolin et al. (1990) compared the performance of a group of dementia patients with that of a group of patients with nominal aphasia on two tests: the Boston Naming Test (Kaplan et al. 1983), in which the subject is shown pictures and asked to name the objects portrayed, and the Controlled Oral Word Association Test (COW; Benton et al. 1994), in which subjects are asked to make a list of words beginning with specified letters of the alphabet. Both groups of patients did worse than nonimpaired control subjects on both tests. Patients with dementia did better

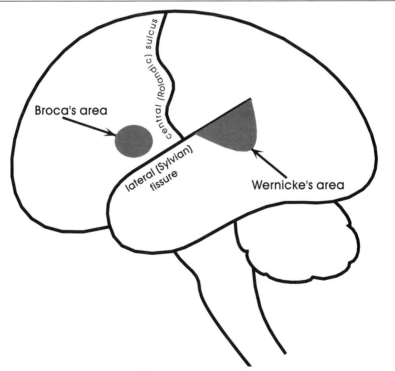

Figure 6–2.   Broca's area and Wernicke's area in left hemisphere.

on the Boston Naming Test than on the COW, whereas the converse was true for those with nominal aphasia.

Posterior Aphasias

The posterior (or "fluent") aphasias are receptive aphasias. They are thought to result from lesions of the cortex behind the central sulcus, although some have been described with other localized brain lesions. Although, in this group of aphasias, the production of speech is not primarily affected, speech becomes incoherent because of the inability to understand speech. The predicament is analogous to that of a deaf person trying to talk without the feedback needed to produce understandable speech. Speech in patients with these aphasias, especially in those with "jargon aphasia" and "word salad," can be similar to the speech produced by patients with dementia or psychosis.

Receptive (Wernicke's) Aphasia

Receptive, or Wernicke's, aphasia consists of the inability, in the absence of dementia, to understand or repeat spoken or written speech. The capacity to talk and write is retained. Wernicke's original patients were regarded as suffering from a psychiatric illness. Wernicke found that they had lesions in the left temporal cortex, impinging on the parietal lobe, below and behind Broca's area (see Figure 6–2).

This localization is generally accepted, and has been confirmed via computed tomography (CT) scan by Mazzocchi and Vignolo (1979). Karbe et al. (1990), however, found that among 26 patients with infarcts in the area of the left middle cerebral artery, 5 of whom had Wernicke's aphasia, there was no relation between the site of the infarct and the type of aphasia present.

Theoretically, a patient with Wernicke's aphasia should be able to give an exact account of his or her situation in fluent written or spoken speech, but this is rare. Some authors have stated that patients with severe Wernicke's aphasia are liable to anxiety, agitation, and paranoia (Damasio 1992), but in the presence of severe psychiatric disturbance, the diagnosis of receptive aphasia can be problematic.

Transcortical Sensory Aphasia

Transcortical sensory aphasia is similar to Wernicke's aphasia except that the patient remains able to repeat words or phrases spoken to him

or her. Because the patient can talk and repeat but has difficulty understanding, this disorder can resemble a psychiatric condition. Transcortical sensory aphasia is traditionally held to be caused by cortical damage
behind Wernicke's area; however, the area in question is less well defined than Wernicke's area, and localization has not been confirmed by
statistically based imaging studies (Karbe et al. 1990; Mazzocchi and
Vignolo 1979).

Auditory Agnosia

Auditory agnosia is a condition distinct from deafness and receptive
aphasia in which there is inability to recognize sound or to understand
spoken speech. The theoretically ideal auditory agnosia patient would be
distinguished from receptive aphasia patients by the ability to understand writing and by the production of understandable speech. This patient would have a lesion affecting Heschl's area (Figure 6–3).

Buchtel and Stewart (1989) described a patient with auditory agnosia
who could not understand spoken speech, although he could understand
written commands. The patient claimed to be deaf, but the audiogram
did not confirm this. In addition to his inability to understand spoken
speech, he also could not recognize sounds—he described the noises of

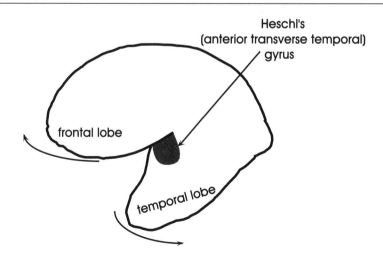

Figure 6–3.   Temporal lobe pushed downward to show Heschl's area.

a shower or an automobile engine as "music." If several drawings of common objects were put before the patient and someone said the name of one of the objects, he could point to the picture containing it. A CT scan showed evidence of two infarcts—one in the left frontotemporal area and another in the right posterior temporal region.

Shindo et al. (1991) found that patients with auditory agnosia could be trained to read lips and could then improve their understanding of speech by a combination of lipreading and listening.

Phonagnosia is difficulty in distinguishing voices, and *auditory sound agnosia* is difficulty in recognizing nonverbal sounds. Findings of right-side temporal or parietal lesions have been described in case reports of these conditions (Fujii et al. 1990; Van Lancker et al. 1989).

The two lateral lemnisci, which bring hearing sensation from the cochlear nuclei, are connected across the middle of the pons by the trapezoid body (*corpus trapezoideum*), so that sound heard in one ear is bilaterally represented above that level (Figure 6–4). Because of these cross-connections, it is unusual for stroke to cause deafness, and damage to one side of the brain does not affect the ability to hear sound from all directions. In a few rare instances, stroke has caused sudden deafness (Huang et al. 1993). One case has been reported of a nondeaf patient with a left lenticular hemorrhage who could not understand speech heard by his right ear (Pasquier et al. 1991).

Conduction Aphasia

In conduction aphasia, spontaneous speech is retained but makes no sense because the patient cannot "hear" what he or she is saying. Such speech resembles that produced in other mental disorders, such as the disorganized type of schizophrenia. Theoretically, the distinctive feature of conduction aphasia is that the patient can perform actions in response to commands but cannot reply to questions. However, this phenomenon can also occur in patients with schizophrenia, who may talk incoherently but can follow instructions.

Conduction aphasia is traditionally held to result from subcortical white-matter lesions that cut off connections between Broca's area and Wernicke's area. This theory has not been confirmed by modern imaging studies, although an association of conduction aphasia with left cortical damage has been reported (Mazzocchi and Vignolo 1979).

A patient described by Mendez and Rosenberg (1991) was able to handle her own affairs and to maintain her own activities of daily living

(ADL), such as housework and crocheting. She had apparently been diagnosed as having dementia because of a complaint that "something is wrong with my mind" and because she could not understand the speech of others or be understood by them. Her speech was "loquacious and rambling." She was unable either to follow spoken commands or to answer spoken questions. An audiogram showed no hearing loss; however, a CT scan revealed a lesion "deep in the medial aspect of the [left] temporal lobe" (p. 209).

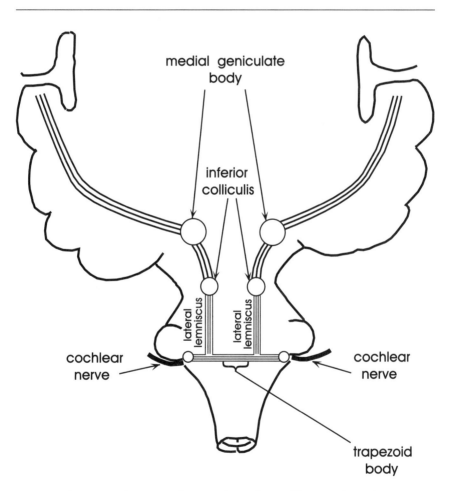

Figure 6–4.   Coronal section, showing the pathway of hearing from the cochlear nerve to the cortex.

Global Aphasia

Global aphasia is a combination of expressive and receptive aphasia. The patient's situation is akin to that of someone set down in the middle of a foreign country, unable to speak, understand, or read a word of the language. Distinguishing global aphasia from dementia can be problematic, as the following case vignette illustrates.

> Mr. J, a patient referred for management of dementia, had become unable to utter understandable speech, although he remained able to dress himself and even to drive a car. He had recently driven from New York to Florida, finding his way and remembering the exits for the motels he was used to staying in.
>
> Mr. J's CT and MRI scans showed dilation of the inferior horn of the left lateral ventricle and left temporal lobe atrophy.
>
> When examined in my office, Mr. J was well groomed and clean, with no movement or gait disturbance. He was unable to respond directly to spoken questions or simple commands, and on any formal test he would have scored as having dementia. He could not repeat any words or point to named objects. He leafed through a magazine shown to him, but he was unable to read any words aloud. As his wife and I conversed in his presence, he interjected short sentences relevant to the situation, frequently using the word "area" to substitute for any noun. Seeing a picture of my family in the office, he pointed and said "Is that your area?" When the picture was put in his hands, he smiled. He then took some family pictures out of his wallet and began to talk in short, complete sentences about his children and grandchildren, but he could not answer any questions I asked him about them.

The traditional view ascribes global aphasia to damage affecting both Broca's and Wernicke's areas, and subcortical lesion sites have been described, but De Renzi et al. (1991) were unable to confirm these locations in their clinical and CT study of 17 cases.

Effects of Right-Brain Damage on Speech

Left-handed people become aphasic from lesions in the right side of the brain, and right-handed people do so from lesions in the left side of the brain. This rule, however, is not universal: one-fifth of stroke patients with weakness on the left side studied by Anderson (1992) had speech problems.

Attempts to attribute particular speech defects to right-hemisphere lesions in right-handed patients encounter the usual problems of adequacy of controls and reliability of measurement of the variables. Ross (1981; Ross and Rush 1981) has suggested that those with right-hemisphere damage lack emotional inflection and humor in their speech.

Occasionally a crossed aphasia occurs, in which a right-handed person becomes aphasic from a right-hemisphere lesion. Alexander et al. (1989) presented evidence that the cerebral localization of speech in such individuals is not a mirror image of the normal localization; however, the number of cases studied has been too small to allow definite conclusions.

Differentiating Dementia and Psychosis From Aphasia

Stroke is a condition that commonly results in dementia or aphasia. Often those who love the patient attempt to protect the patient or to preserve his or her integrity by insisting to the clinician that the patient's mind is intact and that it is only the speech that is damaged. Most of us would feel that there is a certain injustice in misdiagnosing aphasia as a mental disorder, and stroke patients have reported being severely distressed by the failure of caregivers to appreciate that they retained full understanding despite their impaired speech. Although in most cases, fluent aphasia can be differentiated from dementia through an adequate psychiatric examination, in some patients the distinctions can be blurred. One answer to the question of how a mental disorder can be distinguished from a communication disorder has been to claim that there is essentially no difference between the two.

Rogers (1985) has used the expression "conflict of paradigms" to describe the situation in which the same phenomenon may be labeled as either a mental disorder or a brain disorder, depending on the context in which it is seen. If a patient says his wife is his umbrella, for example, he might be recorded as having a delusion, a disorientation-to-person condition suggestive of dementia, or paraphasia. The patient might also be joking, or speak English as a second language and be mixing up words.

I recently asked three patients in the same institution to state where they were. A schizophrenic patient replied, "I haven't seen that place. I'm tired of Mrs. Smith. A new administration." A patient with dementia answered, "Puerto Rico—New York and PR." A patient with a residual right hemiplegia responded, "This is hard right now—everything is good—I can't say it."

Distinctions might be made among these three types of reply, but they would be largely intuitive. One possible conclusion is that patients with dementia have lost the semantic representation of words but retained the lexical-phonological representation. This interpretation implies that the speech disorders of dementia result from interference with the higher and intellectual aspects of language, whereas the speech disorders of aphasia have a mechanical basis.

Speech Content

Methods of making the distinction based on the content of the speech produced have been described by Nicholas et al. (1985). Using a measure of "empty speech" based on linguistic principles, these researchers found that patients with dementia produced more empty phrases and conjunctions and fewer neologisms and "verbal paraphasias" than did those with Wernicke's aphasia.

Ability to Perform Activities of Daily Living

Another point of differentiation among dementia, psychosis, and aphasia is that psychotic patients and aphasic patients retain their ability to perform ADL—tasks such as dressing themselves and finding their way around—but dementia patients lose this ability. Some schizophrenic patients lose hygiene skills and become disheveled but remain able to carry out certain complex activities such as going to a store to buy cigarettes.

Communicative Fluctuation

Psychotic patients are more likely than those with aphasia or dementia to snap out of noncommunication upon occasion but then relapse back into that state.

> An elderly Polish inhabitant in a residential care home was reported to be suspicious and reclusive and to speak no English. On interview, she responded only to gestures and mimed commands. No one in the home spoke Polish. Strenuous efforts were made to relieve her social isolation by contact with Polish groups and a Polish church, but she refused these. Eventually it was found that she was regularly picking up her spending allowance and going to local stores to buy personal items. Subsequent interviews with the aid of a Polish-speaking volunteer led to a diagnosis of paranoid schizophrenia.

First-Person Reports

Some of the most powerful evidence for the existence of a sharp distinction between mental disorders and aphasia comes from patients' first-person narratives. Wender (1987) described her experience as follows:

> In the beginning my native language (English) was badly shattered, and like many aphasics I spoke "fluently" (that is, using sentences) but using many words which were either nonsense or ridiculously incorrect. For example, when I was asked to talk about Ronald Reagan's job I said something like "she's the kitchen of Imerca." Many people, even some neurologists and speech pathologists, would consider this "speech" as gibberish—that is, sounds without meaning. They would be wrong. I understood this question and "knew" the answer in my mind: he ("she")—a male—is the leader ("kitchen") of this country ("Imerca"). If I had been asked whether I would vote for Reagan I would definitely have shaken my head vigorously; if I had been asked to draw a symbol for Imerca I would have drawn a correct sketch of the flag or the eagle; every word I said meant something. (p. 1595)

Stocklin (1989) said,

> I tried to speak then but the words seemed to tumble around in my mouth and I could not make them come out right. . . . When I went to sign my name, I couldn't remember it. So I had to sign with an X. I could remember my first name Alyce, but it was late November or 5 months later before I could remember Stocklin. (pp. 23, 30)

Both of these patients are obviously giving clear accounts of an experience in which language was the primary disturbance, although they recall severe emotional upsets on account of it, and sometimes describe their defect as one of memory.

Tests for Aphasia

Many tests for aphasia have been developed (see Table 6–2). In these, the patient is asked to do things such as name objects, point out specific objects in pictures shown to him or her, read, repeat sentences, write, sing, draw, or mime. Much excellent work has been done in devising and validating tests, but they have drawbacks for use in clinical practice.

A criticism of some tests is that they do not adequately allow for concurrent deafness, blindness, or neurological impairment. For example, if objects in a test involving naming objects are presented to one side, a stroke patient with a visual field defect may fail to see them. The more a test is constructed to avoid such errors, the more prolonged and elaborate it becomes, raising considerations of time and expense. Administration of the Boston Diagnostic Aphasia Examination (Goodglass and Kaplan 1972), for example, takes 3 hours.

Many test drawbacks can be overcome by making the tester part of an interdisciplinary team and ensuring good communication among team

Table 6–2.   Tests for aphasia

Test	Comments
Porch Index (Porch 1967)	Most widely used and standardized
Boston Diagnostic Aphasia Examination (Goodglass and Kaplan 1972)	Gives result in terms of traditionally named types of aphasia
Whurr Aphasia Screening Test (Whurr 1984)	British; intended to be used by speech therapists in planning treatment and measuring change
Speech Questionnaire (Lincoln 1982)	
Grober Test for Nonlinguistic Memory (Grober 1984)	Assesses dementia in presence of aphasia
Western Aphasia Battery (Kertesz 1982)	Gives result in terms of traditionally named types of aphasia
Token Test (De Renzi and Vignolo 1962)	
Functional Communication Profile (Sarno 1969)	Records behavior outside the test situation
Communication Abilities in Daily Living Test (Holland 1980)	
Aachen Aphasia Test (Huber et al. 1983)	German language
Neurosensory Center Comprehensive Examination for Aphasia (Spreen and Benton 1969)	
Boston Naming Test (Kaplan et al. 1983)	

members. Whereas most tests record behavior only during the testing situation (the Functional Communication Profile [Sarno 1969] is an exception), often the vital clue to a patient's communicative ability is observation of his or her behavior over time.

Tests for aphasia may be more useful after brain injury than after stroke. Such tests are most valuable for documenting the severity and extent of a patient's impairment for legal purposes, for assessing the usefulness of a method of treatment, and for keeping track of the progress of patients in an institutional setting, where many have speech problems.

Management of Aphasia

Few conditions require the team approach more than aphasia does. No one person can take undisputed responsibility for every aspect of aphasia management; the efforts of many types of specialists are needed. The patient is the arbiter of the effectiveness of treatment and will reject stereotyped treatment approaches not individualized to his or her needs and preferences. The patient may ultimately assert autonomy by getting better without (or apparently without) treatment.

Spontaneous Improvement Versus Therapy

Most stroke-related aphasia improves, and most such improvement occurs within 10 weeks after the stroke, but improvement may continue for up to 18 months. Neither age nor sex affects outcome (Lendrem and Lincoln 1985; Nicholas et al. 1993). This tendency for improvement has raised questions about the effectiveness of therapy, despite claims of positive results in controlled trials of speech therapy (Basso et al. 1979; Shewan and Kertesz 1984).

Wender (1989), in her first-person account, was critical of those who cite the negative results of controlled trials as an argument against using speech therapy. She noted that many of the study trials are trials of inadequate treatment. Her narrative also illustrated that an effect of therapy is to improve morale, which may be a worthwhile benefit that trials fail to consider.

To generalize from Wender's experience, however, would be to make the assumption that all stroke patients are motivated to participate in speech therapy. Many practitioners have had the experience of organizing therapy for a patient who seems to be a good candidate but is not enthusiastic.

One aspect of Wender's (1989) experience provides interesting evidence that the recovery of speech is dependent on a patient's decision to learn. She had previously been a teacher of Greek and Latin, but found, on recovering from her stroke, that she had forgotten these languages. She deliberately applied herself to relearning Greek. There was recovery of her knowledge of Greek, but no spontaneous return of her knowledge of Latin.

Stocklin (1989) described both negative and positive experiences with her speech therapy. She complained, of work with one therapist, that "it was the same every day. I could feel no progress. I knew she thought I could never learn." Of another therapist she said, "It was only a job to her." However, in subsequent therapy at a university clinic, she found that "they always had something new and we were practicing reading, writing and talking. I was never bored. The enthusiasm of the student teachers was refreshing and I felt that I had to work harder than ever because I was in some way responsible for the grades received by the students" (p. 45).

Speech Therapies

Several professionals may be involved in speech therapy. The role of the speech pathologist in the treatment team in aphasia is as much in diagnosis as in direct treatment (Griffiths and Baldwin 1989). The primary emphasis is assessment, followed by explaining to other caregivers and family members how to communicate with the patient. The line between speech therapy and aphasia education is not sharply drawn. Many family relationships benefit from family education about aphasia (Williams 1993).

Several specific types of speech therapy are typically chosen, and are conducted by trained speech pathologists. Although not all have been subjected to rigorously controlled trials, a review by Albert and Helm-Estabrooks (1988a, 1988b) was optimistic about the effectiveness of such interventions. Table 6–3 lists some of the more widely used speech therapies.

Music therapy, which capitalizes on the ability of some aphasic patients to sing, is incorporated into some forms of speech therapy. There are also registered music therapists who specialize in this work (see Appendix B).

Areas of strength and ability to communicate are often found. As mentioned, some patients remain able to sing; others can sign "yes" or "no" to suggestions, repeat sentences or speak very short sentences, write with the opposite hand, and shout obscenities when angry.

Once a patient's areas of strength and remaining communication skills have been elucidated, programs for daily practice can be set up. Even when based on careful assessment, however, such programs do not always work. Lyon (in press) points out that "if an aphasic adult is fixated on the return of his speech, even when your clinical knowledge and expertise would suggest otherwise, it is NOT an appropriate time to begin with demonstrations of how gestures or drawing might aid a functional return of expression." If the patient has an interested family and is cooperative, the daily practice can be continued by unskilled caregivers or family members. Unfortunately, in many cases, islands of ability do not live up to their apparent promise. The abilities do not generalize, and measurable improvement cannot be attained.

Communicative Partners (Lyon 1992) is a program in which nonaphasic volunteers (communication partners) bring patients with aphasia into a variety of social and recreational settings to practice their communication skills. Each volunteer is matched up with a patient and that pa-

Table 6–3.   Types of speech therapy

Therapy	Use
Syntax Stimulation Program (Helm-Estabrooks et al. 1981)	Agrammatic aphasic patients, who are able to produce words but not sentences
Visual Action Therapy (Helm-Estabrooks et al. 1982)	Global aphasia
Tri-Model System (Glickstein and Neustadt 1993)	Dementia
Melodic Intonation Therapy (Sparks and Holland 1976)	Patients with no understandable speech but preserved auditory comprehension
Treatment of Aphasic Perseveration (TAP) (Helm-Estabrooks et al. 1987)	Patients with perseveration rather than linguistic errors
Language Oriented Approach (Shewan 1976)	Broca's aphasia (for facilitating sentence formulation)
Naeser's Structured Approach (Naeser 1975)	Based on methods for teaching English as a second language; for patients with good verbal output and auditory input scores on Porch Index

tient's primary caregiver. The treatment plan begins with weekly 2-hour sessions in the patient's place of residence. After 2–6 weeks, the patient, volunteer, and primary caregiver go out together to places such as stores, taverns, theaters, or baseball games. The major improvements have been in measurements of psychosocial wellness.

Medication

The place of medication in the treatment of aphasia has yet to be established. Patients with aphasia who have recovered full fluency may still complain of a lack of vocal volume and intonation. Loss of these modulating functions is marked in patients with thalamic infarcts, and resembles the voice changes of Parkinson's disease, pointing to a dopaminergic deficiency. Based on the hypothesis that dopamine deficiency can affect speech, Albert et al. (1988) used bromocriptine successfully for treatment of hesitancy and impaired initiation of speech in a patient with long-standing transcortical motor aphasia.

The Team Approach

To succeed, the approach to management of aphasia must be multidisciplinary, eclectic, pragmatic, and highly individualized. Suggested tasks for each treatment team member are outlined in Table 6–4.

Patients have a strong tendency to choose their own communication methods. Some tend to insist on a nonverbal method and resist attempts at speech. Others set themselves a goal of return to full verbal fluency and become despondent or angry if any lesser goal is substituted. They may insist on prolonged speech therapy and establish a relationship with the therapist in which transference phenomena occur and must be addressed.

A great deal devolves upon the family, even if the patient is institutionalized. In the institutional situation, many family visits are virtually speech therapy sessions; therefore, it can be helpful for the family to look on the visits in this way and to agree on a plan for what they will try to accomplish in the visits. The demands on the family may be exorbitant. Untreated aphasic individuals tend to be unaware of the extent of their impairment and the burdens they impose (Shewan and Cameron 1984). Some patients set up a family member (most commonly the spouse) as the interpreter of their private language, becoming angry and frustrated if he or she is remiss in this appointed role.

The Noisy Patient

Noisiness and shouting are especially common in the nonambulant stroke patient who has both dementia and aphasia. In nursing homes, 30% of residents are nuisance noisemakers, mostly engaging in perseverative shouting (Ryan et al. 1988).

The noisy aphasia patient is often making an effort at communication, and one of the first points to consider is whether the patient is attempting to express a need. Sometimes such patients have developed private languages, understandable to certain caregivers, which they use in lieu of speech. It could be argued that they should be forced to drop their private language in favor of regular speech; however, the history of the attempts to suppress American Sign Language suggests that attempts to wipe out useful communication in favor of "correct" language are misguided.

> A nursing-home patient with a right hemiplegia utters no formed words. He can write his name with his left hand but throws away the felt marker and paper angrily after doing this once. He spends much of the day grunting and barking. When this noise gets louder, he usually attracts the attention of a staff member and tries to communicate his needs to him or her by gestures

Table 6–4.   Team roles in management of aphasia

Team member(s)	Diagnostic/treatment task(s)
All	Find areas of strength and ability to communicate
Speech pathologist, music therapist	Conduct specific speech therapies
Speech pathologist, MD, RN, psychologist	Explain to other caregivers and family members how to communicate with patient
MD, occupational therapist, social worker, government agencies	Assess work capability and provide vocational rehabilitation
MD, RN	Perform neurological examination and investigations; prescribe medication
Psychologist	Conduct neuropsychological testing
Family, volunteers, occupational therapist, music therapist	Carry out daily practice program based on patient's areas of strength and ability to communicate

with his left hand. Certain staff members have become adept at understanding these hand gestures, and are called on to "interpret" when he gets too noisy.

Clearly, those involved in stroke treatment should be prepared to develop treatment plans for noisy patients. Such plans should be flexible, and the specifics will vary. As with all nonviolent antisocial behaviors, it is useful to begin by finding out who is bothered by the behavior and why, and to consider the option of tolerating it.

In institutional settings, those who are affected are commonly other residents, such as hospital patients in the same ward, and their opinions should be sought. Often the primary caregivers are the ones who are most bothered. They may be concerned about the noise representing distress, and feel conflict and guilt about ignoring it. They may need to discuss these feelings. Expressions of concern about noise by the primary caregivers may also represent an appeal for sympathy with their burden. They may simply want to be listened to and appreciated, or they may want more help from another family member or from the administration of the hospital or nursing home.

Noise may be better tolerated in some settings than in others. Sometimes the patient can be moved within the same institution, or a deaf roommate can be found. Relocating the patient may involve some of the wider aspects of placement in the spectrum of care (to be discussed in Chapter 19).

Medications are seldom helpful unless given in doses high enough to cause drowsiness. This point should be discussed with the primary caregivers. They may feel that the prescriber is withholding medication that might help, and this feeling may constitute a partial justification for initiating a time-limited trial of an antipsychotic medication.

Mobilization is the most effective single remedy. Noisemaking practically always diminishes if the patient can walk about. The more mobile patients can be, the less noisy they will be, possibly because they can then attend to some of their own needs that could not be verbally expressed.

Summary

Speech disorders interact with psychiatric disorders to such an extent that complete distinction may not be possible. In expressive aphasias, the limitation of the disturbance to speech rather than to other aspects of memory and intellect can be detected. Receptive aphasias can result in unintelligible speech resembling that characteristic of psychosis or dementia. Although receptive and global aphasias may mimic dementia, there is preservation of the capacity for complex skills, although these may be impaired by neurological defects. Various tests for aphasia may be useful, but their application demands patience and skill. The services of a speech pathologist are helpful in diagnosis and in identification of communication skills that can be built upon by the family and treatment team. There is a tendency for spontaneous improvement of aphasia to occur. The results of controlled trials of speech therapy have been ambiguous, but many patients report considerable benefits. Managing shouting and noisemaking requires a team approach, with identification and involvement of those who are disturbed by the activity.

References

Albert ML, Helm-Estabrooks N: Diagnosis and treatment of aphasia, I. JAMA 259:1043–1047, 1988a

Albert ML, Helm-Estabrooks N: Diagnosis and treatment of aphasia, II. JAMA 259:1205–1210, 1988b

Albert ML, Bachman DL, Morgan A, et al: Pharmacotherapy for aphasia. Neurology 38:877–879, 1988

Alexander MP, Fischette MR, Fischer RS: Crossed aphasias can be mirror image or anomalous. Brain 112:953–973, 1989

Anderson R: The Aftermath of Stroke. Cambridge, UK, Cambridge University Press, 1992, p 46

Basso A, Capitani E, Vignolo L: Influence of rehabilitation on language skills in aphasic patients: a controlled study. Arch Neurol 36:190–196, 1979

Benson DF: Psychiatric aspects of aphasia. Br J Psychiatry 123:555–566, 1973

Benton AL, de S Hamsher K, Sidon AB: Multilingual Aphasia Examination: Manual of Instructions, 3rd Edition. Iowa City, IA, AJA Associates, 1994

Bruyn RPM: Thalamic aphasia. J Neurol 236:21–25, 1989

Buchtel HA, Stewart JD: Auditory agnosia: apperceptive or associative disorder. Brain Lang 32:12–25, 1989

Corina DP, Poizner H, Bellugi U, et al: Dissociation between linguistic and non-linguistic gestural systems: a case for compositionality. Brain Lang 43:414–417, 1992

Damasio AR: Aphasia. N Engl J Med 326:531–539, 1992

De Renzi E, Vignolo L: The token test: a sensitive test to detect receptive disturbances in aphasics. Brain 85:665–678, 1962

De Renzi E, Colombo A, Scarpa M: The aphasic isolate. Brain 114:1719–1730, 1991

Eggert GH: Early Sources in Aphasia and Related Disorders. New York, Mouton, 1977

Fujii T, Fukatsu R, Watabe S, et al: Auditory sound agnosia without aphasia following a right temporal lobe lesion. Cortex 26:263–268, 1990

Glickstein JK, Neustadt GK: Speech-language interventions in Alzheimer's disease. Clinics in Communication Disorders 3:15–30, 1993

Goodglass H, Kaplan E: The Assessment of Aphasia and Related Disorders. Boston, MA, Lea & Febiger, 1972

Griffiths H, Baldwin B: Speech therapy for psychogeriatric services. Psychiatric Bulletin 13:57–59, 1989

Grober E: Nonlinguistic memory in aphasia. Cortex 20:67–73, 1984

Helm-Estabrooks N, Fitzpatrick PM, Barresi B: Response of an agrammatic patient to a syntax stimulation program for aphasia. Journal of Speech and Hearing Disorders 46:422–427, 1981

Helm-Estabrooks N, Fitzpatrick PM, Barresi B: Visual action therapy for global aphasia. Journal of Speech and Hearing Disorders 47:385–389, 1982

Helm-Estabrooks N, Emery P, Albert ML: Treatment of aphasic perseveration (TAP) program: a new approach to aphasia therapy. Arch Neurol 44:1253–1255, 1987

Holland AL: Communication Abilities in Daily Living. Baltimore, MD, University Park Press, 1980

Huang M-H, Huang C-C, Ryu SJ, et al: Sudden bilateral hearing impairment in vertebrobasilar occlusive disease. Stroke 24:132–137, 1993

Huber W, Poeck K, Weniger D, et al: Aachener Aphasie Test. Gottingen, Germany, Verlag für Psychologie, 1983

Kaplan E, Goodglass H, Weintraub S: The Boston Naming Test. Philadelphia, PA, Lea & Febiger, 1983

Karbe H, Szelies B, Herholz K, et al: Impairment of language is related to left parieto-temporal glucose metabolism in aphasic stroke patients. J Neurol 237:19–23, 1990

Kertesz A: Western Aphasia Battery. New York, Grune & Stratton, 1982

Lazzarino LG, Nicolai A, Valasi F: Aphonia due to paramedian thalamo-subthalamic infarction: remarks on two cases. Ital J Neurol Sci 12:219–225, 1991

Lendrem W, Lincoln NB: Spontaneous recovery of language in patients with aphasia. J Neurol Neurosurg Psychiatry 48:743–748, 1985

Lincoln NB: The speech questionnaire: an assessment of functional language ability. Int Rehabil Med 4:114–117, 1982

Lyon JG: Communicative partners. Be Stroke Smart 9:9–11, 1992

Lyon JG: Optimizing communication and participation in life for aphasic adults and their prime caregivers in natural settings: a use model for treatment, in Adult Aphasia: Clinical Management for the Practicing Clinician. Edited by Wallace G. Newton, MA, Butterworth-Heinemann, in press

Margolin DI, Pate DS, Friedrich FJ, et al: Dysnomia in dementia and stroke patients: different underlying cognitive deficits. J Clin Exp Neuropsychol 12:597–612, 1990

Mason PL: The long road to my full recovery. Be Stroke Smart 9:12, 1992

Mauss-Clum N, Cole M, McCort T, et al: Locked-in syndrome: a team approach. J Neurosci Nurs 23:273–285, 1993

Mazzocchi F, Vignolo LA: Localisation of lesions in aphasia: clinical–CT scan correlations in stroke patients. Cortex 15:627–654, 1979

Mendez MF, Rosenberg S: Word deafness mistaken for Alzheimer's disease: differential characteristics. J Am Geriatr Soc 39:209–211, 1991

Naeser MA: A structured approach teaching aphasics basic sentence types. Br J Disord Commun 10:70–76, 1975

Nicholas ML, Obler LK, Albert ML, et al: Empty speech in Alzheimer's disease and fluent aphasia. Journal of Speech and Hearing Disorders 28:405–410, 1985

Nicholas ML, Helm-Estabrooks N, Ward-Lonergan J, et al: Evolution of severe aphasia in the first two years post onset. Arch Phys Med Rehabil 74:830–836, 1993

Pasquier F, Leys D, Steinling M, et al: Agnosie auditive unilatérale droite consécutive à une hémorrhagie lenticulaire gauche. Rev Neurol (Paris) 147:129–137, 1991

Porch BE: The Porch Index of Communicative Ability. Palo Alto, CA, Consulting Psychologists Press, 1967

Rogers D: The motor disorders of severe psychiatric illness: a conflict of paradigms. Br J Psychiatry 147:221–232, 1985

Ross ED: The aprosodias: functional-anatomical organization of the affective components of language in the right hemisphere. Arch Neurol 38:561–569, 1981

Ross ED, Rush JA: Diagnosis and neuroanatomical correlates of depression in brain-damaged patients. Arch Gen Psychiatry 38:1344–1354, 1981

Ryan DP, Tainsh SM, Kolodny V, et al: Noise-making amongst the elderly in long-term care. Gerontologist 3:369–371, 1988

Sarno MT: The Functional Communication Profile. New York, New York University Press, 1969

Segarra JM: Cerebral vascular disease and behavior. Arch Neurol 22:408–418, 1970

Shewan CM: Facilitating sentence formulation: a case study. J Commun Disord 9:191–197, 1976

Shewan CM, Cameron H: Communication and related problems as perceived by aphasic individuals and their spouses. J Commun Disord 17:175–187, 1984

Shewan CM, Kertesz A: Effects of speech and language treatment on recovery from aphasia. Brain Lang 23:272–299, 1984

Shindo M, Kaga K, Tanaka Y: Speech discrimination and lip reading in patients with word deafness or auditory agnosia. Brain Lang 40:153–161, 1991

Skelton-Robinson M, Jones S: Nominal dysphasia and the severity of senile dementia. Br J Psychiatry 145:168–171, 1984

Sparks RW, Holland AL: Method: melodic intonation therapy for aphasia. Journal of Speech and Hearing Disorders 41:287–297, 1976

Spreen O, Benton A: Neurosensory Center Comprehensive Examination for Aphasia. Victoria, British Columbia, University of Victoria Press, 1969

Stocklin A: My Stroke, My Blessing. Aurora, CO, Charles Delperdang, 1989

Van Lancker DR, Kreiman J, Cummings J: Voice perception deficits: neuroanatomical correlates of phonagnosia. J Clin Exp Neuropsychol 11:665–674, 1989

Wender D: "Craziness" and "visions": experiences after a stroke. BMJ 295:1595–1597, 1987

Wender D: Aphasic victim as investigator. Arch Neurol 46:91–93, 1989

Whurr R: The Whurr Aphasia Screening Test. London, Whurr Publishers, 1984

Williams SE: The impact of aphasia on marital satisfaction. Arch Phys Med Rehabil 73:361–367, 1993

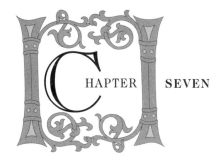

CHAPTER   SEVEN

Seeing and Believing

The visual disturbances of stroke can often be explained organically in terms of damage to the pathways carrying light sensations from the eye to the cortex (Figure 7–1), but sometimes visual disturbances occur that cannot be fully accounted for in this way. The stroke-related disorders of vision have therefore afforded fertile ground for speculation about the nature of our knowledge of the external world. At a practical level, an accurate diagnosis can reassure a patient that his or her disabilities are circumscribed, and can help in planning treatment. In some cases, the most effective treatment of a disorder involving perception may be psychological rather than medical, even if the neuro-ophthalmic syndrome is caused by an infarct.

Damage from stroke affects the visual pathways coming after visual stimuli have reached the lateral geniculate bodies. The visual pathways from the lateral geniculate bodies go next to the occipital cortex. Damage to this part of the visual pathways causes defects of the visual fields. Visual field defects have psychiatric implications, but their exact organic etiology is well established.

The results of damage to the pathways of the visual impulses become less definite, and more likely to be regarded as psychiatric, after the impulses leave the occipital cortex. Somehow the visual impulses arise to

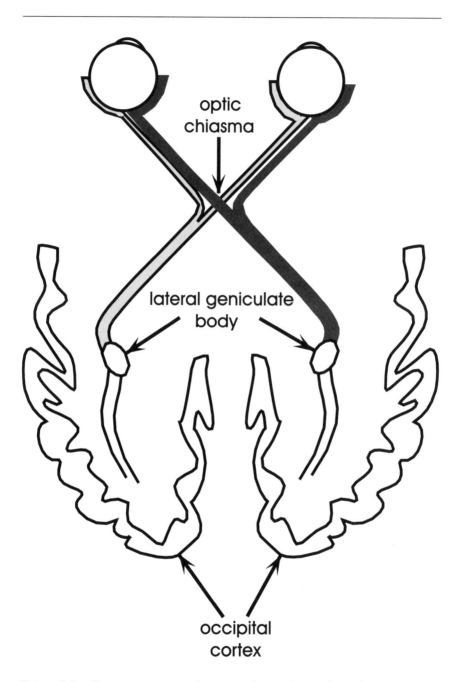

Figure 7–1.   Transverse section, showing pathway of vision from the retina to the occipital cortex.

consciousness; we translate them into pictures and words, and we become aware of seeing. The existence of a center for organizing visual impulses into images in the occipital cortex, and of a center for remembering the images in the temporal cortex, is generally accepted (Damasio et al. 1982). Damage to the pathways connecting these causes a set of disorders called *disconnection syndromes*.

According to Iwata (1990), there are two main pathways forward from the occipital cortex. The upper one (superior longitudinal fasciculus) carries the visual input to the parietal lobes (Brodmann's area 7). The lower one (inferior longitudinal fasciculus) carries visual input to the temporal lobes (Brodmann's area 37). There is also in the left hemisphere a third pathway, in between the other two, that carries visual information to the angular gyrus (Brodmann's area 39). Damage to the upper pathway causes optic ataxia and visuospatial disturbances, with difficulty in tasks such as drawing. Damage to the lower pathway results in disturbances of object recognition, with manifestations such as prosopagnosia and inability to read written symbols such as those in Japanese kanji. Damage to the third pathway causes disturbances in letter recognition, manifested by inability to read characters such as those in European languages or in Japanese kana.

Visual Field Defects

In strokes with right hemiplegia, damage has occurred to the left side of the brain (including the left optic radiation or occipital cortex), causing loss of the right visual field. The patient is often not subjectively aware of the visual field defect because vision can be perfect for objects the patient looks at directly. Detection of visual field defects can be difficult. The procedure for doing so involves having the patient look straight ahead while letting the examiner know when the patient can see an object being brought in from the periphery. For such an examination to yield accurate information, the patient must be cooperative and alert.

Visual fields can also be charted by using a target and perimeter. This approach involves mapping the points at which the patient notices the target coming into view. The points mapped are then joined together on a chart so as to make an outline of the visual field. Patients with mild dementia may begin to cooperate with this procedure but then fail to understand the instructions, so that when the points are connected together into an outline, the result is a jagged spiral.

As the result of these difficulties in examination, the presence of a visual field defect can go undetected, representing an unrecognized obstacle to rehabilitation. Unawareness of the defect may also yield inaccurate results from psychological testing and other kinds of assessment if stimuli are presented to the patient's impaired side.

The fully alert patient who has become used to and has received instruction about a visual field defect can compensate for it, but under some circumstances patients may develop what is called *visuospatial neglect*. The combination of defects in the left (or right) visual field and loss of sensation from the same side of the body can cause the patient to behave as if what is on that side does not exist (hemineglect). This condition is especially likely to occur in patients with dementia.

Management of Visual Field Defects

Recognizing that a visual field defect is present is the most important part of management. The patient and his or her caregivers must develop an understanding of the impairment and organize items needed for tasks so that they will be seen in the visual field. Much of the treatment of visual field defects thus falls to the occupational therapist. Vance (1993) pointed out that nonverbal cues, such as gestures and body language, may be distracting to patients with visual field defects. His suggestion to therapists: "If necessary, put your hands in your pockets while talking, so that you may concentrate on the words."

Part of the treatment task can seem negative and thankless. The therapist needs to make patients aware of their deficiencies. For example, visual field defects constitute a particularly grave handicap in driving a car. Some patients, especially young men, may resent and ignore the advice not to drive, and may resist both social work help in organizing transportation and rehabilitation help in using public transportation. The therapist must be psychologically prepared to receive anger instead of gratitude, and may need positive support from other members of the treatment team.

"Blindsight" and "Hysterical" Blindness

Most ophthalmologists, and many other practitioners, have seen patients who state that they cannot see, but who can be persuaded or tricked into providing evidence that they *can* see. When confronted with this evidence, such patients' inability to comprehend their inconsistency suggests deliberate deception or emotional illness. The condition is commonly called *hysterical blindness,* although this term does not conform to DSM-IV (American Psychiatric Association 1994) or ICD-10 (World Health Organization 1992) nomenclature. Ophthalmologists will sometimes use the term *functional blindness* to avoid distinguishing between hysteria and malingering (Newman 1993).

When a patient with such blindness is found to have an infarct in the posterior part of the brain, a quandary arises as to whether the illness is physical or emotional. The psychiatrist may be asked to give an opinion on which one of the two it is, on the assumption that a complete dichotomy must exist. Nineteenth-century theories of hysteria allowed for the possibility of concomitant neurological and emotional causes for such conditions. According to Pierre Janet (1907/1965), patients with this type of blindness lacked the capacity to organize incoming sensory data into a logically coherent view of the world, and this lack of capacity could be physical or mental. Although such theories no longer command widespread support, recent studies of the phenomenon called "blindsight" (Weiskrantz 1991) provide some evidence in their favor.

Blindsight has been studied in patients with visual field defects. Sometimes, although the patient is apparently blind to what is going on in the area of a visual field defect, events in this area can affect behavior. There is thus a kind of knowledge of events in the defective visual field without a consciousness of them. This knowledge, called *implicit* or *covert* knowledge, is knowledge that is present without the knower's awareness of it. Dissociation between explicit, conscious knowledge and implicit knowledge is called *disconnected awareness.* Such awareness can result in unconscious learning, which apparently takes place without involving the cortex.

Management of "Hysterical" Blindness

There is no purely psychiatric method of distinguishing cases of apparent "hysterical" blindness with infarcts from those without. The patient's behavior may be the same in both cases. Indeed, no studies have statistically shown that occipital infarcts are associated with the condition, but when such an infarct is found, a causal relationship is assumed, and this results in a shift in the practitioner's attitude toward the patient. This shift in attitude is generally an improvement, because the presence of the infarct relieves the patient of blame, whereas psychodynamic theories of hysterical blindness, and the pejorative connotation of the word *hysterical,* can be construed to suggest that the illness is some-how motivated and the symptom somehow simulated.

Even when caregivers say that they accept that the blindness is genuine, the patient's behavior does not always improve. These patients often resist all attempts at rehabilitation and insist on being waited on and helped, as if willfully emphasizing their disability. This behavior could be interpreted as seeking the secondary gain of the subservient attention of others. It may also be that such patients detect, and need to resist, their caregivers' skepticism of the genuineness of their blindness. This skepticism may in turn be a manifestation of negative countertransference.

Treatment is primarily psychotherapeutic, and any summary would do an injustice to the many complex theories that have arisen from and contributed to the therapy of hysteria. Results are slow and uncertain, and the family should be prepared for this. Counseling the family on how to deal with chronic illness may be more useful in the initial stages than insight-oriented therapy.

Anosognosia and Anton's Syndrome

At the opposite extreme we have anosognosia, the denial of illness. This again is familiar to ophthalmologists. Most of us who resist wearing our bifocals have indulged in some degree of it. This kind of inability to ac-knowledge change, especially change for the worse, is sometimes called cognitive dissonance. It has usually been explained in terms of behavior-ism and learning theory rather than psychodynamics. Individuals who are totally blind may resist acknowledging their impairment to the point of insisting that they can drive a car. A stroke may cause complete blind-ness by damage to the occipital cortex on both sides (with the pupils continuing to react to light because the damage is above the midbrain level where the pupillary reflexes are mediated). When this cortical blind-ness is denied, the condition is called *Anton's syndrome* (although An-ton's original papers in 1898 and 1899 covered other entities). In prac-tice, it is difficult to establish this diagnosis, because brain damage ex-tensive enough to be bilateral is often accompanied by dementia that impedes or precludes visual testing.

Agnosia

The patient with a pure and simple case of visual agnosia is unable to recognize objects seen, in the absence of speech disorder or blindness

(Lissauer 1890/1988). According to traditional localization, such a patient should be right-handed and should have a lesion in the left parieto-occipital area of the cortex.

Tagawa et al. (1990) found that lesions of the right occipital cortex cause spatial agnosia in the left visual field; lesions of the left occipital cortex cause pure alexia and color agnosia; and bilateral lesions in both occipital cortices cause prosopagnosia, color blindness, and object agnosia.

The validity of the diagnosis of agnosia in the presence of severe mental disorder or multiple neurological impairment may be doubtful. The more esoteric the agnosia, the more difficult it is to separate from a visual field defect, an aphasia, an emotional disturbance, or dementia. If patients with dementia are shown various objects and asked to name them, they may fail to do so correctly. Is this phenomenon just another example of pervasive mental disability, or is it nominal aphasia or visual agnosia? Rochford (1971), in an ingenious attempt to answer this question, showed that the ability to name was improved if the object to be named was a body part of the patient touched by the examiner, and concluded that visual agnosia was a primary defect in dementia.

In some cases of agnosia without dementia, there is disconnected awareness (Cowey 1991). The patient cannot name objects or tell them apart, but positions the fingers correctly for the objects' size and shape (accurate prehension) when asked to pick up those objects. Such a phenomenon might suggest that the agnosia was psychogenic or simulated, but is another example of covert knowledge, with a neurological basis for a "hysterical" symptom.

Simultanagnosia

In addition to seeing what is within our field of vision with our eyes kept still, we have an ability to move our eyes rapidly over something, such as a line of print or a picture, and grasp its totality. Simultanagnosia (also called *Balint's syndrome* or *optical ataxia*) is a condition in which this ability is lost. The person can see only one thing at a time, or can see parts of things but not the wholes, although the visual fields are normal. One letter of a word can be seen, for example, but not the word.

Cognitive psychologists have been very interested in this disability, and through studying it have obtained evidence of ways in which the brain processes information like a computer (Coslett and Saffran 1991). The causative lesion is in the occipitoparietal region, and is bilateral in most cases, but sometimes is only on the left (Rizzo and Robin 1990).

Prosopagnosia

Prosopagnosia is an inability to recognize faces that is not due to eye problems, visual field defects, or dementia. There have been striking case reports of patients with complete prosopagnosia who have retained the ability to make other fine distinctions (Bodamer 1947).

There is an emotional aspect to the ability to recognize faces. Occasional difficulty in fitting the name to a face happens to most people; it is a familiar experience that conscious efforts to remember the name, especially under stress, render the task more difficult, but the name can later be remembered effortlessly. This phenomenon has been termed *affective prosopagnosia* (Harrington et al. 1989) and can become distressing to individuals who tend to be obsessive, whereas others with severe face recognition impairment may be unconcerned and unaware of the disability (Young et al. 1990).

In some cases of prosopagnosia there is an apparent ability to remember faces and to use the remembered knowledge without being able to bring the name to full consciousness. This phenomenon is called *covert face recognition* (Bruyer 1991). In most patients with the condition, the problem is that of remembering faces in social situations, not of distinguishing between two portraits set side by side. Some authors (e.g., De Renzi et al. 1991) therefore divide prosopagnosia into two forms: *mnestic* (or associative) prosopagnosia, in which there is trouble remembering faces, and *perceptual* (or apperceptive) prosopagnosia, in which there is trouble distinguishing between faces (as with portraits set side by side). This classification is disputed by neuropsychologists (McNeil and Warrington 1991).

Classically, the lesion in prosopagnosia is occipital, and is associated with color blindness (or difficulty in naming colors). The lesion is bilateral in most cases, but on the right if unilateral (Benton 1990; Walsh 1990). Some authorities on the subject believe that prosopagnosia is caused by damage to a connection between a center for seeing in the occipital lobe and a center for remembering in the temporal lobe, and classify it as a disconnection syndrome (Damasio et al. 1982). The particular nerve fiber bundle thought to be damaged is the inferior longitudinal fasciculus.

There have been no controlled trials of treatment of prosopagnosia. In practice, the patient's emotional state is of greatest concern, and recognizing and explaining the alarming syndrome to the patient can be helpful.

A 67-year-old patient was referred who complained of inability to remember faces. He had been hospitalized on a psychiatric floor because of depression with psychotic and suicidal features. He had undergone open-heart surgery and was in atrial fibrillation. A computed tomography (CT) scan of the head several months before had been negative. On interview he was in emotional distress with some of his complaints being somatic. Staff reported that he needed encouragement with his activities of daily living and with eating, and became worried over minor decisions. He complained that his memory was bad, but it was not possible to find defects on any of the usual questions. He was fully oriented in space and time, stated the date of Pearl Harbor as "December 7, 1941," and was able to supply his telephone number and the names and ages of family members. However, he became visibly upset if he had to hesitate in answering, so that testing of his cognitive function had to be curtailed.

Asked what his memory problem was, he said that he could not remember faces. His trouble was in fitting the name to the face. This did not happen with family members or close long-term friends, or with celebrities seen on television.

In view of the strong stroke risk factors, the possibility of a visual scotoma or of a localized infarct causing prosopagnosia could not be ruled out, but repeating the CT scan was not thought justified. The patient asked about medication for his memory, but it was explained to him that his forgetfulness was circumscribed and not due to senility or Alzheimer's disease. Antidepressant medication had been started.

A program of training to recognize faces was discussed with the patient, including trying to remember faces by the presence of specific features such as eyeglasses, beard, or hair color, rather than relying on the gestalt. Discussions were also held with the nursing and occupational therapy staff, and a program of occupational therapy with practice in recognizing faces from pictures was devised.

Alexia

In pure word blindness, or alexia without agraphia, the patient remains able to write but cannot read. There is usually a right homonymous hemianopsia. When there is also difficulty in naming colors, the term *Poetzl's syndrome* is sometimes used. The cases described of this syndrome have involved lesions of the left occipital lobe and the splenium (Walsh 1990).

Hallucinations

Hallucinations can occur in any modality of sensation. When there is damage to a peripheral sense organ, the result is mostly a simple sensory experience, such as flashes of light with a blow to the eye, although eye pathology can sometimes result in a formed visual hallucination if there is dementia (Berrios and Brook 1984). More central damage is more likely to cause hallucinations that are more formed (White 1980). Some authors use the term "pseudohallucinations" for abnormal sensory experiences that the subject knows do not correspond to anything in the real world. It might be expected that a psychotic patient would think visual hallucinations were real, whereas a patient with eye disease would know they were not real, but the degree of insight does not relate to the cause of the hallucinations in a straightforward way. Visual hallucinations can occur in patients with functional psychosis, with dementia, with occipital infarcts, and with various kinds of eye disease. When the degree of insight in patients in these four different categories is compared, those with infarcts are most likely to claim that their hallucinations are real (Jeste and Harris 1992).

Hallucinations may result from severe sensory deprivation. Sudden and complete loss of hearing from any cause, for example, is often accompanied by elaborate, frequently musical, auditory hallucinations (which are not helped by antipsychotic medications). Such sensory-deprivation hallucinations have been called *release hallucinations* by Cogan (1973). It seems that the parts of the brain concerned with vision or hearing may activate spontaneously when they are deprived of input from the eyes or ears.

According to Cogan, visual release hallucinations are due to loss of sensory input to the visual area of the cortex and are more changeable, but also more continuous, than "irritation" hallucinations, which are due to damage within the brain center for vision rather than loss of input to it. (Few of Cogan's cases were stroke patients.) Irritation hallucinations occur in paroxysmal attacks and are less well formed, sometimes merely consisting of flashes of light.

Visual Versus Auditory Hallucinations

Visual symptoms in general are more strongly associated with organic brain disease, whereas hearing voices is commonly due to functional psychosis. Auditory hallucinations figure among the first-rank Schneiderian symptoms of schizophrenia.

The reason for this difference has not been established. It may reflect differences in the anatomical structure of the pathway to the brain from the ears and from the eyes. There is, for example, no exact auditory parallel to the visual field defect. Another dissimilarity is that, in schizophrenia, the auditory hallucinations have a motor component. They are often accompanied by muttering of the words being heard.

Lanska et al. (1987) reviewed cases of "brain stem auditory hallucinosis" and described a patient with a left-side dorsal pontine hemorrhage who heard noises "like people talking" and "rain falling on a roof" bilaterally, but more intensely in the left ear. The hallucinations continued over weeks, varied in content, and were associated with moderate hearing loss.

Geriatric Hallucinations

Hallucinations, often accompanied by delusions, are so common in geriatric psychiatric practice that geriatric psychiatrists are not always convinced of the significance of focal lesions found on brain scan. Eastwood and Corbin (1983) found hallucinations in 15% of hospitalized geriatric psychiatry patients. Of these, less than half had an organic etiology. These geriatric hallucinations may occur in any modality, and may be tactile or olfactory.

Hallucinations and Hemianopsia

There is a tendency for visual hallucinations to be associated with damage to the occipital cortex, and for the hallucinations to occur in the area of the visual field defect.

These hallucinations are often recurrent or persistent visual images, all of the same kind. Such images are sometimes called *palinopsia*, although the definition of this term varies (Gates et al. 1988). In *visual allesthesia*, images are transposed from the intact field of vision to the area of the field defect.

Wender (1987), in her first-person account of her stroke, described hallucinations with a right hemianopsia, which consisted of children or cars coming from the right, and were annoying rather than frightening. She said, "These rapid visions do not seem insane but merely physical problems in my eyes, much like ordinary people's dreams" (p. 1595).

Kolmel (1985) found that 16 out of 120 patients with homonymous hemianopsia experienced complex visual hallucinations in the hemianopsic field. The hallucinations appeared after a latent period and were "weak in color, and stereotypical in appearance." In three cases of occipital lobe infarction described by La Mancusa and Cole (1988), there were visual hallucinations, visual field defects, and inability to name colors. Visual hallucinations associated with giant cell arteritis have also been described (Hart 1967).

Peduncular Hallucinosis

Peduncular hallucinations are vivid visual hallucinations of strange animals or beings caused by damage to the cerebral peduncles. Two weeks after a stroke, the patient described by Lhermitte (1922) began to see cats and chickens with staring eyes walking across the floor of her room. She was able to touch them, and they felt like real animals, but they disappeared through the floor when touched. She was aware that they were not real, and did not expect others to be able to see them. Subsequently, the animals changed to strangely dressed human figures, which would change form as she watched. Although she experienced disturbances of sleep and memory, her only other psychiatric symptom was her reaction to the hallucinations.

Lhermitte described only this one case, and there was no autopsy follow-up. He deduced the location of the lesion from the presence of eye-movement paralysis due to involvement of the oculomotor (third) nerve in the midbrain (Figure 7–1). Geller and Bellur (1987) found 10 more published cases of peduncular hallucinosis and confirmed the localization in their own case by magnetic resonance imaging (MRI).

Management of Visual Hallucinations

It is important in treatment of stroke-related visual hallucinations to make sure that they are not due to anything other than the stroke. The presence of a cerebral infarct, even of an occipital one, does not reduce this necessity. Delirium tremens caused by drug or alcohol withdrawal is life-threatening if not promptly treated. Stroke can be accompanied by—and can obscure the signs of—other illness. Hallucinations may be part of a delirium due to concomitant infectious or metabolic disease, and the patient's temperature should be checked. Prescriptions should be reviewed for drugs (especially anticholinergics) that can cause visual hallucinations.

Reassurance should be attempted, although explanation of the organic origin is not always enough to resolve distress caused by organically induced hallucinations. If there is a history of previous psychosis responsive to medication, antipsychotic drugs may be tried. These drugs can also be useful in some geriatric patients who have hallucinations accompanied by delusions. The elderly stroke patient is, however, likely to be vulnerable to adverse medication effects, and supervision by the primary care physician is important. The question of whether antipsychotics can be used as nonspecific antihallucinogenic medication remains open. Good results can sometimes be seen, but there have been no adequate controlled trials (Hall 1993).

In a case described by Gates et al. (1988), the patient became depressed and experienced weight loss and sleep disturbance. It was found on psychiatric interview that he was upset by persistent hallucinations of "Pac-Man" figures, which appeared in the center of his visual field and marched off to his right. He was found to have a right homonymous hemianopsia, and CT scan showed a large left occipital lobe infarct. His distress immediately resolved when he was given this explanation for his condition.

Miller et al. (1987) described a patient with distressing visual hallucinations, seen primarily in the left visual field. This 82-year-old woman, who was widowed and had depression and dementia, saw "four Spanish men sitting on the dining room table." She had a left visual field defect and a right parieto-occipital infarct on CT scan. Antipsychotic medications and phenobarbital made her worse, but she got much better on Dilantin (phenytoin).

Misidentification Syndromes

The taxonomic place of the misidentification syndromes is in doubt. They have been classified as disorders of perception, a designation supported by the fact that they sometimes have an organic etiology, usually a cerebral infarct; however, these syndromes are equally likely to occur in psychoses, where there is no structural brain damage.

The main symptom in misidentification syndromes is a belief that a place or person exists in two forms, and that one form has been substituted by the other. There is general agreement on the existence of four basic types of delusion: intermetamorphosis, the syndrome of subjective doubles (doppelgänger), and the syndromes of Capgras and Fregoli (Christodoulou 1991; Cutting 1991).

Because no official definition exists for the misidentification syndromes, the category could conceivably be widened, and Joseph (1986), who was largely responsible for recognizing the syndromes as a group, listed 11 entities. Mere disorientation to person or space is not included among these entities, but the distinction is not always easy in cases with fluctuating cognitive impairment. Most of the phenomena of the misidentification syndromes can be observed at some stage in dementia patients with no neurological evidence of a focal lesion (Neitch and Zarraga 1991). Prosopagnosia and reduplicative paramnesia are sometimes included in the misidentification syndromes on the grounds that their central feature is mistaking one thing for another. Other possible candidates include image animation ("picture sign"), autoscopy, and a syndrome described by Steiner et al. (1987) in which the patient saw the world upside down (the patient had vertebrobasilar ischemia).

The Capgras syndrome, or *délusion des Sosies,* is the delusion that a familiar person is an impostor and has been replaced by an identical-looking double. This syndrome is relatively common (Förstl et al. 1991). Intermetamorphosis and the syndrome of Fregoli are rare. In Fregoli's syndrome, the patient believes that a stranger is really a familiar person in disguise. In intermetamorphosis, there is no disguise; rather, one person has been completely replaced by another. A doppelgänger is a ghostly counterpart that has taken on the appearance of the patient. Reduplicative paramnesia is a condition in which the patient believes that he or she is in several different places at the same time (Patterson and Mack 1985). Image animation, object animation, and picture sign are terms used to describe a condition in which the patient addresses and treats a picture or inanimate object as if it were alive (Weinberg 1992).

Patients whose misidentification syndrome has an organic origin are generally less likely to have had paranoid symptoms preceding the syndrome's onset, less likely to have misidentification of person, and more likely to have delusional misidentification of place (Fleminger and Burns 1993).

Among 100 cases reviewed by Fleminger and Burns (1993), there were 12 patients who had had a cerebrovascular accident, and another 14 with a clinical diagnosis of dementia. These researchers found that the combination of bilateral frontal damage and right parietal damage was especially common.

Of 260 cases reviewed by Förstl et al. (1991), 18 patients had a clinical diagnosis of cerebrovascular disease and another 19 had a clinical diagnosis of dementia. Of the 80 patients who had had CT scans, 9 showed infarcts, mostly on the right. Cerebral infarction was most common among those with reduplicative paramnesia and least common among those with delusions that their own form or identity had been affected.

Fregoli's syndrome was too rare to figure in these surveys. The patient described by De Pauw et al. (1987) had a posterior temporoparietal infarct on the right side.

Psychological Explanations

Several psychological explanations of the misidentification syndromes have been advanced. The person replaced in Capgras' syndrome is characteristically one with whom the patient is closely involved emotionally, and there is hostility toward the impostor. Freudian theories link this syndrome to emotional ambivalence about the person being replaced. Assuming that the formerly loved one is effectively gone allows the expression of previously repressed anger (De León 1993). The fact that dualism is a feature of many religions and that many folktales and legends—such as that of Leda and the swan—contain doubles and impersonations has led to a Jungian theory in which the etiology of misidentification syndromes is linked to reversion to archaic types of thinking (Todd 1957).

Neuroanatomical Explanations

The three major neuroanatomical explanations advanced for the misidentification syndromes have been those of Cutting (1991), of Joseph (1986; Ellis et al. 1993), and of Ellis and Young (1990). Cutting suggested that the syndromes are due to loss of a distinction-making faculty located in the right cerebral hemisphere. Joseph postulated that they result from an absence of integration between the right and left hemispheres. Ellis and Young theorized that they are caused by a loss of connections between visual receptor areas in the occipital cortex and visual organizing areas in the parietal cortex, thus relating them to prosopagnosia. There is not yet enough evidence to provide firm neuropathological and statistical support for any of these explanations, although the preponderance of right-hemisphere infarcts in the cases so far described probably favors Cutting's theory.

Management of Misidentification Syndromes

Even if an infarct is present, the diagnosis of schizophrenia or paranoid disorder must be considered. These disorders may require appropriate psychiatric treatment, probably involving antipsychotic medication. The place of antipsychotic medications in cases caused solely by infarcts has not been established by controlled trials, but there is evidence from single case reports that such drugs are useful.

Beliefs that amount to delusions are, by definition, impervious to rational argument, and reassurance in these cases may have to be within the framework of the delusion, but the phenomenological status of the misidentification syndromes is often ambiguous. When there is associated confusion, reassurance and reorientation are often helpful. For example, a patient with reduplicative paramnesia who insists she is not in her own home can be taken for a walk around the block and may then realize where she is.

Caution must be exercised in managing patients with either Capgras' or Fregoli's syndrome because of a risk of homicide. The therapist who is aware of expressed homicidal intent against the supposed impostor may incur a *Tarasoff* liability by failure to take appropriate precautions.

Summary

The distinction between neurological and psychiatric causes of visual disturbance may be incomplete or impossible. The presence of dementia can impair diagnosis. Exact diagnosis and explanation of a neuro-ophthalmic disorder may be therapeutic, although in some cases the patient may resent having the disability pointed out. Patients with occipital infarcts may mimic "hysterical" blindness and need the same kind of management. Agnosia patients may respond to reeducation and training, and some cases may need treatment for depression. Hallucinations tend to occur in the blind areas of visual field defects. Hallucinations are so common and have so many possible causes that the presence of an infarct should not prevent a search for other treatable causes, including delirium and psychosis. Misidentification syndromes may be due either to organic brain damage or to functional psychosis.

References

American Psychiatric Association: Diagnostic and Statistical Manual of Mental Disorders, 4th Edition. Washington, DC, American Psychiatric Association, 1994

Anton G: Über Herdekrankungen des Gehirns welche vom Patienten selbst nicht wahrgenommen werden. Wiener Klinische Wochenschrift 11:227–229, 1898

Anton G: Über die Selbswahrnehmungen der Herderkrankungen des Gehirns durch den Kranken bei Rindenblindheit und Rindentaubheit. Archiv für Psychiatrie und Nervenkrankheiten 32:86–127, 1899

Benton AL: Facial recognition. Cortex 26:491–499, 1990

Berrios GE, Brook P: Visual hallucinations and sensory delusions in the elderly. Br J Psychiatry 144:662–664, 1984

Bodamer J: Die Prosop-Agnosie. Archiv für Psychiatrie und Nervenkrankheiten 179:6–53, 1947

Bruyer R: Covert face recognition in prosopagnosia: a review. Brain Cogn 15:223–235, 1991

Christodoulou GN: The delusional misidentification syndromes. Br J Psychiatry 159 (suppl 14):65–69, 1991

Cogan DG: Visual hallucinations as release phenomena. Albrecht Von Graefes Archiv fur Klinische und Experimentelle Ophthalmologie 188:139–150, 1973

Coslett HB, Saffran EM: Simultanagnosia: to see but not two see. Brain 114:1523–1545, 1991

Cowey A: Grasping the essentials. Nature 349:102–103, 1991

Cutting J: Delusional misidentification and the role of the right hemisphere in the appreciation of identity. Br J Psychiatry 159 (suppl 14):70–75, 1991

Damasio AR, Damasio H, Van Hoesen GW: Prosopagnosia: anatomic basis and behavioral mechanisms. Neurology 32:331–341, 1982

De León OA: El sindrome de Capgras; estudio clinico de nueve casos. Revista Médica de Panamà 18:128–139, 1993

De Pauw KW, Szulecka TK, Pollock TL: Fregoli syndrome after cerebral infarction. J Nerv Ment Dis 175:433–437, 1987

De Renzi E, Faglioni P, Grossi D, et al: Apperceptive and associative forms of prosopagnosia. Cortex 27:213–221, 1991

Eastwood MR, Corbin S: Hallucinations in patients admitted to a geriatric psychiatry service. J Am Geriatr Soc 31:593–597, 1983

Ellis HD, Young AW: Accounting for delusional misidentification. Br J Psychiatry 157:239–248, 1990

Ellis HD, de Pauw KW, Christodolou GN, et al: Responses to facial and nonfacial stimuli presented tachiscopically in either or both visual fields by patients with the Capgras delusion and paranoid schizophrenics. J Neurol Neurosurg Psychiatry 56:215–219, 1993

Fleminger S, Burns A: The delusional misidentification syndromes in patients with and without evidence of organic cerebral disorder: a structured review of case reports. Biol Psychiatry 33:22–32, 1993

Förstl H, Almeida OP, Owen AM, et al: Psychological, neurological and medical aspects of misidentification syndromes: a review of 260 cases. Psychol Med 21:905–910, 1991

Gates TJ, Stagno SJ, Gulledge D: Palinopsia posing as psychotic depression. Br J Psychiatry 153:391–393, 1988

Geller TJ, Bellur SN: Peduncular hallucinosis: magnetic resonance confirmation of mesencephalic infarction during life. Ann Neurol 21:602–604, 1987

Hall CJ: The EEG and visual hallucinations in old age. International Journal of Geriatric Psychiatry 8:529–530, 1993

Harrington A, Oepen G, Spitzer M: Disordered recognition and perception of human faces in acute schizophrenia and experimental psychoses. Compr Psychiatry 30:376–384, 1989

Hart CT: Formed visual hallucinations: a symptom of cranial arteritis. BMJ 3:643–644, 1967

Iwata M: Visual association pathways in human brain. Tohoku J Exp Med 161 (suppl):61–78, 1990

Janet P: The Major Symptoms of Hysteria (reprint of 1907 edition). New York, Hafner, 1965

Jeste DV, Harris MJ: Visual hallucinations in non-psychotic elderly. American Association for Geriatric Psychiatry Newsletter 12:6–7, 1992

Joseph AB: Focal central nervous system abnormalities in patients with misidentification syndromes. Bibl Psychiatr 164:68–79, 1986

Kolmel HW: Complex visual hallucinations in the hemianopic field. J Neurol Neurosurg Psychiatry 48:29–38, 1985

La Mancusa JC, Cole AR: Visual manifestations of occipital lobe infarction in three patients on a geriatric psychiatry unit. J Geriatr Psychiatry Neurol 1:231–234, 1988

Lanska DJ, Lanska MJ, Mendez MF: Brainstem auditory hallucinosis. Neurology 37:1685, 1987

Lhermitte J: Syndrome de la calotte du pedoncule cérébral (les troubles psycho-sensoriels dans les lésions du mésencéphale). Rev Neurol (Paris) 29:1359–1365, 1922

Lissauer H: Ein Fall von Seelenblindheit nebst einen Beitrag zur Theorie derselben (1890; translated by Jackson M). Cognitive Neuropsychology 5:157–192, 1988

McNeil JE, Warrington EK: Prosopagnosia: a reclassification. Quarterly Journal of Experimental Psychology 43A:267–287, 1991

Miller F, Magee J, Jacobs R: Formed visual hallucinations in an elderly patient. Hosp Community Psychiatry 38:527–529, 1987

Neitch SM, Zarraga A: A misidentification delusion in two Alzheimer's patients. J Am Geriatr Soc 39:513–515, 1991

Newman NJ: Neuro-ophthalmology and psychiatry. Gen Hosp Psychiatry 15:102–114, 1993

Patterson SH, Mack JL: Neuropsychological analysis of a case of reduplicative paramnesia. J Clin Exp Neuropsychol 7:111–121, 1985

Rizzo M, Robin DA: Simultanagnosis: a defect of sustained attention yields insights on visual information processing. Neurology 40:447–455, 1990

Rochford G: A study of naming errors in dysphasic and demented patients. Neuropsychologia 9:437–443, 1971

Steiner I, Shahin R, Melamed E: Acute "upside down" reversal of vision in transient vertebrobasilar ischemia. Neurology 37:1685–1686, 1987

Tagawa K, Nagata K, Shishido F: Occipital lobe infarction and positron emission tomography. Tohoku J Exp Med 161 (suppl):139–153, 1990

Todd J: The syndrome of Capgras. Psychiatr Q 31:250–265, 1957

Vance B: An open letter to family, relatives and friends of stroke survivors. Be Stroke Smart 10:15–16, 1993

Walsh KW: Two posterior neuropsychological syndromes revisited. Tohoku J Exp Med 161 (suppl):121–130, 1990

Weinberg EL: Image animation (letter). J Am Geriatr Soc 40:640, 1992

Weiskrantz L: Disconnected awareness for detecting, processing, and remembering in neurological patients. Proceedings of the Royal Society of Medicine 84:466–470, 1991

Wender D: "Craziness" and "visions": experiences after a stroke. BMJ 295:1595–1597, 1987

White NJ: Complex visual hallucination in partial blindness due to eye disease. Br J Psychiatry 136:284–286, 1980

World Health Organization: International Statistical Classification of Diseases and Related Health Problems, 10th Revision. Geneva, Switzerland, World Health Organization, 1992

Young A, De Haan EHF, Newcomb F: Unawareness of impaired face recognition. Brain Cogn 14:1–18, 1990

CHAPTER EIGHT

Pain, Touch, and Stroke

etection of the effects of stroke on sensation is impeded by several factors, including the subtle nature of some of the alterations of sensations in proportion to the overwhelming obviousness of the motor disabilities. Because of the patient's communication difficulties, others often do not realize that stroke may be painful.

In general, sensations of pain, temperature, and touch, and awareness of the body's position in space (proprioception) from the left side of the body travel, if from below the neck, up to the posterolateral ventral nucleus of the right thalamus, and, if from the face, to the posteromedial ventral (arcuate) nucleus. Sensations from the right side of body go to the left thalamus.

Theories of the brain based on the hierarchical structure of the nervous system assume that the cerebral cortex is the location of complex conscious thought. In this view, sensations arriving in the thalamus are not yet conscious, and, in order for them to rise to consciousness, the thalamus must pass them up to the parietal cortex. However, pain and temperature sensations are seldom lost in infarcts of the cortex, and the clinical evidence could be interpreted to mean that pain sensations become conscious at the thalamic level.

Thalamic Pain Syndrome

The thalamic pain syndrome consists of spontaneous pain on the affected side following a stroke with mild hemiplegia, often with choreoathetoid movements on the affected side. It does not usually present until a few weeks or months after the initial stroke, and is relieved if either full recovery occurs or the stroke extends (Pearce 1988; Wilton 1989). The recovery upon a second stroke is thought to be due to the cutting off of pathways carrying messages from the thalamus to the parietal cortex (Soria and Fine 1991).

Normal pain and touch sensation on the affected side are lost, but there is a phenomenon called *thalamic overreaction* in which stimuli that usually are not painful are experienced with extreme discomfort. Some describe the pain as having a special quality called *allodynia*. Nuzzo and Warfield's (1985, p. 32d) patient said that he had a constant burning pain "as if my hand were stuck in a hot griddle," and when a sheet was placed over his body, he said it "felt like lead."

Like many pain syndromes, thalamic pain syndrome has a subjective element. Déjerine and Roussy (1906), who discovered the syndrome, suggested that personality factors are involved. Agnew (1984) found that patients with poststroke pain are younger than most stroke patients and "almost uniformly have a more chaotic, strained or unsatisfactory, perhaps ambivalent, relationship with their spouse or significant other" (p. 96).

In some cases, a further symptom that can appear to be psychogenic is the "ease of falling" syndrome, or *astasia,* in which there are slow, stereotyped falls to the painful side without loss of consciousness (Nair 1990).

Although the syndrome is described as thalamic, and the lesions found at autopsy by Déjerine and Roussy were in the thalamus, modern imaging techniques have shown that most patients with the classical syndrome do not have damage to the thalamus (Agnew 1984). Several authors have described a similar syndrome associated with damage to the parietal lobe of the cortex, especially the postcentral gyrus (Demierre and Siegfried 1985). In the cases reported by Schmahmann (1992), the area of involvement was in the white matter deep to the parietal cortex.

Pure Sensory Stroke

In most cases in which stroke affects sensation on one side, there will be paralysis on that side also. However, it is possible for infarcts to affect only sensory pathways and to cause loss of sensation without paralysis, and these sensory abnormalities may be diagnosed as psychogenic.

The hallmark of *hysterical anesthesia* is sometimes stated to be that it does not correspond to the distribution of anesthesia caused by interference in any anatomical pathway, but anesthesia produced by infarcts can cover a wide variety of distributions. Infarcts in the thalamus or midbrain can cause loss of all sensation from one side of the body, or from one side of the face and the hand of the same side (cheiro-oral syndrome).

Damage to the thalamus can sometimes cause loss of deep sensation in the limbs of one side, with retention of the ability to feel light touch, painful pinpricks, and heat and cold. Patients with such damage cannot tell where their limbs on one side are in space unless they can see them. As a result, they become clumsy (Dobato et al. 1990). This condition is theoretically, but not practically, distinguishable from the parietal lobe syndromes discussed later in this chapter.

Yang Yi-jie (1991) has described five cases of pure sensory stroke in patients, none of whom complained of severe spontaneous pain, although they were aware of numbness and tingling.

Paresthesias and Parasitosis

Abnormal sensations such as tingling on one side of the body may be due to infarcts affecting the thalamus or parietal lobe on the opposite side. Such sensations may be accompanied by anxiety and hyperventilation (Scialdone 1990) or by delusions of creeping skin parasites (Flynn et al. 1989).

These psychiatric symptoms can obscure the diagnosis if the patient cannot provide a good account of his or her symptoms. Careful questioning may be required to elicit the fact that the symptoms affect all of one side of the body, thus furnishing a clue to their central organic origin.

Other Causes of Stroke-Related Pain

Headache

Headache occurs in one-fourth of patients with acute stroke, often ipsilateral to the stroke lesion (Kawamura and Meyer 1991), and is believed by most authorities to be of organic rather than psychogenic origin (Vestergaard et al. 1993), although Pintoff (1992), in his first-person account, described the throbbing headaches he suffered as being associated with anxiety. Pintoff's headaches were relieved by a medication containing codeine, but this raised concerns by his nurse and doctor that he would become addicted.

Patients with dementia are less likely than those without dementia to complain of headache (Takeshima et al. 1990). The relationship between migraine and stroke and the association of headache with the antiphospholipid antibody syndrome (APLAS) are discussed in Chapter 3.

One of the most notorious medical pitfalls is the subarachnoid hemorrhage, which often presents as a severe headache. Because judgments of the severity of pain are subjective, social and cultural factors are involved. The more a patient's actions emphasize the severity of the pain, the more negatively the physician may react, especially if the behavior is accompanied by demands for addictive drugs for the relief of pain. A full and careful examination of the patient should reveal the diagnosis. The classical sign in subarachnoid hemorrhage is the presence of neck rigidity, but this may be hard to assess if the patient is cringing and writhing in agony. Often what is conveyed to the physician is emotional distress, to which the physician may respond by attempting to resist getting caught up in the emotion and to maintain professional detachment. Such an attempt can lead to a stance of apparent aloofness, disdain, or hostility.

Bendor (1991) has given a harrowing firsthand account of such an error:

> The doctor saw me immediately, but was unable or unwilling to hear what I was saying. He insisted that this was just a tension headache, or a different version of migraine. Ignoring my plea that this pain was qualitatively and quantitatively different from any pain I had ever experienced and was located in a very different place, he sent me home with a new pain medication. Later that evening the pain became so explosive that I thought I was having a stroke and may die. We drove to the emergency department of the nearest teaching hospital. There I was sent home again with a careless diagnosis of tension headache and another prescription. My frightened but emphatic insistence that this was no ordinary headache was dismissed by young interns and residents who may already have been inducted into a view of medicine that arrogates all knowledge to the physician and relegates patients to a passive role as the unlearned objects of the physician's diagnosis and intervention. (p. 6)

Muscle Spasm and Spasticity

A common cause of pain on a paralyzed side is what are generally called cramps or spasms. *Muscle spasm* is an imprecise term, often used as a "diagnosis of destitution" in cases of obscure pain that are suspected of being psychological in origin (Ciccone and Grzesiak 1990). There is, however, a specific organic basis for the muscle spasm diagnosis when the patient has spasticity due to an upper motor neuron lesion, such as from a stroke.

Spasticity is an exaggeration of the normal tendency for muscle that has been stretched to contract. When muscles are stretched, the muscle spindles pass messages back along afferent nerve fibers of group Ia. These incoming messages stimulate the alpha motor neurons in the spinal cord to send efferent messages back to the muscle telling it to contract. Normally, this simple reflex arc is modified by impulses that come down from the motor areas of the brain. Failure of this modification results in increased and uncoordinated muscle contraction, which may be painful.

Prolonged contraction can cause *contracture*—a loss of the normal balance between extensors and flexors—that results in permanent deformity and wasting. Steps taken to prevent this condition can cause conflict situations. Physical therapists and occupational therapists may see their primary duty as maintaining function by preventing development of contractures. This can be done by measures such as splinting to keep the limbs from bending into dysfunctional positions. Patients are sometimes intolerant of these measures, and splints put on at night are often off by the next morning. Some patients seem to find it more comfortable to allow the spastic muscle to contract than to wear the splints, even if they do not specifically complain of pain from the splints. The patient's awareness of the rationale for the treatment is crucial, and discussions by the other treatment team members, such as physicians and nurses, with the physical therapist, occupational therapist, and orthotist are useful in promoting such awareness.

Shoulder Pain

The cause of shoulder pain in stroke is not always clear (Griffin 1986). Sometimes the contraction of a muscle affected by spasticity is painful. Certain muscles, such as the subscapular muscle, which controls some shoulder movements, are especially liable to this, and pain can be relieved by completely paralyzing the muscle (Chironna and Hecht 1990).

Quite often the shoulder on the paralyzed side gets dislocated, although this does not seem to be a physically painful event. Kumar et al. (1990) showed that overvigorous rehabilitation, particularly the use of overhead pulleys, was a cause of shoulder pain in stroke. Many patients develop pain in the shoulder and hand of the affected side for no identifiable reason, a condition sometimes referred to simply as "shoulder-hand syndrome," and they later may develop reflex sympathetic dystrophy (Chalsen et al. 1987).

Reflex Sympathetic Dystrophy

Reflex sympathetic dystrophy refers to a set of changes undergone by a limb that is in pain and is not used. Even if no organic basis for the pain can be discovered, organic changes ultimately occur in the affected area. The skin becomes cold, the muscles become atrophic, and the bones turn osteoporotic. These changes are attributed to overactivity of the sympathetic nerves supplying the limb. Whether the sympathetic overactivity can cause the pain in the first place, or whether it is a result of disuse of the limb resulting from the pain, is not known.

Imaginary Pain

A common situation in practice is that a stroke patient has an ache or pain that cannot be diagnosed. The question asked is whether or not the pain is psychosomatic. Pain of undiagnosed cause is certainly not unique to stroke. Many patients complain of pain for which no organic basis can be found in the area of the professed pain. Even more perplexing are unusual sensations such as feeling "cold" or "numb" in an apparently healthy body part. If the discomfort is unilateral and a contralateral cerebral infarct is found, the connection will suggest itself. If the pain was of sudden onset and the estimated date of the infarct coincides with the onset of the pain, a relationship is even more strongly suggested.

Complete proof of such connections is rare, and they may be hypothesized because inability to find an organic cause for a symptom is felt to be a failure. There is often a hierarchy in diagnosis. Most physicians and patients want to find something wrong in the part where the discomfort is felt. Failing this, a physician may resort to "pinched nerves" and "root pain." Only if all else fails will the pain be considered what in DSM-IV (American Psychiatric Association 1994) is called a "pain disorder associated with psychological factors."

Treatment of Stroke-Related Pain

Psychiatric practitioners are involved at several points in the treatment of stroke-related pain. Management of stroke-related pain presents some dilemmas that are common to the treatment of all chronic pain. The use of narcotics can entail the need to increase the dose as time goes on, and can arouse concern about possibly prescribing improperly to a person with an addiction. Withholding narcotics from a patient is equally untenable, especially when there is no prospect of cure. One of the functions of mental health practitioners on the stroke treatment team is therefore to provide and document an assessment of addiction potential. If the mental health practitioner feels insecure about fulfilling this function, further consultation can be sought with another clinician who has special experience in dealing with addiction. If the risk of addiction is minimal or manageable, the use of morphine is limited primarily by its possible effects on respiration and its other potential adverse physical effects (e.g., nausea, vomiting, constipation). The adverse effects of synthetic narcotics are often mental, and include hallucinations and confusion.

A further consideration in stroke is that if the pain is of central origin, it may be amenable to psychiatric treatment methods such as antidepressant drugs, relaxation, hypnosis, or psychotherapy.

Treatment of Thalamic Pain Syndrome

Treatments tried for the thalamic syndrome have included antidepressants, anticholinesterase drugs, anticonvulsants, and a variety of neurosurgical techniques. Déjerine and Roussy (1906) noted that the pain was not suppressed by any medical or analgesic treatment but did not specify the types and dosages. The statement sometimes made that narcotics are ineffective is apparently based on this original account.

Koppel (1986) described two patients treated with the tricyclic antidepressant drug amitriptyline. One patient was a 44-year-old woman whose pain was relieved by 75 mg/day of amitriptyline. Another was a 73-year-old man whose pain was partially relieved by 25 mg twice a day but worsened when the dose was increased. Tricyclic blood levels and severity of depression were not measured.

Leijon and Boivie (1989) carried out a double-blind, three-phase, crossover, placebo-controlled trial of amitriptyline against carbamazepine in cases of central poststroke pain. Of the 23 patients included, only 9 were known to have a lesion of the thalamus, but all had a disturbance of cutaneous sensibility. Depression was assessed by rating scales, and tricyclic blood levels were monitored. The dose of amitriptyline was gradually increased to 75 mg/day. Amitriptyline proved superior to both placebo and carbamazepine. The superiority in pain relief was not secondary to any measurable change in depression. The pain relief effect began in the second week, and was greatest in those patients whose plasma levels of combined tricyclics rose about 300 nmol/L.

Demierre and Siegfried (1985) reported that significant relief was obtained in only 3 out of 10 patients treated with intermittent stimulation of electrodes implanted in the ventroposterior thalamic nuclei. In Tsubokawa et al.'s (1991) study of seven cases, anticonvulsants and antidepressants were tried with no effect, whereas the participants experienced relief from implantation of electrodes under the skull over the motor cortex. Levin et al. (1983) described three patients in which narcotics and antidepressants (the doses and blood levels of which are not stated) failed to provide relief, and the pain was relieved following hypophysectomy. In one of the three, there was complete relief within 48 hours of hypophysectomy. All patients needed lifelong hormone replacement therapy.

In summary, evidence exists that antidepressants may sometimes be helpful in relieving the pain of thalamic syndrome. The management of pain is ultimately a matter for individual medical judgment based on clinical experience and good rapport with the patient. Pain management must include the search for treatable causes of pain outside the central nervous system and consideration of analgesic medications such as nonsteroidal antiinflammatory agents.

Treatment of Muscle Spasm Pain

Muscle spasm pain has been treated with surgery, medication, application of heat or cold, and massage. Purely psychological methods have received little attention in stroke-related muscle spasm pain, although such methods have been used for muscle spasm pain of other etiologies. Communication impairment and dementia may limit the usefulness of relaxation techniques and hypnotic suggestion.

Drugs used for the relief of spasticity include dantrolene (Dantrium), baclofen (Lioresal, Atrofen), clonidine (Catapres), and the benzodiazepines. Sindou (1989) described treatment of pain associated with spasticity by posterior rhizotomy in 25 patients with upper-limb spasticity and pain due to hemiplegia; 85% of the patients obtained relief with this treatment.

Massage and application of heat and cold all bring some relief to this kind of pain, although it is intrinsically difficult to carry out controlled trials on such methods. Major disadvantages are that they are labor-intensive and the relief is often temporary.

It is important that the individuals doing the treatments not feel that they are wasting their time. Team meetings can be used to discuss the placebo effect and its place in pain management, and to ensure that the work of each team member is properly valued and appreciated.

Parietal Lobe Syndromes

Various syndromes traditionally associated with parietal infarcts can be understood fundamentally as stemming from problems in receiving sensory information. These syndromes include apraxia and some kinds of anosognosia, which may overlap, or be confused with, dementia and emotional disorders. Their diagnosis is not easy. Because it is often tedious and difficult to test sensation accurately in patients who cannot communicate, losses of sensation can go undetected. In the parietal lobe syndromes, the sensation loss is especially subtle and unobvious, because patients will commonly retain sensitivity on the affected side to pain, heat, cold, and some forms of touch. The sensory handicaps can be an unrecognized obstacle to rehabilitation.

Anatomically, the loss of two-point discriminations and somatosensory function following damage to one parietal lobe should be on the opposite side. However, in some studies it has been found that if one parietal lobe is severely damaged, there may be loss of these functions on both sides (Caselli 1991). Dysfunction on both sides is especially likely if the left parietal lobe is the one that is damaged (Mayer-Gross et al. 1960).

Ataxia and Apraxia

Ataxia and *apraxia* both refer to clumsiness of movement. The distinctions between them are not consistent. Ataxia is more commonly used to describe difficulties in standing and walking and is associated with damage to the cerebellum. Apraxia commonly refers to clumsiness in carrying out tasks with the upper limbs, is associated with parietal lobe damage, and is due to a disturbance of sensation. The term *constructional apraxia* denotes difficulty in performing tasks such as copying designs. *Dressing apraxia* is sometimes defined as a separate entity that is due to left parietal lobe lesions. The term *ideational apraxia* has been applied to deficits in tool selection and use (Ochipa et al. 1988).

Ambiguities in defining apraxia arise because so many kinds of impairment—for example, dementia, drowsiness, bad eyesight—can lead to difficulty in tasks such as dressing. Hier et al. (1983) suggested, perhaps tautologically, that apraxia should be defined as the inability to do well on tests for apraxia, regardless of the presence of other impairments.

Several tests exist for detecting apraxia. Some are essentially tests for dexterity, and patients do poorly on them because of visual impairment or paralysis. Practitioners are sometimes left to speculate that apraxia may exist as an obstacle to rehabilitation, without being able to isolate it from other mental and physical disabilities. The results of testing must therefore be considered along with assessment for visual field defects, for dementia, and for other possible factors. This is best done in consultations by the person doing the testing with the team responsible for treatment.

Anosognosia

Anosognosia, the denial of illness, is discussed here on the grounds that it is primarily a defect of sensation, but its taxonomic place is arguable. It could be classified as a delusion, but it also resembles phenomena such as "phantom limb" that occur because of peripheral neurological damage without any psychiatric illness. Anosognosia is more common if there is sensory loss on the affected side or if there is dementia, but it may also occur in the absence of either of these. Psychiatrists encounter psychotic patients who have had paralytic strokes but deny or seem oblivious to their physical illness. Babinski (1914) excluded patients with psychosis and dementia from his definition of anosognosia. Anosognosia can occur in several conditions, but most typically, as in Babinski's original description, it involves denial of weakness of a limb, usually a left limb, in stroke.

Anosognosia can cause considerable management problems, among them the risk of accidents. Patients with a right parietal lobe infarct and left hemiplegia may not recognize their deficits, and may want to walk although half of their body is paralyzed.

Theories of anosognosia were reviewed by Ellis and Small (1993). According to the "discovery" theory (Levine et al. 1991), the condition is caused by the combination of loss of proprioceptive sensation (awareness of the position of the limb in space) on the paralyzed side and cognitive impairment, which makes the patient unable to understand what has happened, so that the patient does not discover the paralysis. According to the "defensive" theory, anosognosia is due to a need to deny one's imperfections and is associated with a tendency to be compulsive. In the theory of Gerstmann (1942), a mechanism for converting impulses outside central consciousness to conscious cognition becomes deranged. Gerstmann combined psychodynamic with neurological concepts, and suggested that this mechanism, while having affinities with those involved in repression, was organic and located in the parietal area.

Astereognosis

Loss of the ability to recognize objects by their feel, *astereognosis,* is sometimes called *tactile agnosia.* This condition is distinguished from the inability to name the object, which has been called *tactile aphasia* or *tactile anomia* (Caselli 1991). *Amorphagnosia* is the inability to recognize size and shape; *ahylognosia,* the inability to recognize weight and texture; and *allocheiria,* the inability to tell which side of the body has been touched. Obviously, any of these disabilities might be a component of a peripheral anesthesia due to peripheral nerve damage, and could be impossible to test for in a patient with dementia.

Hemineglect

Hemineglect is a condition of refusal to acknowledge that one side of the world exists. If it is associated with hemiplegia, the paralysis may improve, but recovery may be complicated by the patient's lack of awareness of sensations coming from the affected side.

Hemineglect was originally associated with lesions of the parietal lobe, usually the right, but there have been several examples of its association with other lesions (Daffner et al. 1990). Although it is associated with visual field defects on the affected side, with sensory loss for two-point discrimination and sense of limb position on the affected side, and with anosognosia for hemiplegia, examples exist in which these defects have been absent (Ellis and Small 1993).

Testing for the presence of hemineglect demands some degree of patient cooperation and the ability to give accurate replies. This requirement hinders diagnosis in patients with dementia, although tests have been devised to detect hemineglect in such patients (Stone et al. 1991).

Treatment of Parietal Lobe Syndromes

Treatment of parietal lobe syndromes begins with the process of diagnosis. The physician or neuropsychologist will be among the first to detect the condition, and will discuss its implications with the patient and with other members of the treatment team. Treatment involves making the patient aware of the extent of the disabilities so as to learn to compensate for them. The kinds of sensation that are lost, such as proprioception, are explained to the patient and his or her caregivers. They learn to anticipate activities that involve proprioception and are instructed in how to compensate for its absence. This approach is a reversal of the process of learning to type. Actions such as those involved in dressing and grooming, which are typically done without looking, must now be done under visual control.

Dementia or impaired communication can impede this process. Another impediment is that awareness may be a negative experience that leads to resentment, because the patient initially feels worse as additional defects are pointed out.

Programs for treatment of hemineglect usually involve training the patient to deliberately scan the affected side. Zoccolotti (1991) and Butter and Kirsch (1992) have shown that such training often fails to generalize. A patient can be reminded to check the left side more carefully when crossing the street, but will quickly forget.

In the program described by Zoccolotti (1991) and by Pizzamiglio et al. (1990), patients were trained, using computer screens, to direct attention to phenomena on the neglected side. Although results were generally good, they tended to be poor in those with marked anosognosia. Those patients who were not aware of their problems tended to forget the instructions.

Butter and Kirsch (1992) used visual stimulation in the periphery of the neglected areas of the visual field, and a program of patching the eye on the side of the lesion. They found that both treatments were effective. Combining the two yielded significantly greater benefits than using either alone. The authors noted that the condition tends to improve spontaneously.

Ice-water irrigation of the external auditory canal contralateral to the brain lesion has been claimed to produce transient complete remission of denial of illness (Vallar et al. 1990).

Summary

Thalamic pain syndrome consists of spontaneous pain on the affected side following a stroke with mild hemiplegia, often with choreoathetoid movements on the affected side. It is sometimes treated with antidepressant medications.

Subarachnoid hemorrhage often presents as a severe headache. Negative physician-patient relationships can delay the correct diagnosis.

Pain without a clear anatomical basis may be regarded as psychogenic but may not be amenable to specific psychiatric treatment. Infarcts affecting only sensory pathways can cause loss of sensation without paralysis, and these sensory phenomena may be diagnosed as psychogenic. Unusual sensations on one side of the body may be due to infarcts affecting the thalamus or parietal lobe on the opposite side.

Parietal lobe syndromes, including apraxia and some kinds of anosognosia, are due to disturbances in awareness of body sensation. These syndromes may overlap, or be confused with, dementia and emotional disorders. Loss of sensation is difficult to detect if communication is impaired, which can lead to difficulties in rehabilitation. Treatment involves increasing the patient's awareness of the handicap.

References

Agnew DC: Thalamic pain. Bull Clin Neurosci 49:93–98, 1984

American Psychiatric Association: Diagnostic and Statistical Manual of Mental Disorders, 4th Edition. Washington, DC, American Psychiatric Association, 1994

Babinski J: Contribution a l'étude des troubles mentaux dans hémiplegie organique cérébrale (anosognosie). Rev Neurol (Paris) 27:845–847, 1914

Bendor SJ: You are just the patient: a consumer's perspective on preventing medical malpractice suits. Medical Malpractice Prevention 6:6–8, 1991

Butter CM, Kirsch N: Combined and separate effects of eye patching and visual stimulation on unilateral neglect following stroke. Arch Phys Med Rehabil 73:1133–1139, 1992

Caselli RJ: Rediscovering tactile agnosia. Mayo Clin Proc 66:129–142, 1991

Chalsen G, Fitzpatrick K, Bean S: Prevalence of the shoulder-hand pain syndrome in an inpatient rehabilitation population. Journal of Neurological Rehabilitation 1:137–141, 1987

Chironna RL, Hecht JS: Subscapularis motor point block for the painful hemiplegic shoulder. Arch Phys Med Rehabil 71:428–429, 1990

Ciccone DS, Grzesiak RC: Chronic musculoskeletal pain: a cognitive approach of psychophysiologic assessment and intervention. Advances in Clinical Rehabilitation 3:197–214, 1990

Daffner KR, Geoffrey LA, Weintraub S, et al: Dissociated neglect behavior following sequential strokes in the right hemisphere. Ann Neurol 28:97–101, 1990

Déjerine J, Roussy G: Le syndrome thalamique. Rev Neurol (Paris) 14:521–532, 1906

Demierre B, Siegfried J: Le syndrome douloureux thalamique. Corrélations radiologico-cliniques et traitement par la stimulation intermittente des noyaux sensitifs du thalamus. Neurochirurgie 31:281–285, 1985

Dobato JL, Villanueva JA, Giménez-Roldán S: Sensory ataxic hemiparesis in thalamic hemorrhage. Stroke 21:1749–1753, 1990

Ellis SJ, Small M: Denial of illness in stroke. Stroke 24:757–759, 1993

Flynn FG, Cummings JL, Scheibel J, et al: Monosymptomatic delusions of parasitosis associated with ischemic cerebrovascular disease. J Geriatr Psychiatry Neurol 2:134–139, 1989

Gerstmann J: Problems of imperception of disease and of impaired body territories with organic lesions. Archives of Neurology and Psychiatry 48:890–913, 1942

Griffin JW: Hemiplegic shoulder pain. Physical Therapy 66:1884–1893, 1986

Hier DB, Mondlock J, Caplan LR: Behavioral abnormalities after right hemisphere stroke. Neurology 33:337–344, 1983

Kawamura J, Meyer JS: Headaches due to cerebrovascular disease. Med Clin North Am 75:617–630, 1991

Koppel BS: Amitriptyline in the treatment of thalamic pain. South Med J 76:759–761, 1986

Kumar R, Metter EJ, Mehta A, et al: Shoulder pain in hemiplegia: the role of exercise. Am J Phys Med Rehabil 69:205–208, 1990

Leijon, Boivie J: Central post-stroke pain—a controlled trial of amitriptyline and carbamazepine. Pain 36:27–36, 1989

Levin AB, Ramirez LF, Katz J: The use of stereotaxic chemical hypophysectomy in the treatment of thalamic pain syndrome. J Neurosurg 59:1002–1006, 1983

Levine DN, Calvanio R, Rinn WE: The pathogenesis of anosognosia for hemiplegia. Neurology 41:1770–1781, 1991

Mayer-Gross W, Slater E, Roth M: Mental disorders in trauma, in Clinical Psychiatry. Edited by Mayer-Gross W, Slater E, Roth M. Baltimore, MD, Williams & Wilkins, 1960, pp 419–476

Nair KR: Ease of falling syndrome associated with unilateral thalamic lesion. Journal of the Association of Physicians of India 38:872–873, 1990

Nuzzo JA, Warfield CA: Thalamic pain syndrome. Hospital Practice (office edition) 20:32c–32d, 32h–32j, 1985

Ochipa C, Roth LJG, Heilman KM: Ideational apraxia: a deficit in tool selection and use. Ann Neurol 25:190–193, 1988

Pearce JMS: The thalamic syndrome of Déjerine and Roussy. J Neurol Neurosurg Psychiatry 51:676, 1988

Pintoff E: Bolt From the Blue. Salt Lake City, UT, Northwest, 1992

Pizzamiglio L, Anonucci G, Guariglia C, et al: La Rieducazione Neurocognitiva dell'eminattenzione in pazienti con lesione cerebrale unilaterale. Milan, Italy, Masson Ed, 1990

Schmahmann JD: Parietal pseudothalamic pain syndrome—clinical features and anatomic correlates. Arch Neurol 49:1032–1037, 1992

Scialdone AM: Thalamic hemorrhage imitating hyperventilation. Ann Emerg Med 19:817–819, 1990

Sindou M: La zone d'entrée des racines postérieures dans la moelle: cible chirurgicale pour le traitement de la douleur et de la spasticité. Bull Acad Natl Med 173:1039–1045, 1989

Soria ED, Fine EJ: Disappearance of thalamic pain after parietal subcortical stroke. Pain 44:285–288, 1991

Stone SP, Halligan PW, Wilson B, et al: Performance of age matched controls on a battery of visuo-spatial neglect tests. J Neurol Neurosurg Psychiatry 54:341–344, 1991

Takeshima T, Taniguchi R, Kitagawa T, et al: Headaches in dementia. Headache 30:735–738, 1990

Tsubokawa T, Katayama Y, Takamitsu Y, et al: Treatment of thalamic pain by chronic motor cortex stimulation. Pace 14:131–134, 1991

Vallar G, Sterzi R, Bottini G, et al: Temporary remission of left hemianesthesia after vestibular stimulation: a sensory neglect phenomenon. Cortex 26:123–131, 1990

Vestergaard K, Andersen G, Nielsen MI, et al: Headache in stroke. Stroke 24:1621–1624, 1993

Wilton LM: Thalamic pain syndrome. J Neurosci Nurs 21:362–365, 1989

Yang Yi-jie: Pure sensory stroke confirmed by CT scan. Chin Med J (Engl) 104:595–598, 1991

Zoccolotti PL: La rieducazione neurocognitiva dell'eminattenzione in pazienti con una lesione emisferica destra. Minerva Med 82:381–385, 1991

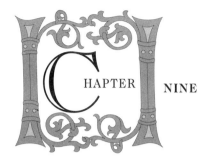

CHAPTER NINE

Sex and Stroke

Neuroanatomy of Sex

Autonomic Nervous System

The effects of stroke at the autonomic level are mostly indirect. For example, antihypertensive medications may be used in treatment of the stroke, or diabetes mellitus may be a causative factor in the stroke, and these may affect the autonomic nervous system.

The motor side of the sex act is relatively well understood. The efferent side of the reflex travels along both sympathetic and parasympathetic autonomic nerves. The sympathetic nerve impulses exit from the spinal cord at level T12–L1, then go to the hypogastric plexus and thence by way of the hypogastric nerves. The parasympathetic impulses travel in the nervi erigentes. During sexual excitement, these nerves constrict venous return from the penis or clitoris and increase blood flow to it.

Male erection is largely cholinergic, and ejaculation is noradrenergic. Complete ejaculation also depends on contractions of the striated muscle of the pelvic floor.

Central Nervous System

Because the autonomic nervous system and spinal cord contain all the elements of the reflex chain that can lead to sexual activity, erections and orgasms may occur in paraplegic patients. However, in order to consciously desire, initiate, and consummate a sexual act, there must be a link between consciousness and autonomic function, although the autonomic system is outside the direct control of the will.

A variety of conscious sensations may cause sexual arousal. Incoming stimuli probably all journey to conscious awareness through the thalamus. Ascending sensory inputs from the genitalia relay in the ventrolateral and intralaminar nuclei of the thalamus and then travel to the parietal cortex in the same way that other somatic sensations do.

The cerebral cortex is probably linked with the autonomic system through the limbic system and the hypothalamus. There is some evidence from neurophysiology and animal experiments that the limbic system is a center for sexual behavior, but the clinical implications of this localization remain speculative. Stimulation of the septal nuclei (see Figure A–17 in Appendix A) has been found to produce a pleasure sensation in animals, although this pleasure cannot be proven to be sexual. The Papez circuit, in the limbic system, consists essentially of the pathways from the hippocampus (Figure 9–1) through the hypothalamus to the cingulate gyrus and back to the hippocampus. Part of these pathways is the mammillothalamic tract (see Figure A–16 in Appendix A) connecting the hypothalamus with the anterior nucleus of the thalamus, which projects to the cingulate gyrus. The medial forebrain bundle and dorsal longitudinal fasciculus connect the hypothalamus with the autonomic nervous system. It is theoretically possible that a strategically located infarct might damage these connections that link the cortex with the autonomic nervous system, thereby affecting sexual function. This mechanism has not yet been proven clinically.

The hypothalamus mediates between the central nervous system and two systems not under conscious control: the autonomic nervous system and the endocrine system. Its control of the endocrine system is mediated by its production of "releasing factors." One of these polypeptide releasing factors is gonadotropin-releasing factor (GnRH), which regulates the release of the pituitary hormones (gonadotropins) that control the production of testosterone and prolactin. Increase of prolactin and decrease of testosterone may reduce male potency (Weizman et al. 1983). Hypothalamopituitary disorders in women have been associated with lack of sexual desire and with problems with lubrication or orgasm, but the prevalence of these problems does not correlate with prolactin and testosterone levels (Hulter and Lundberg 1994).

In tumors and traumatic brain injuries, endocrine disorders resulting from hypothalamic damage are well recognized, and sexual disorders have been linked to such disorders (Mitiguy 1992). In stroke, on the other hand, it has not been possible to relate sexual dysfunction to any localization of the infarct in the brain or to blood levels of serum testosterone (including response to human chorionic gonadotropin [HCG] stimulation), luteinizing hormone (LH), follicle-stimulating hormone (FSH), or prolactin (Sjögren et al. 1983). It may be that this difference relates to the different age groups of patients with stroke and patients with brain injury.

Diminished Sex Drive

Stroke is often associated with old age, with diabetes, with dementia, and with the use of drugs for hypertension. All of these conditions can affect sex drive. The direct neurological effects of a stroke cannot always be separated from its psychological consequences. Stroke is a devastating life event, and any devastating life event can reduce interest in sex.

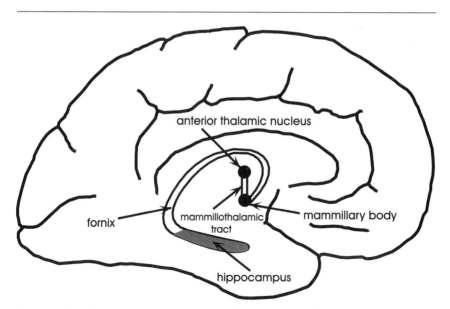

Figure 9–1.   Hippocampus in relation to the structures of the limbic system.

For many patients, a stroke comes at a time of declining sexual function. In one study (Diokno et al. 1990) of married adults 75 years of age and older in Washtenaw County, Michigan, half of the men and one-third of the women reported that they were no longer sexually active.

Antihypertensive Drugs

Antihypertensives are commonly considered to be among the drugs most likely to interfere with sexual function ("Drugs That Cause Sexual Dysfunction," 1992), but the evidence is contradictory. Sjögren et al. (1983) did not find any relationship between use of blood pressure medication and loss of sexual function after stroke. Often, it is not until a new drug has been on the market for some time that sexual side effects become apparent. Traditionally, it has been a medication's effects on male potency that have been the best documented.

Drug manufacturers' studies mention reduced libido as a possible effect of several beta-blockers, but not of calcium blockers. Raftos et al. (1973) found that clonidine (Catapres), which acts on central nervous system control of autonomic sympathetic activity, did not affect potency, and that several male patients who had previously become impotent on methyldopa treatment recovered potency when switched to clonidine. In other studies, however, clonidine has caused impotence. Diuretics and low-sodium diets have also been associated with impotence (Wassertheil-Smoller et al. 1991).

Direct Effects of Vascular Disease

Stroke patients often have multiple manifestations of vascular disease. In men, vascular disease may affect the penile arteries; sexual fantasy and desire persist, but there is loss of capacity for erection. Presumably, clitoral engorgement could be similarly affected by vascular disease, although this topic has not been separately studied.

Impotence was found to be vasculogenic, as determined by Doppler examination, in one-fourth of impotent men studied by Kaiser et al. (1988). Impotence was associated with other evidence of vascular disease, including heart disease, peripheral vascular disease, and stroke.

Surveys of Stroke Patients

Most of the surveys reported in the literature have concerned male potency. Orgasmic capacity in female stroke victims has not been extensively studied, but the literature reviewed by Emick-Herring (1985) indicated that it is as frequently lost as is erectile potency in males.

In Sjögren's (1983) Swedish studies, the greatest predictor of loss of a man's sexual activity was becoming dependent on his wife. She interpreted this finding as due to psychological feelings about role reversal and male dominance. Sjögren did not find that the side of the stroke mattered in regard to sexual function. Boldrini et al. (1991), who studied Italian patients with hemiparesis, also found a decline in sexual functioning, which was due to psychological and interpersonal factors related to the stroke rather than to any organic factor.

Coslett and Heilman (1986), on the other hand, found that men with right-hemisphere infarcts had significantly more sexual dysfunction than those with left-hemisphere infarcts. They measured sexual function by self-report, confirmed by spouses when available, of interest in sexual activity and frequency of intercourse. Only one of their 26 subjects had increased sexual activity.

Coslett and Heilman (1986) suggested that the discrepancy between their results and those of Sjögren (1983) was due to their more rigorous exclusion criteria: They excluded "patients who refrained from sexual activity because of feelings that sexual activity was inappropriate, concern about the consequences of sexual activity for their health, or their perception that the spouse had lost interest because of their medical condition" (Coslett and Heilman 1986, p. 1036); those with depression, debilitating illness, and preexisting epilepsy; and those who used drugs known to affect sexual function.

Habot et al. (1989) studied 35 men, one-third under the age of 60 and one-third over the age of 70, who had had a stroke with hemiplegia within the previous 2–3 months. All of the subjects had been sexually active before their stroke, and one-third (including one of those over 70) claimed to have been having sexual intercourse more than once a week. One-third of the men reported complete cessation of sexual activity after their stroke, and none continued to have sex more than once a week. No differences were found relating to right versus left hemiparesis, duration of marriage, country of origin, educational level, functional ability, or medical condition. The most common reason reported for decline in sexual activity was problems with physical movement (36%). Other reasons given were lack of libido (22%), lack of cooperation from spouse (16%), lack of satisfaction (13%), and fear (9%). Impotence was not a stated reason.

Bray et al. (1981) investigated sexual interest and function in 24 men and 11 women before and after a stroke. Although they found no general loss of sexual desire or inclination following stroke, in the men there was frequent loss of the ability to achieve erection and ejaculation. The five women in Bray et al.'s series who were premenopausal reported major alterations in their menses. Only one of the 11 female patients reported attaining orgasm after her stroke.

Management of Diminished Sex Drive

Tact and restraint are virtues, but a common failing of health care practitioners is not discussing sex at all. Rehabilitation staff members usually agree that sexual adjustment is important but do not feel comfortable discussing it; often the topic is addressed only if a patient specifically asks about it (Ducharme and Gill 1990).

Loss of sexual activity may be accepted as a normal consequence of aging by some patients, and some clinicians may not regard intervention as necessary (Muckleroy 1977). Other patients may regard loss of sexual pleasure as a deprivation equal to severe physical handicap (Angeleri et al. 1993).

A knowledge of the patient's culture and religion is important. Although the practitioner need not have the same cultural background as the patient, he or she should have been trained to communicate in ways the patient can understand and accept. In dealing with the sexually reticent, it is easiest to incorporate a sexual history, along with such matters as weight and appetite, in a medical history taken by a practitioner of the same sex.

For male patients, it should be determined whether erections occur at all, such as by masturbation or during rapid eye movement (REM) sleep. Erections in the course of REM sleep are often present as morning erections. Various strain gauges and transducers are available to determine whether erections occur during sleep, but it is often simpler to get the patient's sleeping partner to find out if this is happening. (The process can be made part of therapy.) If no erections occur at all, an organic cause such as vasculogenic impotence becomes more likely.

Sometimes a patient has a concern, which should be discussed, that sexual activity may raise his or her blood pressure (see "Coitus-Related Stroke," later in this chapter), and that this may precipitate a second stroke. Fear of soiling or wetting the bed is a deterrent for some patients.

Burgener and Logan (1989) recommend that a nurse discuss with the patient the management of care tasks that the patient finds particularly demeaning or distressing. They provide the example of 64-year-old stroke patient who found that having his wife help him with toileting activities was upsetting and affected his willingness to initiate sex. The nurse was able to design a way for him to carry out these activities without his wife's assistance.

Positions for coitus may also need to be discussed with stroke patients. Most couples discover through trial and error what positions work best for them. Extra pillows, side rails on the bed, and a handle on the headboard may help. Sensation changes on the affected side should be taken into consideration (Ellis 1986). Stroke patients should avoid coital positions in which they are on top. Side-by-side positions are recommended, with the stroke patient lying on his or her affected side. More detailed positioning instructions are given by Conine and Evans (1982), and McCormick et al. (1986) provide diagrams, but there the danger in getting too explicit is that the couple may take the instructions so seriously that they become inhibited from experimentation.

Coitus-Related Stroke

Heart rate and blood pressure increase by about 40% in men during coitus with man-on-top positions, and less during other sexual activities. The rate-pressure product increases by more than 90% (Bohlen et al. 1984; Mann et al. 1982).

Although these increases suggest that sexual activity may present cardiac risks, the few accounts of strokes related to sexual intercourse suggest that such phenomena are likely to occur only in the presence of an aneurysm or a vascular malformation (Finelli 1993; Okura et al. 1993). There may be a specific connection of recent coitus with transient global amnesia (see Chapter 16). Benign coital cephalgia does not seem to be related to stroke (Nick and Bakouche 1980).

Aberrant Sexual Behavior

Loss of both desire and potency are not the only sexual dysfunctions seen after stroke. Hyperactivity and inappropriate behaviors can also occur; in one recent series (Angeleri et al. 1993), such behaviors were found in 2% of the subjects. In some stroke patients, a preexisting sexual predilection may be uncovered by the disinhibiting effect of the brain damage.

Whether increased sexual activity in stroke truly represents hypersexuality rather than simply disinhibited behavior is difficult to determine. The latter is probably more common. Disinhibited sexual behaviors may result from dementia or other types of mental disorder, may be specifically associated with localized brain damage, may be a manifestation of preexisting antisocial inclinations, or may represent a cultural clash of differing views of acceptable sexual behavior.

In many cases, sexual misbehavior is associated with some degree of dementia. The onset of dementia frequently coincides with loss of erectile capacity in men (Zeiss et al. 1990), but poor judgment and loss of sense of sexual propriety can also occur in the early stages.

In the disinhibited type of frontal lobe syndrome, "socially inappropriate actions, such as sexual indiscretions, may be engaged in with little concern for the consequences" (American Psychiatric Association 1987, p. 114). Such behavior might also occur as a result of stroke, although no association of infarct location with particular sexual proclivities has been proven. Hypersexuality has been attributed to ablation of the amygdala (Kupfermann 1991), but infarcts of this area have not been associated with hypersexuality in stroke patients.

Uninhibited sexual behavior can occur in mania. The manic patient typically also exhibits other symptoms of a manic episode, such as euphoria or grandiosity (American Psychiatric Association 1994). Stroke and mania are both common enough conditions that they may coincide with cerebral infarction by chance. When a stroke patient becomes manic, a useful clue to the diagnosis is a previous history of manic episodes, but the onset of mania for the first time in late life is being increasingly recognized (see Chapter 12).

At least one of the cases described by Monga et al. (1986) seemed to have true hypersexuality. Following a stroke with left hemiparesis, this patient began having intercourse three to six times a day, and regarded this as an improvement. Cummings and Mendez (1984) described a 63-year-old patient with a right thalamic infarct who developed increased and socially inappropriate sexual activity with manic behavior. Spontaneous orgasmic sensations have been reported in a patient being treated with fluoxetine for poststroke depression (Morris 1991).

An association has been found between cocaine addiction and risk-taking promiscuity. The original cause-and-effect relationships among poverty, social deprivation, drug addiction, and prostitution may not be clear by the time a cocaine-related stroke has occurred.

What constitutes inappropriate sexual behaviors may be a matter of opinion. There may be an element of ageism in the attitudes of disapproval of sexuality in the elderly patient occasionally seen in younger family members and caregivers. Sometimes hypersexuality may be inappropriate and socially handicapping even in the most liberal of environments.

Management of Aberrant Sexual Behavior

Guidelines for dealing with disapproval of sexual behavior on the part of the stroke patient's family have been offered by McCartney et al. (1987) and Costello-Smith (1991), but flexibility and intuition, perhaps honed by training in psychotherapy, are as important as such rules. Sometimes liberalism and tolerance may be the answer, but it is best not to suggest this bluntly to the family. The ideal approach is to hold a session with several family members, if there are time and staff available for this, during which a family member will bring up the toleration option spontaneously, or can be encouraged to do so. The subject can then be discussed in a nonjudgmental way.

In institutions, something of the same approach can be followed. Although staff members' attitudes about sex will vary, nursing-home employees tend to have very conservative sexual attitudes (Paget 1991), which may lead them to restrict sexual activities that would be acceptable to many people. Opinions based on sincerely held convictions must be respected. Too much emphasis on tolerance may lead to acquiescence in sexual harassment. A female nursing aide who quits her job because of sexual molestation by male patients could be considered a harassment victim.

It is important to establish whether mania is present because of the great efficacy of lithium. Other psychotropic medications suggested to manage sexual hyperactivity include trazodone (Desyrel), propranolol (Inderal), pindolol (Visken), and all of the antipsychotics (Jensen 1989); however, there have been no placebo-controlled trials of the use of these drugs for sexual hyperactivity.

Progestogens and testosterone antagonists such as medroxyprogesterone acetate (Provera) and cyproterone have been advocated to control sexual hyperactivity (Kyomen et al. 1991). Byrne et al. (1992) stated that their experience with using cyproterone in sexually aggressive elderly men was unfavorable because of adverse effects that included muscle atrophy.

Homosexuality and Stroke

Literature about the effects of stroke on sexuality in homosexual patients is sparse. Most of what little has been written concerns patients with accidental brain injury (Mapou 1990).

In some cases, brain damage will cause disinhibition, and an individual previously regarded as heterosexual will come out of the closet. Miller et al. (1986) suggested, on the basis of four cases, that changes in sexual preference are the result of local damage to the limbic system rather than of a nonspecific disinhibiting effect.

In cases of severe brain damage, legal questions may arise about the status of a long-term homosexual companion who regards him- or herself as the patient's spouse and wishes to become guardian. In the *Kowalski* case (Thompson and Adrzejewski 1988), the Minnesota courts initially ruled against the patient's lesbian lover but later reversed this decision. The points raised were that the lover showed greater concern for and interest in the patient than were demonstrated by the patient's spouse, and the patient was subsequently found able to express her own wishes in the matter.

Information Sources

Many resources are available for staff or family members who want more training or information about sexual matters, or direct referrals. These include the Sexual Information and Education Council of the United States (SIECUS); the Sexuality and Disability Training Centers at Boston University Medical Center and the University of Michigan Medical Center; and the American Association of Sex Educators, Counselors, and Therapists (AASECT) (see Appendix B for addresses and telephone numbers of these organizations).

Summary

The emotional effects of stroke, together with such factors as blood pressure medications, diabetes, and vascular disease, may reduce sexual activity. Vascular disease may affect the penile arteries. In vasculogenic impotence, sexual fantasy and desire persist, but there is loss of capacity for erection. Orgasmic capacity is frequently lost in female stroke patients. The fact that most strokes occur in elderly patients affects expectations of sexual function.

Stroke patients should avoid coital positions in which they are on top. Changes in sensation on the affected side should be taken into consideration.

Aberrant sexual behavior may be caused by disinhibition resulting from dementia or by coincidental mania. True hypersexuality from stroke is rare. Management of disinhibited behavior includes involvement of the family and consideration for potential victims.

References

Angeleri F, Angeleri VA, Foschi N, et al: The influence of depression, social activity, and family stress on functional outcome after stroke. Stroke 24:1478–1483, 1993

American Psychiatric Association: Diagnostic and Statistical Manual of Mental Disorders, 3rd Edition, Revised. Washington, DC, American Psychiatric Association, 1987

American Psychiatric Association: Diagnostic and Statistical Manual of Mental Disorders, 4th Edition. Washington, DC, American Psychiatric Association, 1994

Bohlen JG, Heid JP, Sanderson MO, et al: Heart rate, rate-pressure product, and oxygen uptake during four sexual activities. Arch Intern Med 144:1745–1748, 1984

Boldrini P, Basaglia N, Calanc MC: Sexual changes in hemiparetic patients. Arch Phys Med Rehabil 72:202–207, 1991

Bray GP, Defrank R, Wolfe TL: Sexual functioning in stroke survivors. Arch Phys Med Rehabil 62:286–288, 1981

Burgener S, Logan G: Sexuality concerns of the post-stroke patient. Rehabilitation Nursing 178:178–181, 195, 1989

Byrne A, Brunet B, McGann P: Cyproterone acetate therapy and aggression (letter). Br J Psychiatry 160:282–283, 1992

Conine TA, Evans JH: Sexual reactivation of chronically ill and disabled adults. Journal of Adult Health 11:261–270, 1982

Coslett HB, Heilman KM: Male sexual function impairment after right hemisphere stroke. Arch Neurol 43:1036–1039, 1986

Costello-Smith P: The sexual recovery of the stroke patient. Sexual Medicine Today 5:6–11, 1981

Cummings JL, Mendez ME: Secondary mania with focal cerebrovascular lesions. Am J Psychiatry 141:1084–1087, 1984

Diokno AC, Brown MB, Herzog AR: Sexual function in the elderly. Arch Intern Med 150:197–200, 1990

Drugs that cause sexual dysfunction: an update. Medical Letter 34:73–78, 1992

Ducharme S, Gill KM: Sexual values, training, and professional roles. Journal of Head Trauma Rehabilitation 5:38–45, 1990

Ellis K: What to say about sex. RN 49:54–55, 1986

Emick-Herring B: Sexual changes in patients and partners following stroke. Rehabilitation Nursing 10:28–30, 1985

Finelli PF: Coital cerebral hemorrhage. Neurology 43:2683–2685, 1993

Habot B, Rabinowitz H, Friedman JB, et al: Sexual function among male hemiparetic post-CVA patients (letter). J Am Geriatr Soc 37:1003, 1989

Hulter B, Lundberg PO: Sexual function in women with hypothalamo-pituitary disorders. Arch Sex Behav 23:171–183, 1994

Jensen CF: Hypersexual agitation in Alzheimer's disease (letter). J Am Geriatr Soc 37:917, 1989

Kaiser FE, Viosca SP, Morley JE, et al: Impotence and aging: clinical and hormonal factors. J Am Geriatr Soc 36:511–519, 1988

Kupfermann I: Hypothalamus and limbic system, in Principles of Neural Science, 3rd Edition. Edited by Kandel ER, Schwartz JH, Jessell TM. Norwalk, CT, Appleton & Lange, 1991, pp 732–750

Kyomen HK, Nobel KW, Wei J: The use of estrogen to decrease aggressive physical behavior in elderly men with dementia. J Am Geriatr Soc 39:1110–1112, 1991

Mann S, Craig MW, Gould BA, et al: Coital blood pressure in hypertensives: cephalgia, syncope, and the effects of beta-blockade. Br Heart J 47:84–89, 1982

Mapou RJ: Traumatic brain injury rehabilitation with gay and lesbian individuals. Journal of Head Trauma Rehabilitation 5:67–72, 1990

McCartney JR, Izeman H, Rogers D, et al: Sexuality and the institutionalized elderly. J Am Geriatr Soc 35:331–333, 1987

McCormick GP, Riffer DJ, Thompson MM: Coital positioning for stroke afflicted couples. Rehabilitation Nursing 11:17–19, 1986

Miller BL, Cummings JL, McIntyre H, et al: Hypersexuality or altered sexual preference following brain injury. J Neurol Neurosurg Psychiatry 49:867–873, 1986

Mitiguy J: Neurological damage to the anatomical substrate for sexual functioning. Headlines 3:4–5, 1992

Monga TN, Monga M, Mehar S, et al: Hypersexuality in stroke. Arch Phys Med Rehabil 67:415–417, 1986

Morris PL: Fluoxetine and orgasmic sexual experiences. Int J Psychiatry Med 21:379–382, 1991

Muckleroy RN: Sex counselling after stroke. Medical Aspects of Human Sexuality 11:115–116, 1977

Nick J, Bakouche P: Les cephalées déclenchées par l'acte sexuel. Semaine des Hôpitaux (Paris) 56:621–628, 1980

Okura M, Nakayama H, Ikuta T: Sexual intercourse as a precipitating factor of transient global amnesia. Jpn J Psychiatry Neurol 47:13–16, 1993

Paget D: Sex in the nursing home. Contemporary Senior Health 3:22, 1991

Raftos J, Bauer GE, Lewis RG, et al: Clonidine in the treatment of severe hypertension. Med J Aust 1:786–793, 1973

Sjögren K: Sexuality after stroke, II: with special regard to partnership adjustment and to fulfillment. Scand J Rehabil Med 15:63–69, 1983

Sjögren K, Damber EJ, Lilliequest B: Sexuality after stroke with hemiplegia, I: aspects of sexual function. Scand J Rehabil Med 15:55–61, 1983

Thompson K, Adrzejewski J: Why Can't Sharon Kowalski Come Home? San Francisco, CA, Spinsters/Aunt Lute, 1988

Wassertheil-Smoller S, Blaufox MD, Oberman Al: Effect of antihypertensives on sexual function and quality of life. Ann Intern Med 114:613–620, 1991

Weizman A, Weizman R, Hart J, et al: The correlation of increased serum prolactin levels with decreased sexual desire and activity in elderly men. J Am Geriatr Soc 31:485–488, 1983

Zeiss AM, Davies HD, Wood M, et al: The incidence and correlates of erectile problems in patients with Alzheimer's disease. Arch Sex Behav 19:325–331, 1990

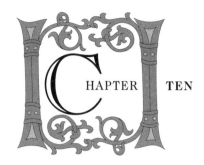

CHAPTER TEN

Apathy and Failure to Rehabilitate

Unmotivated patients who fail to take part in their own rehabilitation are often described as *apathetic*. When used in connection with the rehabilitation and recovery of the stroke patient, the word usually refers as much to the patient's manifest behavior as it does to his or her mood, and covers several clinical entities that have the same end result.

The interaction between the physical and the mental control of movement is especially complex in stroke, because the characteristic paralysis of stroke is upper motor neuron paralysis, which is less complete than lower motor neuron paralysis. In lower motor neuron paralysis, no amount of willpower or effort can make the muscle move, whereas in upper motor neuron paralysis, it remains possible to move the affected part under certain circumstances—for example, strong motivation on the part of the patient. The movement disabilities of upper motor neuron paralysis include weakness, slowness, clumsiness, spasticity, and abnormal movement synergies (Corcos 1991).

The phrase "lack of motivation" usually implies a certain willfulness on the part of the patient, and is slightly pejorative. The patient who seems unmotivated may actually lack capacity, perhaps because of a factor such as confusion or apraxia that is not immediately obvious from physical examination. The patient may be perfectionistic and unwilling to accept the compromise of working toward any goal lower than return to full function. The patient may be pessimistic and unwilling or unable to believe that anything can be done. The patient may have become comfortable at a dependent level and not want to change to more independence (Hesse and Campion 1983).

Among the entities that may cause or mimic apathy are inobvious neurological defects, fatigue, depression, other concurrent mental disorders, concurrent medical disorders, medications, dementia, and social factors fostering dependency. Some authors recognize a *syndrome athymhormique* due to cerebrovascular disease (Habib et al. 1991). It is also possible that apathy is due to a specific localized lesion.

Localization of Brain Lesions Associated With Apathy

Apathy has been attributed to lesions of a specific anatomical area, most commonly the frontal lobes, but also the posterior limb of the internal capsule and parts of the thalamus and caudate nucleus (see Table 10–1).

Self-neglect, or the *Diogenes syndrome,* has been associated with frontal lobe lesions, although not specifically infarcts (Orrell et al. 1989). Neary (1990) gave an anecdotal account of what he called "dementia of frontal lobe type," characterized by reduced initiative; neglect of hygiene and personal responsibilities; and rigid, inflexible behavior. The neuropathology in his cases was spongiform encephalopathy.

Bogousslavsky et al. (1986) found apathy in cases of infarction of the thalamus that had bilaterally affected the ventrolateral and dorsomedial nuclei in the territory supplied by a branch of the posterior communicating artery called the *tuberothalamic artery.* Croisile et al. (1989) referred to their patient—who had damage to the head of the caudate nucleus—as apathetic, although their description is also consistent with obsessive slowness or bradykinesia.

McGilchrist et al. (1993) described a patient with infarcts in the central part of the thalamus, initially in the right hemisphere but later bilateral. The illness began with a transient drowsiness that lasted a day. The patient was subsequently apathetic, sleeping and eating excessively for periods of 3 weeks at a time. These were interspersed with shorter

Table 10–1.   Causes of apathy and failure to rehabilitate in stroke

Cause	Comments
Localized lesions	
Frontal • Diogenes syndrome • Frontal lobe dementia of Neary (1990)	Not reported as resulting from infarcts
Thalamus • Tuberothalamic artery syndrome • Thalamofrontal psychosis of McGilchrist et al. (1993)	Reports of single cases
Caudate • Syndrome athymhormique	Periventricular and caudate rarefactions on MRI
Posterior limb of internal capsule	Statistical correlation with apathy score found by Starkstein et al. (1993)
Inobvious neurological defects	
Sensory defects • Loss of two-point sensory discrimination • Loss of proprioception • Receptive aphasia	Neuropsychological tests may help in making diagnosis
Extrapyramidal disorders • Parkinsonism • Abnormal movements	May be iatrogenic
Cerebellar disorders	Seldom due to infarct, although cerebellar infarcts are frequent
Social factors fostering dependency	
Age Culturally determined expectations Family intervention	
Fatigue	
Sleep changes of aging Tiredness due to stroke	
Concurrent mental disorder	
Depression	May mimic apathy
Dementia	Strongest predictor of failure to rehabilitate
Schizophrenia Personality disorder	So common that chance overlap occurs

(continued)

Table 10–1.   Causes of apathy and failure to rehabilitate in stroke *(continued)*

Cause	Comments
Concurrent medical disorder	
General medical illnesses, especially vascular disease of other systems	
Medications	
Psychotropics	Dementia and aphasia may obscure diagnosis
Antispasmodics with sedative effects	
Anticonvulsants	
Antihypertensives	

periods when he would suddenly become elated, excitable, and sleepless. The authors called this entity "thalamofrontal psychosis."

In the "syndrome athymhormique" described by Habib et al. (1991), a sudden onset of mental changes occurred, with loss of spontaneous activity and initiative, loss of interest in work or recreation, and total flatness of affect. These patients had previous histories of hypertension but were normotensive when examined. They had no focal neurological signs, and were not depressed or demented. Their magnetic resonance imaging (MRI) scans showed multiple rarefactions in the caudate nuclei and periventricular white matter.

Inobvious Neurological Defects

Sensory Defects

Although a hemiplegia is usually obvious, other neurological effects of stroke can be misinterpreted as psychological obstacles to rehabilitation. Disabilities can be caused by loss of proprioception and two-point sensory discriminations, resulting in apraxia; by visual field loss; or by receptive aphasia. These impairments may be difficult for patients to discern and describe, even if they are able to talk and have neither dementia nor depression. If speech disturbance or dementia is present, then the task of identifying the disability can become almost insuperable. No single member of the stroke treatment team can accomplish this task upon one examination.

Testing of sensation is a tedious and difficult process that depends on the patient's ability to cooperate. Such testing is best conducted in a separate session after the patient's degree of paralysis and ability to communicate have been approximately determined. Even if sensation testing cannot be complete, a prediction of probable sensory impairments can be based on the rest of the neurological examination and computed tomography (CT) scan results.

Which neuropsychological tests are performed will depend on the psychologist. The psychologist will normally want to begin by discussing the patient's medical state and neurological condition—especially defects of eyesight and hearing—with the rest of the treatment team. If sensory deficits are deemed likely to interfere with rehabilitation, then parietal function tests (see Table 4–1) will be useful.

Ideally, the results of neurological examination, brain imaging, nurses' observations, and neuropsychological testing will be made available for discussion with the physiotherapists, occupational therapists, recreational therapists, and family caregivers at a team meeting to formulate a treatment plan. Obviously, such an optimal arrangement will not always be achievable under time and financial constraints, but it should remain the goal.

Extrapyramidal System Disorders

Although the concept of the extrapyramidal system as an entity is now questioned by neuroscientists, it remains clinically useful. Damage to this system causes disturbances of movement that may be in the direction of rigidity and slowness or of shaking and jerking.

The corpus striatum and globus pallidus receive input from the sensory cortex, the substantia nigra, and the subthalamic nucleus (*corpus luysii*), and project to the ventrolateral nucleus of the thalamus, from which output goes to the motor cortex. Although this extensive system is hypothetically vulnerable to damage by strategically located infarcts, such infarcts do not often occur. The use of medications and the presence of comorbid degenerative neurological diseases are more common causes of extrapyramidal symptoms than are actual infarcts in this region.

Parkinsonism.   Parkinsonism can complicate diagnosis in stroke because its presentations can mimic those of psychiatric conditions. The clinician should keep in mind that a patient's symptoms might be attributable to parkinsonism, a treatable disorder. The typical manifestations include drooling, slow tremor, and a cogwheel type of rigidity. Parkinsonian patients are often inactive and silent, and they can be misdiagnosed as demented, depressed, or catatonic (McKenna et al. 1991).

Parkinsonism due to primary disease of the substantia nigra is called *idiopathic* Parkinson's disease, or simply Parkinson's disease. It is common in elderly individuals, so that it often happens by coincidence that a patient with Parkinson's disease suffers a stroke.

Drug-induced parkinsonism is common in institutional settings. Dopamine-blocking drugs are used in hospitals as nonspecific sedatives for disturbed or noisy patients, as well as for patients with nausea or esophageal reflux. They include the antipsychotic drugs and prochlorperazine (Compazine) and metoclopramide (Reglan).

An entity of "arteriosclerotic parkinsonism" is recognized by some authors but disputed by others. Unilateral parkinsonism is sometimes seen with infarcts in the corpus striatum but is not common in relation to the frequency of infarcts of this area.

Abnormal movements.   Classification of abnormal movements, which are varied in kind, is often easier in theory than in practice. Even the distinction between what is psychogenic and what is due to structural brain disease is not sharp. Many movement disorders of undisputed organic cause will vary with the patient's mental state.

Clinicians tend to be more convinced of an organic origin, and to look more carefully for it, when abnormal movements are unilateral rather than bilateral. In cases of hemiballismus, the flailing movements of one side of the body are attributed to vascular damage to the subthalamic nucleus. Probably the movements are produced by the influence of the globus pallidus, which normally receives inhibitory input from the subthalamic nucleus. In some cases, the patient has been unaware of these movements (Lazzarino and Nicolai 1991). Ballismus, in which the movements affect both sides of the body, is more likely to be construed as psychogenic.

Tardive dyskinesia is unlikely to be caused directly by stroke, but enters into the differential diagnosis of abnormal movements in any patient who has received dopamine-blocking drugs. Although this condition typically consists of lip and tongue movements, the movements may be more widespread and disabling. The risk of tardive dyskinesia is increased in elderly patients with any kind of brain damage.

Unclassifiable abnormal movements are frequently seen in elderly patients with dementia and in patients with chronic schizophrenia. The relationship of such movements to previously administered drugs or to infarcts found on CT scan can remain questionable.

Cerebellar Disorders

Although small cerebellar infarcts are commonly found at autopsy, the classical cerebellar signs are seldom seen in isolation in long-term stroke survivors. These signs include intention tremor and other movement disturbances, such as a reeling, unsteady gait. It may be that such symptoms are overwhelmed in the clinical examination by the other disorders of movement and gait resulting from stroke. The high death rate in the acute stage of severe cerebellar infarction may also reduce the number of stroke survivors with purely cerebellar signs.

The onset of cerebellar signs in a stroke patient is often attributable to a medication that is being used for treatment of seizures or anxiety. Dilantin (phenytoin) and benzodiazepines are among the most common of these.

Social Factors Fostering Dependency

Assessing whether elderly patients have resumed normal social roles can be difficult, because such roles are less clearly defined in later life. With retirement from work and the independence of children, the goals of rehabilitation—and of life itself—become less clear. Some psychotherapists, therefore, believe that a task of therapy should be to assist in this definition.

Dacher (1989) drew on the theories of Erik Erikson to suggest ways of motivating the elderly stroke patient to adopt a new set of age-appropriate goals. Erikson posited eight ages of man, with goals to be achieved at each stage, the last being the attainment of integrity and wisdom. Despite being intuitively rather than experimentally based, Erikson's work has been validated to some extent by authors, such as Vaillant (1977), who have been able to demarcate stages in the life cycle of the adult with characteristic motives and goals. Erikson's psychology offers inspiration rather than concrete guidelines on how to treat a stroke patient. Pintoff (1992) speaks positively of his experience with an Eriksonian therapist after his stroke:

> Frolich, a disciple of Erik Erikson, simply laid out four points that he thought I should consider: 1) slow down, 2) let go, 3) review life, and 4) transmit wisdom. At first I didn't grasp the meaning or the significance, but the gist felt good to me and I weighed that philosophy as a basis for living. Most significantly, it started me on a new way of thinking: principally, evaluating life at the moment. (p. 132)

Social factors explain why the ability to carry out an activity under prompting and supervision in rehabilitation does not always carry over to the home setting. The findings of Andrews and Stewart (1979) suggest that it is important to demonstrate a patient's capabilities to his or her family. These authors found a difference between what stroke patients could do in a day hospital and what they actually did at home. Although confused and aphasic patients were excluded from their study, they found that "in 52% of cases the chief carer claimed that the patient did not do two or more activities at home which the patient was capable of doing in the day hospital. This was not related to the features of the stroke but more to the attitude of the patient and his chief carer" (Andrews and Stewart 1979, p. 43). One-sixth of those patients who could wash, bathe, and use the toilet by themselves in the day hospital did not do so at home. In some cases, this lack of carryover was because the patient was apathetic or withdrawn; in others, it was because of a negative attitude of the chief caregiver at home. In still other instances, the patient would ask for help and the caregiver felt unable to refuse. A major problem was lack of communication: most of the chief caregivers were unaware of what the patient had been achieving in the day hospital and thus did not expect improvement.

Because it is not socially acceptable to admit to taking pleasure in being an invalid, most people would not tell us if they enjoyed being dependent (Rusin 1990), but the possibility exists that they do. Older patients who accept their impairments with equanimity and complacency may be less emotionally distressed—but also less motivated to engage in rehabilitation.

Fatigue

Sleep Changes of Aging

The changes that occur in sleep with aging include increased daytime napping and more frequent nighttime waking, with a tendency to spend more time in bed. Total sleep time at night is reduced, although this may be compensated for by the daytime naps. The proportion of sleep time spent in the lightest kind of sleep (stage 1 sleep) increases. The deeper kinds of sleep (stages 3 and 4) decrease both absolutely and as a proportion of total sleep time. The amount of rapid eye movement (REM) sleep decreases absolutely but remains the same as a proportion of total sleep. Health care providers should be tolerant of the changes in sleep patterns that come with age, and should know about the different sleep stages and the significance of REM sleep.

Tiredness Due to Stroke

There is persuasive evidence that stroke has a direct effect in causing fatigue. Some authors (Kuhlmey 1989) accept the existence of an entity of *chronische pseudoneurasthenitische Syndrom* in organic brain damage. (The term *neurasthenia* has disappeared from DSM-IV [American Psychiatric Association 1994] but is allowed in the ICD-10 [World Health Organization 1992].) Feelings of tiredness are common in the first year after a stroke, but tend to diminish thereafter (Åström et al. 1992).

Smithells (1978), in his first-person account, related that "one general reaction was a perpetual state of drowsiness and ennui, so that if I took my usual postprandial sleep, it was apt to go on for too long. I used an alarm to control this tendency. After a sleep I was very slow to pick up in vitality of perception and action and would stumble around in an uncoordinated fashion, blundering hither and thither" (p. 397).

Concurrent Mental Disorder

Depression

Although it seems intuitively plausible that depression would adversely affect rehabilitation, proving this is difficult, because rating scales for depression contain objective behavioral items that can be influenced by apathy or physical impairment (Marin et al. 1993). If other negative emotions are present, such as anger or fear, the difficulty is increased. Kotila et al. (1984) found that negative emotions other than depression had the greatest adverse effect on prognosis.

Studies showing that depression is a major factor in failure to rehabilitate from stroke include those of Parikh et al. (1990) and Morris et al. (1992). Parikh et al. compared two groups of clinic outpatients who had suffered strokes—one with depressed subjects and the other with nondepressed subjects. Although the two groups had not differed significantly in their degree of functional impairment in the hospital, at 2-year follow-up, the depressed group was significantly more impaired than the nondepressed group in both physical activities and language function. The disparity in recovery between the initially depressed and nondepressed patients could not be explained by differences in demographic or neurological characteristics, frequency of use of rehabilitative services, cognitive impairment, social function, presence of aphasia, or size or location of the lesion. Lamhut (1991) criticized this study on the grounds that the patients in it were able to return to an outpatient clinic, and half of them had no visible lesions on CT scan.

Cognitive Impairment

Cognitive impairment strongly reduces the prospects for recovery of mobility in stroke. This reduction is independent of age and aphasia (Maehlum et al. 1990) and is produced by even moderate dementia. Moderately demented patients display a range of emotions, and may be euphoric or angry or sad rather than apathetic. In the more advanced stages of dementia, the expression of emotion weakens, but it is unusual for the acute stroke to cause dementia severe enough to cause true emotional apathy.

Other Mental Illness

Even aside from depression, dementia, and cocaine use, the chances of finding mental disorder in a stroke patient are high, simply by coincidence. At any given time, for example, more than 1 million Americans will have schizophrenia. The diagnosis may not be obvious against a background of disability and aphasia. The best clue comes from previous history, and it is important that hospital charts contain adequate background on psychiatric history. This can be difficult in large hospitals where people come in off the street. One-third of homeless people have histories of symptoms such as delusions and hallucinations, and a quarter of them were previously mental hospital patients (Jencks 1994) so that the proportion with schizophrenia is probably high. Previous emergency room records can often help.

Negativism is sometimes a feature of schizophrenia, and some patients may appear apathetic. As Bleuler (1911/1950) pointed out, however, "the large number of schizophrenics who show considerable activity (pseudo-authors, world reformers, workers in hospitals) contradicts this generalizing description" (p. 381).

Personality Disorders

The status of personality disorders as disease entities has often been questioned. DSM-III-R (American Psychiatric Association 1987) classified them as Axis II diagnoses, implying that they were long-standing attributes rather than disease. Patients with types of personality disorders such as the dependent, the avoidant, and the passive-aggressive might be expected not to respond well to rehabilitation, but it is seldom possible to know enough about the premorbid personality of a stroke patient to fit him or her into one of these categories. The assessment of personality remains largely intuitive and descriptive, which does not necessarily mean that it is invalid. A picture of strengths and weaknesses of character builds up gradually from frequent contact with the patient, family, and caregivers.

> A depressed woman recently came to my office, driven by her 78-year-old male friend who had had a stroke with left hemiplegia 6 months earlier. This man was also under treatment for congestive heart failure and cancer of the tongue, and was working at two jobs.

The positive traits that enable people with such character strengths to go on functioning have been studied far less than negative traits. It may be that these qualities are attributes of personality that can be reduced to quantifiable psychological measures, but at present we can only use such unscientific words as *morale* and *spirit* to describe them.

Concurrent Medical Disorder

Medical disorders can be misinterpreted as psychological apathy in stroke for several reasons. Speech disorders and dementia hinder recognition of symptoms of medical illnesses, even when the symptoms are typical. In elderly patients, the symptoms are often not typical. The first sign of pneumonia may be that the patient "looks ill," and the first symptom of congestive heart failure may be fatigue. Stroke is associated with arterial disease, which affects the heart; with swallowing difficulties, which can cause pneumonia; with diabetes; with renal failure; and with many other medical conditions.

Medications

The medication order sheet should be reviewed when a stroke patient is apathetic. Including the pharmacist in the treatment team may be helpful. A large number of potentially sedative medications may be given to stroke patients. Psychotropic medications are given for agitation, and hypnotics are given for insomnia; benzodiazepines are given for spasticity; phenobarbital is given for seizures; propranolol (Inderal) is given for hypertension.

If a drug is suspected of producing oversedation, an alternative nonsedative drug with the same action can often be substituted. If the sedating drug is unique and indispensable, however, the time of administration can sometimes be arranged so that alertness is not impaired during rehabilitation activities.

Management of Apathy

In most cases, the diagnosis of the cause will suggest the treatment. The search for a cause need not be limited to the conditions discussed in this chapter. Valuable clues may come from conversations with the family, caregivers, and the patient (in any communication modality). If there is no treatable cause, then the goal of treatment may have to be adjusted downward. In addition, because some units and some therapists simply "do better" with some patients than others, a change may be beneficial and need not reflect poorly on the original treatment team.

One young hemiplegic patient spent many months in an excellent stroke unit in a well-known rehabilitation hospital. He was rebellious and resented the staff as authority figures. No progress was made, and no funds were available for further treatment on the stroke unit. He was transferred to a nursing home, where he was horrified to find himself among elderly long-term patients. He made vigorous efforts at rehabilitation and walked out a few weeks later.

Indeed, the interaction between the physical and the mental is especially close in stroke rehabilitation. The handicap caused by stroke is physical in origin but remains influenced by an entity—baffling to neuroscientists, philosophers, and psychologists—called willpower.

Summary

Upper motor neuron paralysis is less complete than lower motor neuron paralysis, and return of mobility can be influenced by motivation. It is possible that certain lesions in the frontal lobe, caudate nucleus, and thalamus specifically cause apathy. Entities that may cause or mimic apathy include inobvious neurological defects, fatigue, depression, other concurrent mental disorder, concurrent medical disorder, medications, dementia, and social factors fostering dependency. Inobvious neurological defects include apraxia, receptive aphasia, loss of proprioception, lack of two-point sensory discriminations, visual field loss, parkinsonism, abnormal movements, and cerebellar disorders. Cognitive impairment hinders stroke recovery. It can be hard to determine whether or not older patients have resumed normal social roles, because social roles are less clearly defined in later life. Demonstrating the patient's capabilities acquired in a rehabilitation setting to the family is important to ensure transfer of gain from hospital to home. Young patients are often intolerant of rehabilitation procedures that they do not perceive as immediately leading to desired objectives. Health care providers should be aware of the changes in sleep patterns that come with age. A direct effect of stroke is fatigue. Medical disorders can be misinterpreted as psychological apathy in stroke. Potentially sedative medications given to stroke patients include psychotropics, hypnotics, benzodiazepines, anticonvulsants, and beta-blockers. Valuable clues to the cause of symptoms of apathy may come from conversations with the family or caregivers.

References

American Psychiatric Association: Diagnostic and Statistical Manual of Mental Disorders, 3rd Edition, Revised. Washington, DC, American Psychiatric Association, 1987

American Psychiatric Association: Diagnostic and Statistical Manual of Mental Disorders, 4th Edition. Washington, DC, American Psychiatric Association, 1994

Andrews K, Stewart J: Stroke recovery: he can but does he? Rheumatology and Rehabilitation 18:43–48, 1979

Åström M, Asplund K, Åström T: Psychosocial function and life satisfaction after stroke. Stroke 23:527–531, 1992

Bleuler E: Dementia praecox, oder Die Gruppe der Schizophrenien (1911). Translated by Zinkin J as *Dementia Praecox, or the Group of Schizophrenias*. New York, International Universities Press, 1950

Bogousslavsky J, Regli F, Assal G: The syndrome of unilateral tuberothalamic artery territory infarction. Stroke 17:434–441, 1986

Corcos D: Strategies underlying the control of disordered movement. Physical Therapy 71:25–38, 1991

Croisile B, Tourniaire D, Confavreux C, et al: Bilateral damage to the head of the caudate nucleus. Ann Neurol 25:313–314, 1989

Dacher JE: Rehabilitation and the geriatric patient. Nurs Clin North Am 24:225–237, 1989

Habib M, Royere ML, Habib G, et al: Modifications de la personnalité et hypertension arterielle. Le "syndrome athymhormique." Arch Mal Coeur Vaiss 84:1225–1230, 1991

Hesse KA, Campion EW: Motivating the geriatric patient for rehabilitation. J Am Geriatr Soc 31:586–589, 1983

Jencks C: The Homeless. Cambridge, MA, Harvard University Press, 1994

Kotila M, Waltimo O, Niemi M-L, et al: The profile of recovery from stroke and factors influencing outcome. Stroke 15:1039–1044, 1984

Kuhlmey J: Wie homogen sind klinische Stichproben? Zeitschrift für Alternsforschung 44:363–366, 1989

Lamhut P: Influence of poststroke depression on recovery from functional impairment. Geriatric Medicine Currents 12:1, 1991

Lazzarino LG, Nicolai A: Hemichorea-hemiballismus and anosognosia following a contralateral infarction of the caudate nucleus and anterior limb of the internal capsule. Nuova Rivista de Neurologia 61:9–11, 1991

Maehlum S, Roaldsen K, Kolrud M, et al: Rehabiliterung etter hjerneschlag. Tidskrift for den Norske Laegeforening 110:2657–2659, 1990

Marin RS, Firinciogullari S, Biedrzycki RC: The sources of convergence between measures of apathy and depression. J Affect Disord 28:117–124, 1993

McGilchrist I, Goldstein LH, Jadresic D, et al: Thalamo-frontal psychosis. Br J Psychiatry 163:113–115, 1993

McKenna PJ, Lund CE, Mortimer AM, et al: Motor volitional and behavioral disorders in schizophrenia. Br J Psychiatry 158:328–336, 1991

Morris PL, Raphael B, Robinson RG: Clinical depression is associated with impaired recovery from stroke. Med J Aust 157:239–242, 1992

Neary D: Dementia of frontal lobe type. J Am Geriatr Soc 38:71–72, 1990

Orrell MW, Sahakian BJ, Bergmann K: Self-neglect and frontal lobe dysfunction. Br J Psychiatry 155:101–105, 1989

Parikh RM, Robinson RG, Lipsey JR, et al: The impact of poststroke depression on recovery in activities of daily living over a 2-year follow-up. Arch Neurol 47:785–789, 1990

Pintoff E: Bolt From the Blue. Salt Lake City, UT, Northwest, 1992

Rusin MJ: Stroke rehabilitation: a geropsychological perspective. Arch Phys Med Rehabil 71:914–922, 1990

Smithells P: A personal account by a sufferer from stroke. N Z Med J 87:396–397, 1978

Starkstein SE, Fedoroff JP, Price TR, et al: Apathy following cerebrovascular lesions. Stroke 24:1625–1630, 1993

Vaillant GE: Adaptation to Life. Boston, MA, Little, Brown, 1977

World Health Organization: International Statistical Classification of Diseases and Related Health Problems, 10th Revision. Geneva, Switzerland, World Health Organization, 1992

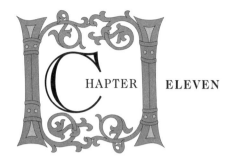

CHAPTER ELEVEN

Anger and Violence

Definitions and Incidence

Outbursts of apparent anger are common in stroke, and violence is not rare. Aggression ranks after depression and memory loss among mental changes causing concern to caregivers (Hanger and Mulley 1993). Isaacs et al. (1976) found that among 35 stroke patients they studied, 3 showed the pattern they termed "aggression," with verbal and sometimes physical hostility, usually directed against the patient's spouse. The "frustration" pattern—characterized by excessive irritability or reluctance to cooperate—was demonstrated by 10 patients.

Mood disturbances in the direction of anger have been less well defined and classified than have anxiety and depression. ICD-10 (World Health Organization 1992) recognizes an organic personality disorder that can be characterized by irritability and outbursts of anger. Yudofsky et al. (1990) proposed the term *organic aggressive syndrome,* but this was not officially adopted in DSM-IV (American Psychiatric Association 1994), which does not include organic disorders as a separate entity. Western psychiatry tends to look at mood disorders in terms of a happiness–unhappiness spectrum—unlike, for example, traditional Chinese medicine (Lee 1992). Patients are often unable to describe angry feelings.

The nuances of antipathy, irritation, hostility, bitterness, frustration, rage, and hatred may be elusive even in the most articulate patients, and even more so in patients with dementia or aphasia.

A mood disturbance typical of stroke (although also seen in multiple sclerosis and motor neuron disease) is *emotional incontinence,* which manifests as a tendency to cry at the least provocation (see Chapter 12). Many patients with this condition find it quite embarrassing, and must continually explain to others that the crying represents not necessarily sadness, but rather an inability to control their emotions. It may be that a slight cause for irritation, therefore, results in an outburst in the stroke patient that is wrongly interpreted as anger. The first-person accounts describe different versions of the emotional state, suggesting that even stroke patients themselves cannot always determine whether their mood was truly angry.

Stocklin (1989) recalled becoming enraged with a much-loved sister-in-law who tried to explain to her that her (Stocklin's) husband had died. Although at the time the rage felt justifiable, Stocklin realized later that it was unwarranted. Anger in stroke could be explained as a reaction to the situation of being ill. Acutely injured young quadriplegic and paraplegic patients may rage against the world, feeling surges of envy and hostility toward those who can get up and walk. In some cases, anger appears to be caused by frustration, as when a stroke patient struggles with a difficult task and gives up in despair.

Goldstein's Catastrophic Reaction

Goldstein (1952) described a phenomenon he termed the *catastrophic reaction:*

> When a patient is not able to fulfill a task set before him, this condition is a frequent occurrence. A patient may look animated, calm, in a good mood, well-poised, collected and cooperative when he is confronted with tasks he can fulfill; the same patient may appear dazed, become agitated, change color, start to fumble, become unfriendly, evasive, and even aggressive when he is not able to fulfill the task. His overt behavior appears very much the same as a person in a state of anxiety. . . . In the catastrophic condition, the patient not only is incapable of performing a task which exceeds his impaired capacity, but he also fails, for a longer or shorter period, in performances which he is able to carry out in the ordered state. For a varying period of time the organism's reactions are in great disorder or are impeded altogether. (p. 247)

Goldstein's catastrophic reaction has been studied experimentally by Gainotti (1970), who presented brain-damaged patients with progressively more difficult tests and observed their reactions at the point of failure. In patients with left-hemisphere damage, there were outbursts of tears, anger toward the examiner, and abandonment of or refusal to continue the task. In those with right-hemisphere damage, reactions tended toward indifference, anosognosia, and joking (e.g., blaming the limb for being paralyzed). Petty et al. (1996) described a patient with bilateral caudate infarctions but no paralysis for whom minor frustrations repeatedly precipitated catastrophic rage reactions. During these episodes, the patient became violent, aggressive, and dangerous.

Agitated Behaviors

Annoying behavior on the part of the patient with dementia or aphasia is often described as "agitation," although those who use this term find it difficult to define. The word is more frequently used by health care professionals than by family members, and implies increased motor activity of some kind, together with a negative mood—anger, irritation, fear, and/or despair. Scales of severity of agitation have been constructed that can be useful in assessing treatment efficacy (Cohen-Mansfield 1989; Rosen et al. 1994).

The troublesome behaviors of noncommunicating patients can take a variety of forms. Some of these suggest disinhibition, as further discussed in Chapter 12. Among such behaviors noted by Zimmer et al. (1984) in nursing-home residents were spitting out medication, refusing to eat, lying on the floor, throwing food or objects, unfastening others' restraints, engaging in dangerous smoking habits, removing catheters, taking others' belongings, urinating in wastepaper baskets, smearing feces, masturbating publicly, and hoarding objects. Although many of these behaviors are not truly aggressive, violent, or based on anger (Cohen-Mansfield 1986), caregivers may find them quite difficult to deal with.

Causes

Location of Infarct

The severity of the patient's motor disability and aphasia will obviously affect the way anger is physically expressed. Apart from this indirect effect of lesion location, several areas of the brain have been proposed as ones in which damage actually causes aggression. These sites include the amygdala, hypothalamus, cingulum, temporal lobes, and frontal lobes (Patel and Hope 1993). Evidence for involvement of the frontal lobe, the temporal lobes, and the hypothalamus has come, respectively, from clinical syndromes seen after injury, observation in seizure disorders, and animal studies.

ICD-10 (World Health Organization 1992) states that although the frontal lobe syndrome may be associated with aggression, "it is now known that this syndrome occurs not only with frontal lobe lesions but also with lesions to other circumscribed areas of the brain" (p. 66).

Several reasons have been suggested for linking the limbic system with the expression of emotions, aggression in particular. One of these has been the association of damage to the temporal lobe with seizures involving violence. Although recent changes in the terminology of epilepsy complicate summarization of the earlier literature on this disorder, it is widely accepted that epilepsy associated with temporal lobe damage is the type most likely to involve aggression (Herzberg and Fenwick 1988). This form of epilepsy is also associated with psychosis (Flor-Henry 1969).

Epilepsy of temporal lobe origin can be of the type often referred to as *psychomotor*, in which the seizure can take the form of complex actions rather than uncoordinated movements, and these actions can be violent. Several mechanisms linking the limbic system with these clinically observed phenomena have been postulated. Devinsky and Bear (1984) proposed that limbic system activity affects the hypothalamus, causing a general deepening of affects and raising the probability of aggressive responses to a variety of environmental stimuli. There is, however, no documented connection between poststroke seizures and violence.

Tonkonogy (1991) compared violent and nonviolent institutionalized patients with evidence of organic brain disease. He found a predominance of lesions in the area of the amygdala in the right anterior inferior temporal lobe in the violent patients. He hypothesized that these patients' violence was due to damage to the amygdala, and that under normal conditions, the amygdala in one hemisphere inhibits the development of aggression-producing brain activity patterns in other parts of the limbic system or in the amygdala of the opposite hemisphere (Figure 11–1). None of the patients with these lesions had definite infarcts. The violent patients who had infarcts had them in various other locations.

Early animal experiments in which the hypothalamus was surgically separated from the rest of the brain produced a condition in which "sham rage" could be elicited by slight stimulation (Bard 1928). Such separation of the hypothalamus has not been shown to occur in stroke, and the relevance of these experiments on the hypothalamus to human aggression is now doubted (Eichelman 1992).

Medina et al. (1974) described a patient who had recovered function after having a left hemiplegia and was "very quiet, stable, and kind," but became suddenly violent, with swearing, biting, and spitting. This patient remained thereafter in a state of agitated delirium, subject to violent bursts of rage provoked by being touched or being asked simple questions. At autopsy, one cerebral infarct was found in the right hemisphere, presumably accounting for the original left hemiplegia, and one in the left hemisphere. The left-hemisphere infarct involved the hippocampus, parahippocampus, and lingual and fusiform gyri. On the basis of this case and 12 previous reports from the literature, Medina and colleagues suggested that a condition of agitated delirium with outbursts of rage can be caused by lesions in two different locations: 1) the cingulate gyrus and orbital areas, and 2) the hippocampus, parahippocampus, and fusiform and lingual gyri.

Neurotransmitter Function

Several neurotransmitters have been implicated in aggressive behavior. Reductions in gamma-aminobutyric acid (GABA) and increases in ace-

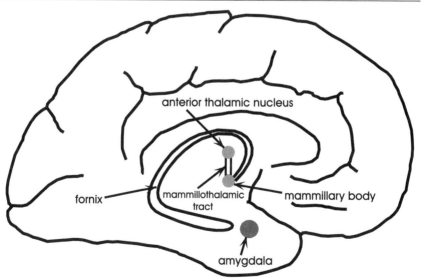

Figure 11–1.   Amygdala in relation to the structures of the limbic system.

tylcholine and catecholamines have been linked to violence in dementia patients (Patel and Hope 1993). Men with histories of aggression have been found to have reduced levels of 5-hydroxyindoleacetic acid (5-HIAA), a serotonin metabolite found in the cerebrospinal fluid (Brown et al. 1982).

A strategically located infarct could hypothetically disrupt pathways from the sites of serotonin production in the raphe nuclei (see Figure A–23 in Appendix A) to the limbic system; however, this mechanism has not been proven as the etiology of violence in stroke patients.

Treatment Environment

Appropriate placement within the spectrum of care is an important factor in preventing violence. The behaviorally disturbed stroke patient is especially vulnerable to errors made in the decision to place him or her in a psychiatric facility, a nursing home, an acute-care medical unit, or even prison. A patient who wanders around tugging at other patients' intravenous lines or oxygen tubes may be dangerous in an intensive care unit but manageable on a psychiatric ward.

Sometimes an individual without any obvious stroke or psychiatric disorder who commits a crime will subsequently be found to have a cerebral infarct. The infarct may be coincidental, but the presence of an organic brain lesion constitutes very convincing evidence to judges, lawyers, and police officers that any criminal behavior engaged in by such a person is due to brain damage and should be dealt with by physicians. Health care facilities thus end up dealing with violent, antisocial individuals who might otherwise be in jail.

The existence of a cerebral infarct is sometimes used by psychiatric facilities as a reason for not accepting a patient, and the presence of mental disorder is similarly cited by general hospitals as a reason for refusing admission. Such restrictive admissions policies can have tragic consequences:

> A patient who had previously had a stroke threatened to kill his wife and was taken to a veterans' hospital for psychiatric admission. He was refused on the grounds that stroke was not a mental disorder. The medical service likewise refused to admit him because he had no acute medical problem. When finally the patient was sent to a nursing home, he walked out, went home, and murdered his wife.

Dementia and Delirium

Cognitive impairment is often associated with violence. On standardized ward-behavior rating scales (e.g., the Brief Psychiatric Rating Scale [BPRS; Overall and Gorham 1962], the Nurses' Observation Scale for Inpatient Evaluation [NOSIE; Honigfeld et al. 1966]), patients with dementia score higher for aggression than do those with nonorganic psychiatric disorders. Acute confusional states or delirium are especially likely to be associated with increased motor activity, which can range from aimless thrashing about to assault on imagined assailants based on delusions or hallucinations.

Episodes of violence in patients with dementia or delirium tend to be brief, without a sustained attack on one person, which limits their damage. Although the likelihood of physical damage is further limited because patients with dementia are often old and relatively weak, the feebleness of their attacks may be counterbalanced by the vulnerability of those who constitute their potential targets—for instance, such patients commonly reside in institutions in which the other residents are also feeble and cannot defend themselves, or live at home with an equally elderly spouse.

A certain amount of what is described as "personality change" in stroke patients is really mild cognitive impairment and corresponding poor judgment. In such patients, the ability to think rationally about a mild irritation, to remember the events leading up to an apparent provocation, or to calculate the consequences of an outburst of temper is impaired, and thus mountains are readily made out of molehills.

Territoriality is at the root of much of the violent behavior manifested by patients with dementia. Ethologists and biosocial philosophers such as Konrad Lorenz (1963/1966) have constructed wide-ranging theories associating territorial defense with evolution. Empty space around the patient provides the most effective protection, especially if his or her mobility is limited. A behavior commonly seen in dementia patients is pushing or punching at anyone who gets too near. In institutions and hospitals, a roommate is a frequent target of such behavior, and sometimes attacks on roommates are accompanied by delusions such as accusations of stealing.

Nonviolent antisocial behaviors can lead to violence by a process of *escalation,* especially in institutions. Some patients with dementia paw and maul at passersby or intrude on the space of others and thus seem to provoke violence. Repetitious shouters may get punched by those they offend; obscenities and ethnic slurs are especially likely to provoke such responses. Quite often, violence occurs as a result of staff members' interventions to prevent a nonviolent offensive behavior.

The phenomenon of *resistance to care* has much in common with escalation. The patient is calm unless touched or moved, such as during washing or changing, at which point he or she launches into punching, kicking, biting, and scratching.

Drugs

Alcohol and cocaine are commonly associated with violence, and both of these may be related to stroke. Some anxiolytic drugs can have a paradoxical effect in the same way that alcohol can; thus, they may cause belligerence at a low dose even though they are sedative at high doses.

Management of Anger and Violence

Medication

The use of drugs to control violent behavior often is, as Lion (1991) pointed out, basically empirical, even if theoretically linked to a concept of behavior as a manifestation of psychosis, epilepsy, mood disorder, or attention-deficit disorder.

Antipsychotic drugs.   Antipsychotic medications are often administered to agitated patients with organic brain conditions (Barnes et al. 1982). A meta-analysis of trials of these drugs in dementia patients revealed that agitation and uncooperativeness tended to improve in most studies, and combativeness, assaultiveness, and hostility were diminished in several double-blind, placebo-controlled trials (Schneider et al. 1990). The patient with violent catastrophic reactions whom Petty et al. (1996) described responded to short-term haloperidol followed by carbamazepine.

The fact that many of the side effects of the antipsychotics are neurological and cardiovascular places limitations on their use in stroke patients; however, experience with these medications has been extensive and their popularity is not unearned.

Trazodone.   Trazodone (Desyrel) is one of several antidepressant medications that inhibit the reuptake of serotonin. Compared with other serotonergic antidepressants, it has a more sedating effect. This combination of properties has led to trazodone's consideration as a drug for managing aggression.

Houlihan et al. (1994) reviewed existing studies on the use of trazodone in dementia and carried out an open trial. They found that the drug produced general behavior improvement in dementia patients but had no specific effect on hostility. Three of their 22 subjects had multi-infarct dementia. Improvement, both in this trial and in that of Pinner and Rich (1988), took several weeks.

Buspirone.   Buspirone (BuSpar) has been shown in animal studies to reduce aggression and to have serotonergic properties. On the basis of these observations, Herrmann and Eryavec (1993) used the drug in 16 psychogeriatric patients with agitation and depression that had not responded to previous treatment. Six of these patients were diagnosed as having multi-infarct dementia; one of these six improved.

Carbamazepine.   The efficacy of carbamazepine (Tegretol) in mania and in episodic violence associated with complex seizures has led to consideration of its use in other forms of violence (Patterson 1987). This drug may also have serotonergic properties, although its primary action on nerve cells is at the voltage-gated sodium channels (see Chapter 5). Carbamazepine's side effects include production of blood, liver, and cardiac abnormalities, as well as dizziness and ataxia.

Marin and Greenwald (1989) suggested that carbamazepine might be particularly useful for dementia patients who resist care. One of the three patients they described had multi-infarct dementia. This man punched, pushed, and otherwise resisted whenever caregivers tried to attend to his needs. His symptoms were unresponsive to trials of haloperidol (Haldol) and lorazepam (Ativan); however, carbamazepine eradicated his symptoms within 10 days.

Emergency sedation.   All emergency psychiatric sedation carries a certain risk, and in the stroke patient this risk is frequently magnified by the presence of cardiovascular disease. Short-acting benzodiazepines such as lorazepam (Ativan) are often used for emergency sedation and can be given either by mouth or by intramuscular or intravenous injection. A phenothiazine or haloperidol is also commonly used, but there is a delay in their onset of action. Intravenous medication produces immediate sedation, and the patient must be kept under close supervision and monitored in a setting where resuscitation is available. This need for close supervision also exists after heavy doses of oral or intramuscular medication. Because the sedation is delayed, the need for supervision may not be immediately obvious to the person giving the medication. Sometimes violent patients who have been given intramuscular medications are then put into seclusion or transported in police care, and this can be dangerous for the patient.

The use of drugs in emergency situations in the home demands special consideration. Family members cannot give injections and are nervous about varying the dose of oral psychotropic medication. If the patient is already established on an antipsychotic or benzodiazepine drug, its dosage can usually be safely increased in increments, depending on the half-life of the drug (Benet and Sheiner 1985). Families often seek telephone advice about dosage changes and the possible adverse effects of psychotropic drugs, and they are sometimes able to manage the patient at home if given reassurance about these issues.

Omnibus Budget Reconciliation Act of 1987 (OBRA '87) regulations. There have been frequent complaints in the past of overmedication of disturbed patients in nursing homes. As a result, nursing homes now operate under stringent federal regulations concerning the use of sedative or psychotropic drugs. Such medications cannot be used simply to control agitated patients but only to treat certain specific conditions, which must be fully documented; they also cannot be ordered "prn." In effect (although the law does not specifically say this), approval for administration of sedative or psychotropic medication requires a psychiatric consultation.

Mental Health Consultation

A mental health professional who is experienced in handling both brain-damaged and elderly patients should be available for consultation. It is helpful if that individual works as an integral member of the stroke treatment team, but the exigencies of time and money do not always permit this. Commonly, he or she must come in as a consultant on particular cases for particular problems. Such a consultation is virtually mandatory if sedative or antipsychotic drugs are to be given, although the consultation should not necessarily be limited to psychopharmacology.

Sometimes a specialist asked to consult on a case of violence will find that the caregivers are already doing all that can be done for the patient. For example, the patient may be institutionalized at the appropriate level of care, be taking the right medication, and be causing no immediate danger but may have a history of violence. The primary caregivers are willing to go on looking after the patient as they have been doing, but they want reassurance and documentation that they are doing everything they can do. In such cases, that documentation should be given. The provision of reassurance may need to include discussions to find out who is frightened of what, explorations of the interpersonal relationships between the various caregivers and between the caregivers and the patient, and expressions of appreciation of the value of the work being accomplished.

Placement of Patients Who Become Angry or Violent

The decision about where a patient can best be managed is often the most important one. Behaviors that may be dangerous on a medical unit can sometimes be easily managed in a mental hospital. However, staff members in such institutions may not feel equipped to handle medical conditions, and the patient's family may be resistant to the patient's transfer to a mental hospital. A psychiatric unit in a general hospital is often the best place for a stroke patient (see Chapter 20).

Within an institution, there should be space—a cushion of air—around the violent patient and plenty of room for him or her to move around. Because the person most in danger is the one closest, a violent patient should be given a single room, and if this is not possible, the reasons should be fully documented.

Aggressive stroke patients are not popular, and often there are disagreements about placement of such patients. A patient advocate is useful when inappropriate placement results in danger to family members or to other residents of an institution. Several volunteer organizations exist that can provide such services, and some state agencies have ombudspersons. A state legislator can also be helpful.

Planning Care

An interdisciplinary care plan is important in the management of patient violence and agitation in institutions. A pragmatic argument in favor of such plans is that they are needed to satisfy the requirements of third-party insurance payers, regulatory agencies, and quality assurance mandates.

Familiarity with applied behavior analysis is helpful in formulating care plans. Burke and Lewis (1986) have provided guidelines for plan formulation using this technique. MacLeod and Mate (1991), on the other hand, have outlined a program of long-term care for stroke patients that is based more on psychodynamic principles. It is useful to follow procedures such as identifying a target behavior, measuring its frequency, and observing what precipitates it. Also important is identifying who is upset by the behavior, and why.

In institutional settings, some team members will object to such a systematic approach. Such objections may arise from various concerns, which should be discussed. Analysis of behavior is based on behaviorist assumptions, and not everyone agrees with these assumptions. Sometimes the objection is a manifestation of frustration at having to cope with a difficult patient and needs to be met with reassurances that the burden on staff members is understood and that their work is appreciated.

Plans for resistance to care.   When a patient's resistance to care is endangering staff, a good basic plan is to begin morning care with two aides present. One of them can serve as bodyguard, protecting the other from blows or punches or going to get a third aide if needed. Often, once care is started, it is safe for the second aide to leave. It will sometimes be found that there is resistance to one aide but not to another, or that feelings of personal modesty are involved.

Modifying medical management.   In the acute-care general hospital, violence often occurs during attempts to restrain a patient in order to carry out a technical procedure or to keep an intravenous line in place. In these cases, the risk-benefit ratio must be carefully considered: it may be better to modify the medical regimen to avoid the need for restraint.

Avoidance of contact.   If violence is directed against a staff member who touches the patient in the course of attempting to stop a nonviolent agitated behavior, ways of dealing with these behaviors without touching the patient should be explored. Tolerating some of these nonviolent behaviors may be the best policy, but adopting such a course must be a team decision.

Summary

Outbursts of apparent anger are common in stroke patients, but we cannot always be sure of the precise emotion felt. Goldstein's (1952) *catastrophic reaction* is a behavioral disturbance with strong negative emotions manifested when a patient is unable to accomplish a task. Specific locations of brain damage have been shown experimentally to cause aggression in some conditions, but the application of these findings to stroke is not yet clear. Risk factors associated with violence include inappropriate patient placement, dementia, delirium, territorial defense, escalation of nonviolent disturbed behavior, resistance to care, cocaine, and preexisting delinquent tendencies. Use of sedative or psychotropic drugs to control violence and agitation in nursing homes is limited by federal law. Short-acting benzodiazepines are often used for emergency sedation. Sedation risks are greater in stroke patients than in other psychiatric patients because of the frequent presence of cardiovascular disease in stroke patients. Treatment measures include reassuring caregivers, placing the patient in the appropriate setting, providing space, avoiding unnecessary physical contact, using a patient advocate, and formulating an interdisciplinary care plan. In planning a program of care, it is useful to identify the target behavior, measure its frequency, observe what precipitates it, and identify those who are hurt by it. Modifying medical treatment regimens and tolerating nonviolent disturbances of behavior may be necessary.

References

American Psychiatric Association: Diagnostic and Statistical Manual of Mental Disorders, 4th Edition. Washington, DC, American Psychiatric Association, 1994

Bard P: A diencephalic mechanism for the expression of rage with special reference to the sympathetic nervous system. Am J Physiol 84:490–515, 1928

Barnes R, Veith R, Okimoto J, et al: Efficacy of antipsychotic medications in behaviorally disturbed dementia patients. Am J Psychiatry 139:1170–1174, 1982

Benet LZ, Sheiner LB: Pharmacokinetics, in Goodman and Gilman's The Pharmacological Basis of Therapeutics, 7th Edition. Edited by Gilman AG, Goodman LS, Rall TH, et al. New York, Macmillan, 1985, pp 3–35

Brown GE, Ebert MH, Goyer PE, et al: Aggression, suicide, and serotonin: relationships to CSF amine. Am J Psychiatry 139:741–746, 1982

Burke WH, Lewis FD: Management of maladaptive social behavior of a brain injured adult. Int J Rehabil Res 9:335–342, 1986

Cohen-Mansfield J: Agitated behaviors in the elderly ill, II. J Am Geriatr Soc 34:711–727, 1986

Cohen-Mansfield J: Agitation in the elderly. Adv Psychosom Med 19:101–113, 1989

Devinsky O, Bear D: Varieties of aggressive behavior in temporal lobe epilepsy: Am J Psychiatry 141:651–656, 1984

Eichelman B: Aggressive behavior from laboratory to clinic: quo vadis? Arch Gen Psychiatry 49:488–492, 1992

Flor-Henry F: Schizophrenia-like reactions and affective psychoses associated with temporal lobe epilepsy. Am J Psychiatry 126:148–152, 1969

Gainotti G: Il comportimento emozionale dei cerebrolesi destri e sinistri in situazione di test neurolopsicologico. Archivio di Psicologia Neurologia e Psichiatria 31:457–480, 1970

Goldstein K: The effect of brain damage on the personality. Psychiatry 15:245–260, 1952

Hanger HC, Mulley GP: Questions people ask about stroke. Stroke 24:536–538, 1993

Herrmann N, Eryavec G: Buspirone in the management of agitation and aggression associated with dementia. American Journal of Geriatric Psychiatry 1:249–253, 1993

Herzberg JL, Fenwick PBC: The aetiology of aggression in temporal lobe epilepsy. Br J Psychiatry 153:50–55, 1988

Honigfeld G, Roderic D, Klett JC: NOSIE-30: a treatment-sensitive ward behavior scale. Psychol Rep 19:180–182, 1966

Houlihan DJ, Mulsant BH, Sweet RA, et al: A naturalistic study of trazodone in the treatment of behavioral complications of dementia. American Journal of Geriatric Psychiatry 2:78–85, 1994

Isaacs B, Neville Y, Rushford I: The stricken: the social consequences of stroke. Age Ageing 5:188–192, 1976

Lee S: The neglect of anger in Western psychiatry (letter). Br J Psychiatry 161:864, 1992

Lion JR: Pitfalls in the assessment and measurement of violence. J Neuropsychiatry Clin Neurosci 3:540–543, 1991

Lorenz K: Das Sogennante Böse. Vienna, Dr. G. Borotha-Schoeler Verlag, 1963. Translated by Latzke M as *On Aggression*. London, Methuen, 1966

MacLeod F, Mate A: Life enrichment for long-stay patients in acute care: an interdisciplinary program. Perspectives Montclair 15:2–6, 1991

Marin DB, Greenwald DS: Carbamazepine for aggressive agitation in demented patients during nursing care (letter). Am J Psychiatry 146:805, 1989

Medina JL, Rubino FA, Ross E: Agitated delirium caused by infarctions of the hippocampal formation and the fusiform and lingual gyri. Neurology 24:1181–1183, 1974

Omnibus Budget Reconciliation Act of 1987 (OBRA), Public Law 100-203

Overall JE, Gorham DR: The Brief Psychiatric Rating Scale. Psychol Rep 10:799–812, 1962

Patel V, Hope T: Aggressive behavior in elderly people with dementia: a review. International Journal of Geriatric Psychiatry 8:457–472, 1993

Patterson JF: Carbamazepine for assaultive patients with organic brain disease: an open pilot study. Psychosomatics 28:579–581, 1987

Petty RG, Bonner D, Mouratoglou V, et al: Acute frontal lobe syndrome and dyscontrol associated with bilateral caudate nucleus infarctions. Br J Psychiatry 168:237–240, 1996

Pinner E, Rich CI: Effects of trazodone on aggressive behavior in seven patients with organic mental disorder. Am J Psychiatry 145:1295–1296, 1988

Rosen J, Burgio L, Kollar M, et al: The Pittsburgh Agitation Scale: a user-friendly instrument for rating agitation in dementia patients. American Journal of Geriatric Psychiatry 2:60–74, 1994

Schneider L, Pollock VE, Lyness SA: A meta-analysis of controlled trials of neuroleptic treatment in dementia. J Am Geriatr Soc 38:555–563, 1990

Stocklin A: My Stroke, My Blessing. Aurora, CO, Charles Delperdang, 1989

Tonkonogy JM: Violence and temporal lobe lesions: head CT and MRI data. J Neuropsychiatry Clin Neurosci 3:189–196, 1991

World Health Organization: International Statistical Classification of Diseases and Related Health Problems, 10th Revision. Geneva, Switzerland, World Health Organization, 1992

Yudofsky SC, Siver JM, Hales RE: Pharmacological management of aggression in the elderly. J Clin Psychiatry 51 (suppl 10):22–28, 1990

Zimmer JA, Watson N, Treat A: Behavioral problems among patients in skilled nursing facilities. Am J Public Health 74:1118–1121, 1984

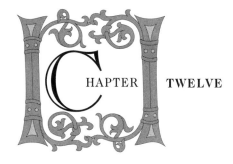

CHAPTER TWELVE

Disinhibition

One group of mental changes in stroke has in common a weakening of the normal social constraints on behavior. The behaviors that result from this condition cause distress to others rather than to the patient. Although not enough experimental work has been done on these behaviors to justify a rigid taxonomy, a tentative arbitrary categorization of the primary phenomena includes negative emotions not classifiable as major mood disorders, euphoria, emotional incontinence, disinhibited behaviors of dementia, and incontinence of urine and feces.

Primary Manifestations

Negative Emotions

Disturbances of mood that do not readily fit into any category of mental disorder are common in stroke. Family and friends will often say of a stroke patient that "his personality has changed" or that "she is not the person I knew." When these expressions are used, usually the change has been for the worse, but sometimes a patient has mellowed or relaxed. Some of these changes are characteristic of brain damage in general and conform to the ICD-10 (World Health Organization 1992) criteria for *organic personality disorder.*

A typical complaint by a spouse is that the patient no longer provides companionship. One of Anderson's (1992) informants said, of her husband, that "He's just not my George, not as he was. His nature has completely changed. You can't get through to him. He's the reverse of what he was" (p. 161).

Dian et al. (1990) compared 20 patients diagnosed as having multi-infarct dementia with a group of 30 control subjects drawn from retirees active in community organizations. The subjects were all men who were living with their wives or at least one daughter, who served as informants. All of the infarct group patients were attendees of a dementia clinic or were inpatients on a psychiatric unit. The informants were asked about changes in the control group subjects since retirement and about changes in the multi-infarct patients since the onset of illness. The multi-infarct patients were reported to have become less energetic, less practical, less mature, less enthusiastic, less happy, less kind, less self-reliant, less generous, less reasonable, less stable, and less talkative. Three of the multi-infarct patients were reported to be severely depressed; none of the control subjects demonstrated this symptom. Some of the adverse changes in the patients may have been due to dementia, but only loss of kindness and generosity were found to correlate with the severity of dementia. Six aspects of personality that remained unchanged in the multi-infarct patients were "affectionateness," cautiousness, fondness for company, irritableness, excitableness, and shortness of temper.

Euphoria

Inappropriate mood may sometimes be elevated, leading to social improprieties such as feeble and repetitive jokes. Inability to contain weeping may sometimes be accompanied by inability to control laughter (although the latter symptom is rarer and is seldom a cause for complaint). In some cases of frontal lobe syndrome and secondary mania (discussed in more detail later in this chapter), euphoria is also present.

Signer et al. (1989) found that, among aphasic patients with behavior disorders, elation was associated with posterior lesions. They described such patients as "happy, ebullient, and unaware of their language impairment" (p. 43).

Bogousslavsky et al. (1988) described a patient with a right-hemisphere thalamic infarct demonstrated on computed tomography (CT) scan that involved the dorsomedian (mediodorsal) nucleus, intralaminar nuclei, and the medial part of the ventral lateral nucleus. The patient had suddenly become somnolent, and on recovery from this condition she produced pressured speech and laughing, although no increased motor activity. She told the physician, "I do not want to be examined by you with your big blue face; your nose is horrible" (p. 116). Single photon emission computed tomography (SPECT) revealed reduced blood flow in the right frontal lobe.

Emotional Incontinence

Some stroke patients suddenly burst into tears at the slightest provocation or no provocation. First-person narratives describe a reaction of social embarrassment associated with the weeping, but no particular severity of depression. Some patients apologize and try to explain that their crying does not represent deep sadness.

Pintoff (1992) gave one of the best first-person accounts of this kind of crying, calling it "annoying" and "humiliating." He said, "The slightest display of sentimentality or a tender emotion provoked me to uncontrollable tears" (p. 84).

Josephs (1992) also gave a good firsthand account of crying, and offered several useful techniques for dealing with the symptom. He felt that his crying, rather than being related to labile mood or depression, was caused by difficulty in controlling the *expression* of the emotion felt.

Jorge et al. (1993) found no correlation between stroke patients' weeping and their scores for depression on the Hamilton Rating Scale for Depression (Hamilton 1960). Goldstein (1952) regarded spontaneous weeping as a manifestation of his *catastrophic reaction,* a phenomenon manifested when a patient is unable to accomplish an assigned task (see Chapter 11). Ross (1981; Ross and Rush 1981) included it in his category of aprosodias.

Efforts have been made to distinguish between pathological crying and emotional lability. Allman et al. (1992) found that the two were not sharply separated. The most common external precipitant of crying in their study was a kind gesture or an expression of sympathy. Although a few patients reported no change in mood with crying, many had difficulty describing their moods. Some patients were not embarrassed by the crying. The symptom tended to diminish gradually over the 6 months following the stroke.

Spontaneous weeping is sometimes said to characterize pseudobulbar palsy (Benson 1973; Black 1994), a condition in which strokes have produced upper motor neuron paralysis on both sides, but the symptom is also commonly seen in stroke patients with unilateral hemiplegia. In one study (Andersen et al. 1994), such weeping was most severe in patients with bilateral pontine lesions. Andersen and colleagues linked this severity to the fact that pontine lesions cause damage to the serotonin-producing raphe nuclei in the brain stem.

Dementia-Related Disinhibition

In fully developed dementia and delirium, it is often obvious that aberrant actions are a direct result of cognitive impairment and that disinhibited behaviors occur because the patient is oblivious of the surrounding world. Some patients may wander as a result of disorientation or be unable to dress themselves properly.

Cohen-Mansfield's (1986) classification of agitated behaviors includes four categories: aggressive-physical, aggressive-verbal, hoarding and stealing, and nonaggressive. The nonaggressive category is characterized by pacing, inappropriate dressing or disrobing, and requests for attention. Using the Cohen-Mansfield classification can be a good first step in analyzing a patient's behavior in order to formulate a plan of care. Hoarding and stealing are complained about more in the institutional setting, perhaps because these behaviors are not as bothersome when the patient is at home. The stealing is done innocently and consists of wandering into other patients' rooms and picking up any objects lying around. The nonviolent agitated behaviors are essentially victimless but can annoy people.

In some cases following a stroke, a patient's judgment may be impaired, an impairment that is noticeable only if compared with the patient's previous functioning. Patients with impaired judgment may insist on resuming their previous business or professional roles and activities, which they may perform at a substandard level even though they do not actually have dementia. The well-studied cases of Woodrow Wilson and other politicians illustrate the problems that can arise in such situations (see Appendix C).

Incontinence of Urine and Feces

Incontinence is a problem in elderly psychiatric patients and stroke patients alike. The overlap of psychiatric and neurological disabilities and incontinence is therefore also common, although incontinence may or may not be, strictly speaking, a psychiatric manifestation of stroke. Dementia must be very severe to be the sole cause of incontinence. Incontinence of urine or feces in elderly persons is not necessarily due to dementia. Because dementia is very common, cases of incontinence due to severe dementia are not rare, but they are not in the majority.

Most strokes cause incontinence at some stage of the illness. Brocklehurst et al. (1985) found that, during the course of the year following a stroke, one-half of their patients were incontinent of urine, and one-quarter were incontinent of feces at some time. Most of this incontinence had disappeared by the end of the year, at which point 15% of the patients were incontinent of urine and 8% were incontinent of feces.

It will sometimes be reported in a hospital or nursing home that a hemiplegic patient with dementia is eating feces. Such patients are found with feces smeared over their faces and mouths. This is seldom a true coprophagia, which is more likely to be seen in functional psychosis. Most of these patients are incontinent of feces. They become aware of the feces in the bed or clothing and then place their hands in it and smear it.

Causes of Disinhibition

The causes of disinhibition are heterogeneous. Similar disinhibited behavior may occur as a result of dementia or specific local brain damage (e.g., as in the frontal lobe and utilization behavior syndromes) or as part of a general mood disorder.

Frontal Lobe Syndrome

Descriptions of this syndrome go back to the large numbers of patients with head injuries studied after the First World War, and perhaps to the earlier case of Phineas Gage (Harlow 1868). Some of the war-wounded patients with frontal injuries had *witzelsucht*; that is, they were shallow, uncaring, cheerful, facetious, and mildly delinquent. Lishman (1968), in his studies of brain-injured soldiers, found that although the disinhibited type of frontal lobe syndrome was a distinct entity, it was relatively rare, showing up in only a minority of those with frontal lobe injury.

Many of the cerebrovascular patients with frontal lobe syndrome have had subarachnoid hemorrhage from a ruptured congenital aneurysm. Such an aneurysm often arises at the region where the two anterior cerebral arteries are joined by the anterior communicating artery (see Figures 12–1 and 12–2). For this reason, the front of the brain is the part most vulnerable to damage.

Storey (1970) followed 261 patients after subarachnoid hemorrhage. Most were impaired in functioning, and 8 had severe dementia, but 13

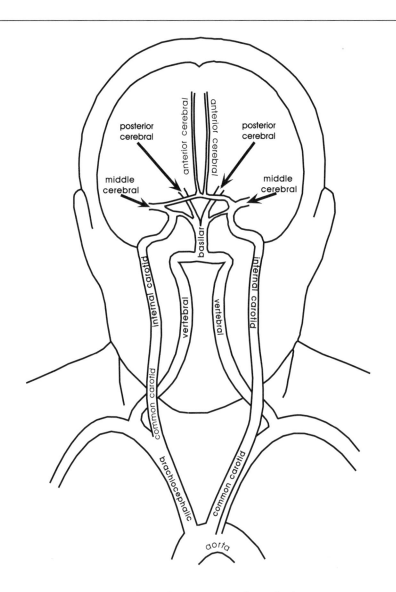

Figure 12–1.   Arteries supplying the brain, seen from the front.

not only were without impairment but were reported by their families to have improved personalities. These individuals became "less sarcastic and irritable, less tense and anxious, less fussy and over-meticulous, and more pleasant to live with generally" (p. 137). Because most of these "improved personality" patients had anterior cerebral artery aneurysms, Storey suggested that the changes may have been caused by a naturally inflicted prefrontal lobotomy. Stenhouse et al. (1991) followed 27 patients who had undergone rupture and repair of an aneurysm of the anterior communicating artery. With regard to outcome, three different groups of patients were identified: one with cognitive deficits, another with good outcome (including return to former activities), and a third with evidence of residual frontal lobe damage. These patient groups were demarcated

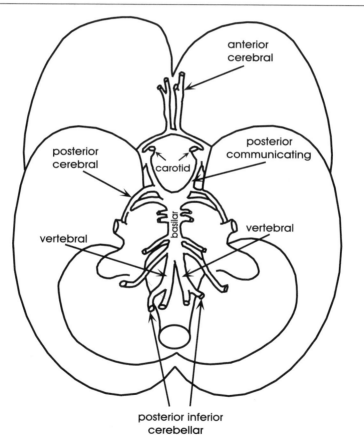

Figure 12–2. Arteries supplying the brain, seen from underneath.

in the published report by neuropsychological testing, and no narrative descriptions of the patients with residual frontal lobe damage were given.

Miller et al. (1989) compared 27 patients with late-onset psychosis with age-matched psychiatrically healthy control subjects. Five of the late-onset patients, and none of the controls, were found to have white-matter lesions in the frontal area (described as caused by vascular disease but not by definite infarcts). The 5 patients with frontal white-matter lesions were distinguished from the others in the late-onset psychosis group by euphoria, disinhibition, and—although the patients were not clinically demented—memory impairment.

Authors who associate depression with right-frontal-lobe infarcts have sometimes suggested that euphoria increases with the distance of the infarct from the right frontal lobe, and that euphoria becomes more likely the farther back the infarct is in the right hemisphere and the farther forward it is in the left hemisphere (refer to Table 14–1).

Utilization Behavior

Utilization behavior is characterized by an inability both to resist a suggestion to perform an action and to stop the action after starting. Patients with this syndrome overreact to any object they see by wanting to pick it up and do something with it. The manipulations performed are instrumentally correct but exaggerated.

When an orange and a knife were put in front of one patient, for example, she immediately proceeded to peel the orange, although not instructed to do so. If she saw a pencil and paper, she immediately began to write. When left alone in her room, she would spend hours preparing her bed, lying in it, and then getting up and remaking it. This patient, described by Eslinger et al. (1991), was found on CT to have bilateral infarcts in the thalamus. These authors characterized her mood as apathetic yet irritable—she would become intermittently aggressive, particularly when fatigued. She improved after treatment with buspirone (BuSpar) and haloperidol (Haldol), but her learning and memory remained poor. After 4 months, this woman still needed supervision by her family and help with her activities of daily living.

When originally reported, utilization behavior was associated with frontal lobe damage (Lhermitte 1986; Lhermitte et al. 1986). Lhermitte described three related syndromes: 1) environmental dependency (seen in two patients, neither with infarcts), characterized by marked behavioral changes in response to environmental changes; 2) imitation behavior, in which the patient inappropriately imitates the examiner; and 3) utilization behavior. He attributed the latter two syndromes to lesions of the inferior half of the anterior part of one or both frontal lobes. Eslinger et al. (1991) suggested that the discrepancy in anatomical location between their cases (thalamus) and Lhermitte's (frontal lobe) might be attributable to the fact that in their case the thalamofrontal tracts in the anterior limb of the internal capsule were involved.

The inconsistencies in localization and the anecdotal nature of the evidence do not provide a strong case for utilization behavior as a discrete entity caused by specific brain lesion. A more exact delineation of this symptom with standardized tests and adequate controls would be needed to establish this.

Hypergraphia.   Okamura et al. (1989) described 10 stroke patients who demonstrated hypergraphia—the sight of a pencil and pad would cause "half-involuntary" writing. The writing was syntactically correct but consisted of loose associations and conveyed little information. All 10 patients were right-handed and had right-hemisphere lesions either in the area supplied by the middle cerebral artery or in the thalamus. Okamura and colleagues also described several cases of hypergraphia associated with temporal lobe epilepsy.

Alien hand syndrome.   Alien hand syndrome is a condition in which one hand seems to have a will of its own. The patient described by Goldstein (1908) found her left hand grabbing her throat, and had difficulty removing it. Corpus callosum infarcts have commonly been implicated in this syndrome (Feinberg et al. 1992), but the number of cases reported is small, and no controlled studies with exact criteria for the syndrome have been done.

Mania

Hyperactivity with an elevated or irritable mood raises the possibility of mania. Episodes of mania are so common that there must be many occasions when they occur in those who also have stroke, which is likewise common.

Sometimes a patient with a well-confirmed diagnosis of recurrent mania becomes demented or aphasic. With knowledge of the patient's previous diagnosis, it is possible to recognize the attacks, but without such prior knowledge, there is no infallible way to distinguish this condition from the agitated behaviors of dementia. Consistent euphoria can be a diagnostic clue, but not every patient with mania is always happy.

Matters can become even more difficult if mania occurs for the first time in late life. The onset of bipolar disorder is most common in the 20s (Loranger and Levine 1978), but the evidence collected by Snowden (1991) shows that late onset is not rare. Thus, although there are several examples in the literature of mania or bipolar disorder following stroke (Cohen and Niska 1980), a causal relationship cannot be assumed. Fujikawa et al. (1995) found magnetic resonance imaging (MRI) evidence of cerebral infarction in most of their patients with late-onset mania.

Locations of infarcts causing mania.   Jeste et al. (1988) found that the literature suggested that lesions in the front of the right hemisphere and at the back of the left hemisphere were associated with mania.

Cummings and Mendez (1984) described two patients who presented with mania and were found to have neurological signs. One patient had diminished pain and temperature sensation on the left side of the body and a left extensor plantar reflex. The other had dense left hemianesthesia, mild left hemiparesis, and left homonymous hemianopsia; no lesion was seen on CT scan. Cummings and Mendez concluded from these cases that right thalamic infarcts may cause mania.

Turecki et al.'s (1993) patient developed mania after an infarct of the left basal ganglia, whereas Berthier's (1992) patient, a man who developed rapid-cycling bipolar disorder after a stroke, had an infarct involving the right temporo-insular and anterior parietal regions. Fujikawa et al. (1995) did not find any consistent relationship between mania and site of infarct.

Shukla et al. (1987) recruited patients who had had a head injury and who subsequently developed an illness that met criteria for mania or schizoaffective disorder. Twenty such patients were found. Their illness was marked by irritability rather than euphoria. They were frequently assaultive and seldom psychotic.

Jorge et al. (1993) found that mania was more likely to follow head injury than stroke. They attributed this tendency partly to the fact that mania was associated in their head-injury patients with damage to the anterior temporal area. Damage to this area was less common in their stroke patients.

Nomenclature.   If mania can indeed result from a stroke, then a question of nomenclature arises. The DSM-IV (American Psychiatric Association 1994) criteria for a manic episode specify that it be "not due to the direct physiological effects of a substance . . . or a general medical condition" (p. 332). The term *mood disorder due to a general medical condition* encompasses cases with an elevated, expansive, or irritable mood, but some authors (e.g., Jorge et al. 1993) have found features more characteristic of mania than of mere mood elevation or irritability in the brain-damaged patients they studied, and therefore prefer to use the term *secondary mania* to describe such cases.

Causes of Incontinence

Incontinence of urine in stroke patients has multiple causes—often an interaction of mental illness and general medical and localized genitourinary problems. Some women, for example, have been incontinent for years because of pelvic-floor weakness, but have cleverly managed to cope with the condition and to conceal it with frequent changes of clothing or by staying close to a bathroom. It is only when an illness reduces their mobility and their intellectual capacity for concealment that the effects of the pelvic-floor condition become apparent.

The disabled and immobile stroke patient is an obvious candidate for functional incontinence. In fact, incontinence is associated more with loss of mobility than with any specific psychiatric or neurological condition (Brocklehurst et al. 1985).

Incontinence of feces can sometimes be due to fecal impaction, especially in patients on psychotropic medications with anticholinergic effects. If no one does a rectal examination, and especially if the patient has dementia or aphasia and thus cannot complain, then the resultant leakage of liquid feces may be mistreated with antidiarrheal medications such as diphenoxylate with atropine (Lomotil) or loperamide (Imodium). In some settings, the excessive and routine use of laxatives is responsible.

Management of Disinhibition

Although these disorders are disparate, their management has a common principle: it must address the concerns of those affected by the behavior, as well as those of the patient. In institutions, this can be accomplished by meetings of the treatment team to formulate multidisciplinary care plans for problems such as incontinence and the nonviolent antisocial behaviors. All staff members should be encouraged to express their ideas and feelings, and should be shown that they are needed and appreciated.

Family caregivers at home must also be encouraged to air their problems, and group sessions are often useful for this. They should be provided
with information and access to community services, and afforded the
opportunity for respite care.

Spontaneous weeping is not upsetting if the patient is alone. Being
told that this is a well-recognized symptom of stroke helps the patient,
and being reassured that it is a disturbance of the *expression* of emotion,
rather than of emotion, helps the family. Support groups are especially
useful for patients with this symptom.

Medications

Several trials of medications in spontaneous weeping have been conducted, including antidepressants and L-dopa (Sandyk 1985). The greatest
success has been reported by Robinson et al. (1993). In a double-blind
placebo-controlled trial, in patients who had requested treatment, using
a rating scale of pathological laughing and crying, they found significant
benefit from nortriptyline. The general applicability of their findings has
been questioned on the grounds that their study population contained
patients with major depression (Allman 1994; Ivan and Franco 1994). In
a study by Andersen et al. (1993), in which there were no patients with
major depression, pathological crying was relieved by the serotonin uptake inhibitor citalopram (not marketed in the United States).

Several cases of secondary mania in the literature are described as
being successfully treated with lithium, which is such a successful medicine in mania that it is probably worth a trial in many cases. However,
lithium in the elderly, in general, and in those with concurrent cardiovascular disease, in particular, causes frequent side effects (Bushey et al.
1983).

There have been no controlled trials of medications for the behaviors
of organic personality disorder. Various psychotropics are often tried empirically, usually phenothiazines, and caregivers may say that these are
beneficial. The use of medications for violence and for the agitated behaviors of dementia is discussed in Chapter 11.

Management of Incontinence of Urine and Feces

The medical and urological aspects of management have been reviewed
in several publications, such as the National Institutes of Health 1988
consensus report. Management is often behavioral despite organic etiol-

ogy. Some women patients with dementia and agitation who constantly demand to be taken to urinate are found, on cystoscopy, to have a low-capacity bladder with trabecular walls. Although this condition suggests a neurogenic bladder, these patients respond better to behavioral than to neurological treatment.

The most effective part of most bladder-training regimens is "prompted voiding." This technique consists of not merely taking the patient to the bathroom frequently, but also talking. Even the patients with severe dementia can report on their continence status (Brandeis 1994). Recording incontinence carefully and discussing it at rounds and team meetings leads to resolution in most cases associated with stroke (Silbert and Stewart-Wynne 1992).

The most effective remedy for smearing of feces and coprophagia is checking frequently for the presence of feces and promptly removing it.

When the patient is at home, the burden of incontinence on caregivers can be so severe that institutionalization may be the ultimate resort.

Nonintervention

Existentialist psychoanalysts such as R. D. Laing (see Ratna 1994), have done a great service by reminding us that the function of medicine is not necessarily to intervene to bring every disorder or idiosyncrasy of behavior into conformity with the norms of society. Tolerating harmless deviations may be a valid option, and uninhibited expressions of emotion may have their place.

> Woodrow Wilson, after his stroke, made a speech in which he mentioned the young men killed in the First World War. When he spoke of them, his behavior became inappropriate by some standards: he burst into tears and could not continue his prepared text.

Summary

Stroke can cause weakening of normal social constraints on behavior. Management must address the concerns both of the patient and of those affected by the patient's behavior. Some stroke patients burst into tears at the slightest provocation. Although this behavior may embarrass them, it does not constitute a sign that they are severely depressed. The ICD-10 (World Health Organization 1992) criteria for organic personality disorder include disinhibited behaviors and changes in mood. Aberrant actions can result from cognitive impairment in dementia and delirium. The Cohen-Mansfield (1986) classification can be used as a valuable first step in analyzing a patient's behavior so as to formulate a plan of care. Frontal lobe damage is often caused by subarachnoid hemorrhage from a ruptured congenital aneurysm. In some cases of frontal lobe syndrome, there are euphoria and disinhibition. Utilization behavior manifests as an inability to resist a suggestion either to perform an action or to stop after starting. The most effective part of bladder-training regimens is taking the patient to the bathroom frequently. Incontinence of feces can sometimes be due to fecal impaction.

References

Allman P: Post-stroke laughing and crying (letter). Am J Psychiatry 151: 291, 1994

Allman P, Hope T, Fairburn CG: Crying following stroke: a report on 30 cases. Gen Hosp Psychiatry 14:315–321, 1992

American Psychiatric Association: Diagnostic and Statistical Manual of Mental Disorders, 4th Edition. Washington, DC, American Psychiatric Association, 1994

Andersen G, Vestergaard K, Riis JO: Poststroke pathological crying treated with the selective serotonin reuptake inhibitor citalopram. Lancet 342:837–839, 1993

Andersen G, Ingeman-Nielsen M, Vestergaard K, et al: Pathoanatomic correlation between poststroke pathological crying and damage to brain areas involved in serotonergic neurotransmission. Stroke 25:1050–1052, 1994

Anderson R: The Aftermath of Stroke. Cambridge, UK, Cambridge University Press, 1992

Benson DF: Psychiatric aspects of aphasia. Br J Psychiatry 123:555–566, 1973

Berthier ML: Post-stroke rapid cycling bipolar affective disorder (letter). Br J Psychiatry 160:283, 1992

Black KJ: Pathological laughing and crying (letter). Am J Psychiatry 151: 456, 1994

Bogousslavsky J, Ferrazzini M, Regli F, et al: Manic delirium and frontal-like syndrome with paramedian infarction of the right thalamus. J Neurol Neurosurg Psychiatry 51:116–119, 1988

Brandeis GH: Behavioral treatment of urinary incontinence in the nursing home. Nursing Home Medicine 2:14–18, 1994

Brocklehurst JC, Andrews K, Richards B, et al: Incidence and correlates of incontinence in stroke patients. J Am Geriatr Soc 33:540–542, 1985

Bushey M, Rathey U, Bowers MB: Lithium treatment in a very elderly nursing home population. Compr Psychiatry 24:155–160, 1983

Cohen MR, Niska RW: Localized right cerebral dysfunction and recurrent mania. Am J Psychiatry 137:847–848, 1980

Cohen-Mansfield J: Agitated behaviors in the elderly ill, II. J Am Geriatr Soc 34:711–727, 1986

Cummings JL, Mendez ME: Secondary mania with focal cerebrovascular lesions. Am J Psychiatry 141:1084–1087, 1984

Dian L, Cummings JL, Petry S, et al: Personality alterations in multi-infarct dementia. Psychosomatics 31:415–419, 1990

Eslinger PJ, Warner GC, Grattan LM, et al: "Frontal lobe" utilization behavior associated with paramedian thalamic infarction. Neurology 41:450–452, 1991

Feinberg TE, Schindler RJ, Flanagan NG, et al: Two alien hand syndromes. Neurology 42:19–24, 1992

Fujikawa T, Yamawaki S, Touhouda Y: Silent cerebral infarctions in patients with late-onset mania. Stroke 26:946–949, 1995

Goldstein K: Zur Lehre von der motorischen Apraxie. Journal für Psychologie und Apraxie 11:169–187, 1908

Goldstein K: The effect of brain damage on the personality. Psychiatry 15:245–260, 1952

Hamilton MA: A rating scale for depression. J Neurol Neurosurg Psychiatry 23:56–62, 1960

Harlow JM: Recovery from the passage of an iron bar through the head. Publications of the Massachusetts Medical Society 2:320–347, 1868

Ivan TM, Franco K: Post-stroke pathological laughing and crying (letter). Am J Psychiatry 151:290–291, 1994

Jeste DV, Lohr JB, Goodwin FK: Neuroanatomical studies of major affective disorders: a review and suggestions for further research. BMJ 153:444–460, 1988

Jorge RE, Robinson RG, Starkstein SE, et al: Secondary mania following traumatic brain injury. Am J Psychiatry 150:916–921, 1993

Josephs A: Stroke: An Owner's Manual. Long Beach, CA, Amadeus Press, 1992

Lhermitte F: Human autonomy and the frontal lobes, II: social situations. Ann Neurol 19:335–343, 1986

Lhermitte F, Pillon B, Serdaru M: Human autonomy and the frontal lobes, I: imitation and utilization behavior. Ann Neurol 19:326–334, 1986

Lishman WA: Brain damage in relation to psychiatric disability after head injury. Br J Psychiatry 114:373–410, 1968

Loranger AW, Levine PM: Age at onset of bipolar affective illness. Arch Gen Psychiatry 35:1345–1348, 1978

Miller BL, Boone KB, Hill E, et al: White matter lesions and psychosis. Br J Psychiatry 155:73–78, 1989

National Institutes of Health: Urinary incontinence in adults. National Institutes of Health Consensus Development Conference Statement, Vol 7, No 5, October 1988

Okamura T, Motomura N, Asaba H, et al: Hypergraphia in temporal lobe epilepsy—compared with stroke of the right cerebral hemisphere. Jpn J Psychiatry Neurol 43:524–525, 1989

Pintoff E: Bolt From the Blue. Salt Lake City, UT, Northwest, 1992

Ratna L: Books reconsidered. Br J Psychiatry 165:420–423, 1994

Robinson RG, Parikh RM, Lipsey JR, et al: Pathological laughing and crying following stroke: validation of a measurement scale and a double-blind treatment study. Am J Psychiatry 150:286–293, 1993

Ross ED: The aprosodias: functional-anatomical organization of the affective components of language in the right hemisphere. Arch Neurol 38:561–569, 1981

Ross ED, Rush JA: Diagnosis and neuroanatomical correlates of depression in brain-damaged patients. Arch Gen Psychiatry 38:1344–1354, 1981

Sandyk R: Nomifensine for "emotional incontinence" of the pseudobulbar type (letter). J Am Geriatr Soc 33:375, 1985

Shukla S, Cook BI, Mukherjee S, et al: Mania following head trauma. Am J Psychiatry 144:93–96, 1987

Signer S, Cummings JL, Benson DF: Delusions and mood disorders in patients with chronic aphasia. Journal of Neuropsychiatry 1:40–45, 1989

Silbert PL, Stewart-Wynne EG: Incontinence after stroke (letter). Lancet 339:428, 1992

Snowden J: A retrospective case-note study of bipolar disorder in old age. Br J Psychiatry 158:485–490, 1991

Stenhouse LM, Knight RG, Longmore BE, et al: Long-term cognitive deficits in patients after surgery on aneurysms of the anterior communicating artery. J Neurol Neurosurg Psychiatry 54:909–914, 1991

Storey PB: Brain damage and personality change after subarachnoid hemorrhage. Br J Psychiatry 117:129–142, 1970

Turecki G, de Mari J, del Porto A: Bipolar disorder following a left basal ganglia stroke. Br J Psychiatry 163:690–701, 1993

World Health Organization: International Statistical Classification of Diseases and Related Health Problems, 10th Revision. Geneva, Switzerland, World Health Organization, 1992

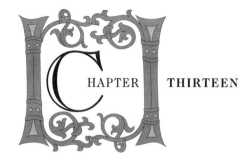

CHAPTER THIRTEEN

Delusions and Paranoia

In general, the presence of delusions suggests a psychosis, in which the brain is physically intact, whereas cognitive impairment and loss of memory suggest physical damage to the brain. Although these are useful generalizations, numerous exceptions exist. These exceptions are of particular concern in dealing with stroke, where the added complications of aphasia and specific neuropsychiatric syndromes interfere with assessment.

Delusions and hallucinations occur commonly in delirium, for example, although in this condition they are accompanied by confusion and disorientation. In addition, on occasion patients with schizophrenia or major affective disorders will seem confused or will fail to give relevant answers to questions meant to test memory and intellect.

Delusions in Organic Conditions

The validity of any division between organic and functional psychiatric disorders is increasingly being questioned (see Chapter 16). The term *organic* will be provisionally used here in its older sense of referring to conditions associated either with a general medical condition of the kind that can be diagnosed by usual clinical methods, or with visible structural brain damage of the kind that can be identified under the microscope.

Phenomenology

The main distinguishing feature of the delusions and hallucinations of disorders associated either with a general medical condition or with visible structural brain damage is that they are commonly accompanied by confusion, but they have certain distinctive features apart from this. The delusions and hallucinations of delirium are often fleeting and variable, and their content is likely to involve imminent danger to others or bizarre happenings in the immediate vicinity. Such delusions are rare in schizophrenia and manic-depressive disorders. In schizophrenia, auditory hallucinations are more common and visual hallucinations less common than in delirium and dementia. A classical "first-rank Schneiderian" symptom of schizophrenia is hearing voices commenting on one's thoughts and arguing or commanding. Hallucinations of this kind are very rare in other conditions (Cutting 1987).

Delusions—believing that one's deceased spouse is still alive or that one has been robbed when one has not—can often be related to memory loss. These are sometimes described as secondary delusions. However, some types of delusion that are especially common in dementia, such as that of the "phantom boarder" (the belief that uninvited guests have taken up residence in one's home), cannot be explained on the simple basis of memory loss.

The phenomenological status of some of the misidentification syndromes and agnosias remains unsettled, as does the question of whether the investigation of these syndromes' subjective content is of practical utility in establishing their etiology. It also remains questionable whether entities such as reduplicative paramnesia and anosognosia should be described as delusions.

Organic Delusional Syndrome

In organic delusional syndrome there are delusions without confusion. DSM-III-R (American Psychiatric Association 1987) noted that the syndrome may result from "certain cerebral lesions, particularly of the right hemisphere" and that "some people with cerebral lesions develop the delusion that a limb of their body is missing" (p. 109). The syndrome is not included in DSM-IV (American Psychiatric Association 1994), which instead has a category for "psychotic disorder due to [a specified general medical condition]" with delusions (pp. 309–310). ICD-10 (World Health Organization 1992, p. 62)) excludes drug-induced psychotic disorders from its category of organic delusional disorder. Although the paranoid states of cocaine-induced psychosis might be expected to occur in cocaine-related stroke, no such cases have been documented.

Late Paraphrenia

Late paraphrenia was defined by Roth (1955) as "a well organized system of paranoid delusions with or without auditory hallucinations existing in the setting of a well preserved personality and affective response" (p. 283), with onset usually after the age of 60. The risk factors for this syndrome include being deaf and being single. Late-onset paraphrenia patients do not (by definition) have dementia at the onset of the illness, but when followed over time, they have been found more likely to become demented than their same-aged peers in the general population (Holden 1987). It is not known what proportion of this subsequent dementia is vascular in origin.

Flint et al. (1991) studied 33 elderly patients without dementia who had late-onset paranoid disorders and found cerebral infarcts on computed tomography (CT) in 10 of them. They suggested that patients with cerebral infarcts do not have the risk factors for late paraphrenia usually described.

Cerebral Infarcts With Psychiatric Presentations

Cerebral infarcts are sometimes found in patients who present with an illness that has the usual hallmarks of a functional psychosis.

> A 70-year-old man with a delusion that he was being robbed was admitted to a psychiatric hospital. He had no previous history of psychiatric disorder and displayed no confusion on admission. The patient remained grossly delusional, continuing to make whimsical and extravagant assertions, such as that he had grown a new pair of lungs.
>
> When examined 13 years later at the age of 83, the patient was paranoid and delusional but fully oriented. Four months later, he died suddenly of an aortic aneurysm. Autopsy showed an old cystic infarct in the head of the right caudate nucleus.

Such a case arouses suspicion that the infarct was the cause of the patient's psychiatric symptoms—a suspicion that increases if the age of the infarct, as determined at autopsy or on CT, matches the time of onset of the symptoms. However, confirmation is uncertain in the individual case, and attempts to settle the matter by studying larger numbers of cases have not been conclusive. Commonly, the time of onset of the delusions is not exactly known, and the age of an infarct found on CT cannot be ascertained.

Price and Mesulam (1985) used the term *nonobvious stroke* to describe the condition seen in five patients who presented psychiatrically and were found to have right-hemisphere cerebral infarcts. These patients initially manifested symptoms such as agitation, inattention, suspiciousness, paranoid delusions, hallucination, and lack of appropriate concern, but lateralizing signs were found on later neurological examination.

Cummings (1985) studied 20 patients who had had delusions in the course of an organic brain disorder, although they were not depressed and had no previous history of psychiatric illness. Five of these patients had brain infarcts; two had anosognosia, which is considered a delusion according to some definitions; and three had simple delusions of persecution in the context of moderate dementia.

Miller et al. (1991) studied 24 patients who, after the age of 45, developed a nondementing illness of paranoid or schizophrenic type. Patients were excluded from the study if they had a Mini-Mental State Exam (Folstein et al. 1975) score of less than 24, a history of stroke, or evidence of hemimotor or hemisensory deficits. Although no significant differences in the number or size of white-matter lesions were found between these patients and 72 nonpsychiatrically ill control subjects, the paranoid patients had more lesions in the temporal, occipital, and frontal areas. In 6 of the paranoid patients and 5 of the control subjects, the lesions were described as being infarcts. The authors did not find a preponderance of lesions in either hemisphere.

Location of Infarct

Infarcts that have not produced paralysis tend to be in areas of the brain (e.g., the prefrontal) that are isolated from the main motor areas. Other than this finding, there is no firm consensus regarding which locations of infarct are most likely to be associated with delusions or paranoia. Attempts to compare delusions in patients with right-hemisphere versus left-hemisphere infarcts face the obstacles described in Chapter 4 ("Comparing Left-Sided and Right-Sided Strokes"). The presence of aphasia may cause underreporting of delusions in those with left infarcts.

Levine and Grek (1984) compared right-hemisphere cerebral infarct patients with and without delusions. Of the nine delusional patients, none had previous dementia or were taking psychotropic medication. The location of the lesion had no major effect on the presence or absence of delusions. The size of the lesion also had no effect; however, the authors cautioned that the latter finding may have been due to the fact that they excluded subjects with small lesions.

Signer et al. (1989) found that among aphasic patients with behavior disturbance, delusions were more common in those with posterior lesions than in those with lesions in other locations.

An extensive literature links pathology of the temporal lobe, especially the left temporal lobe, to schizophrenia-like illness. However, no statistically confirmed connection has been found between infarcts of this area and the presence of paranoid delusions or schizophrenia.

Clinical Features of Psychosis After Stroke

In practice, the patient most likely to have a paranoid psychosis after stroke is one who was previously psychotic. The clinical picture is then dominated by the obstacles to rehabilitation presented by the psychosis.

> A 65-year-old patient with paranoid schizophrenia had a stroke with left hemiplegia. She became ambulant but allowed her left upper limb to become contracted and atrophic, and she refused all rehabilitation measures. Hostile and uncooperative, she was not helped by psychotropic medications. Her wrist became so flexed that her fingernails dug into her palms, producing deep ulcers. She refused surgery for this condition, and a court order had to be obtained.

Several other syndromes involving psychosis have been described in individual case reports. Berthier and Starkstein (1987) told of a patient who, following a stroke with left hemiplegia and an extensive right frontotemporoparietal infarct, developed symptoms suggestive of a functional psychosis, although this patient had several features not typically found in functional psychosis. His hallucinations were mainly visual and were seen in his left visual field, which was hemianoptic. His delusions included reduplicative paramnesia: although he remained in the same hospital room throughout his stay, he insisted he had been moved daily to different hospital rooms with the same number. At times he was euphoric. These symptoms gradually subsided over the next few months. From their review of the literature, Berthier and Starkstein concluded that such symptoms are more likely to arise from strokes affecting the right hemisphere.

In some patients, a hemiplegic side may develop involuntary movements (posthemiplegic dystonia), and this condition has been accompanied by bizarre delusions (Kellner and Strian 1991).

Management of Paranoia and Delusions

Treatment of paranoid delusions is often equated with the use of antipsychotic medication. Such medication is considered a mainstay of treatment. A common obstacle to medication is that the paranoid patient may refuse it, leading to legal and ethical complications. In stroke patients, special consideration in stroke must be given to cardiovascular side effects and to drug-induced sedation and parkinsonism, which may interfere with mobility and rehabilitation.

Flint et al. (1991) found that treatment of paranoid symptoms with phenothiazines was difficult in patients with cerebral infarcts because of the appearance of disabling side effects at relatively low dosages. Higher dosages can usually be tolerated by patients with preexisting paranoid schizophrenia who have been previously stabilized on antipsychotic medications, but even in these patients tolerance may be reduced after a stroke, as discussed in Chapter 5.

Deciding where the paranoid patient is to be treated must often take priority over determining what the treatment will be. Patients who refuse treatment may require care in a protected setting and have to be committed to a psychiatric unit, which is one reason that general medical and neurological professionals should be available in such places.

> A farmer in a remote area of Canada was fending off imaginary intruders with a shotgun. His family physician managed to sedate him and, with the help of the police, got him in an ambulance to the provincial psychiatric hospital, which was a 2-hour drive away. On arrival, the man was found to have a dense hemiplegia.

Summary

In practice, the patient most likely to have a paranoid psychosis after stroke is one who was previously psychotic. The clinical picture is then dominated by the obstacles to rehabilitation presented by the psychosis.

Delusions in organic disorder are commonly accompanied by confusion, but also have certain other distinctive features. In organic delusional syndrome, there are delusions without confusion. The location of the lesion has not been consistently shown to have a major effect on the presence or absence of delusions, but the right hemisphere in general, posterior areas in general, and the left temporal lobe have been suggested as more likely locations. Stroke patients with preexisting paranoid schizophrenia may be especially susceptible to developing psychotic symptoms, which can prevent them from cooperating with rehabilitation. Some patients may need care in a protected setting, but inappropriate placement in such settings is also common. Although antipsychotic medications can be useful in treating symptoms of paranoia, these drugs may be refused by severely paranoid patients, and side effects of drowsiness and parkinsonism may cause special problems for stroke patients.

References

American Psychiatric Association: Diagnostic and Statistical Manual of Mental Disorders, 3rd Edition, Revised. Washington, DC, American Psychiatric Association, 1987

American Psychiatric Association: Diagnostic and Statistical Manual of Mental Disorders, 4th Edition. Washington, DC, American Psychiatric Association, 1994

Berthier ML, Starkstein SE: Acute atypical psychosis following right hemisphere stroke. Acta Neurol Belg 87:125–131, 1987

Cummings JL: Organic delusions. Br J Psychiatry 146:184–197, 1985

Cutting J: The phenomenology of acute organic psychosis. Br J Psychiatry 151:324–332, 1987

Flint F, Rifat S, Eastwood R: Brain lesions and cognitive function in late life psychosis (letter). Br J Psychiatry 158:866, 1991

Folstein MF, Folstein SE, McHugh PR: Mini-Mental State: a practical method for grading the cognitive state of patients for the clinician. J Psychiatr Res 12:189–198, 1975

Holden NL: Late paraphrenia or the paraphrenias: a descriptive study with a ten year follow-up. Br J Psychiatry 150:635–639, 1987

Kellner MB, Strian F: Bizarre delusion and post-hemiplegic hemidystonia (letter). Br J Psychiatry 159:448, 1991

Levine DN, Grek A: The anatomic basis of delusions after right cerebral infarction. Neurology 34:577–582, 1984

Miller BL, Lesser IM, Boone KB, et al: Brain lesions and cognitive function in late-life psychosis. Br J Psychiatry 158:76–82, 1991

Price BH, Mesulam MM: Psychiatric manifestations of right hemisphere infarctions. J Nerv Ment Dis 173:610–614, 1985

Roth M: The natural history of mental disorder in old age. Journal of Mental Science 101:281–301, 1955

Signer S, Cummings JL, Benson DF: Delusions and mood disorders in patients with chronic aphasia. Journal of Neuropsychiatry 1:40–45, 1989

World Health Organization: International Statistical Classification of Diseases and Related Health Problems, 10th Revision. Geneva, Switzerland, World Health Organization, 1992

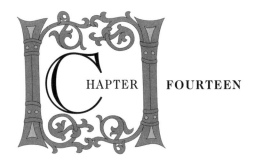

CHAPTER FOURTEEN

Depression

epression following a stroke is a complex and controversial issue. Common sense suggests that so severe and devastating an illness must cause unhappiness, and there are studies that confirm and quantify this. Goodstein (1983) found that one-third of stroke victims became completely dependent. Most distressing was the element of the unexpected and the unpredictable. His subjects feared another stroke and experienced loss of dignity and self-esteem. Isaacs et al. (1976) studied 35 patients, over a period of 3 years, after their discharge from the hospital following stroke. None of them ever used public transport or went to a hairdresser, library, cinema, bingo hall, or other social gathering place. Seven never left their houses. None of the 11 who had been employed full-time returned to work.

Such severe curtailment of activities might well cause poststroke depression. On the other hand, Feibel and Springer (1982) suggested that depression is a cause, rather than a consequence, of reduction of activities after stroke. When they compared stroke patients who stopped social activities with those who kept them up—matched for degree of disability—those who were depressed were more likely to have stopped. Such findings have raised the possibility of something intrinsic to stroke that causes the brain to malfunction and results in a depression.

211

Classification

Official psychiatric nomenclatures, such as DSM-IV (American Psychiatric Association 1994) and ICD-10 (World Health Organization 1992), are in broad agreement about the classification of depression. These diagnostic systems call a depression caused by unhappy events an *adjustment disorder with depressed mood* (DSM-IV, pp. 626–627) or a *depressive reaction* (ICD-10, pp. 150–151). The term *reactive depression* is also commonly used.

Depressions that are not reactive (i.e., not caused by responses to life events) are sometimes called *endogenous*. Several varieties of endogenous depression are recognized. To make the diagnosis of "major depressive episode" in DSM-IV, for example, there must be a depressed mood and at least five symptoms from a list that includes weight loss, sleep disturbance, agitation or psychomotor slowing, feelings of guilt, difficulty in concentrating, and thoughts of death or suicide. There must also be an absence of evidence that the condition is due to a general medical condition.

This last proviso has created a dilemma for those who wish to use the official nomenclature in research. An important research question is whether brain infarcts produce mood change directly, not merely as a result of the misery produced by the disability they cause. If a depression is proved to be due to an infarct, then it must be called a "mood disorder due to a general medical condition, with depressive features" (American Psychiatric Association 1994, pp. 369–370) or an "organic depressive disorder" (World Health Organization 1992, p. 64). Such proof may not be available until the outcome of a study of depression is known; therefore, at the beginning of the study, a provisional nomenclature must be established.

Rating Scales

Another approach to diagnosing depression is to measure it by using rating scales. Some of the special difficulties in using these scales in stroke patients have been reviewed by Primeau (1988). All of the depression rating scales require that patients be able to communicate. In some scales, such as the Zung Self-Rating Depression Scale (Zung 1965) and the Geriatric Depression Scale (Brink et al. 1982), the items consist of questions asked directly to the patient. These obviously have severe limitations for use with patients who have dementia or aphasia.

Attempts have been made to eliminate self-report by devising scales that can be completed from objective observation (Sunderland et al. 1988). Stern et al. (1990) developed scales to measure mood in patients with aphasia. The Center for Epidemiological Studies Depression Scale (CES-D; Radloff 1977) has been validated in populations of nonaphasic stroke patients (Shinar et al. 1986).

The Hamilton Rating Scale for Depression (Hamilton 1960) is the oldest and best-established depression rating scale. It was devised to assess severity of illness in patients already clinically diagnosed as depressed. Based on observation of the patient by a trained administrator, the Hamilton scale contains about 20 questions. Some of the items concerning physical symptoms and ability to provide self-care are difficult to complete accurately for a paralyzed and medically ill patient.

None of the scales add much accuracy to clinical diagnosis by a trained mental health professional (Parmelee et al. 1989) or general practitioner (House et al. 1989). Scales are generally more useful to the researcher than to the practical clinician and are often used to measure the effectiveness of new treatments.

One clinical (or administrative) situation in which a scale may be useful is during the assessment of nursing-home patients. U.S. government rules mandate periodic comprehensive reviews of the physical and mental status of patients in nursing homes (Elon and Pawlson 1992). Completion of a rating scale can provide good documentation of such a review.

Causes of Depression

Relationship to Disability

There are three indications that depression after stroke may not be merely a natural reaction to suffering. The first is that equal amounts of disability from other illnesses may not produce the same degree of depression; the second is that the degree of depression varies with the localization of the brain infarct; and the third is that the mood disorder is not always in the direction of depression, but may instead be characterized by anger, irritability, loss of normal affect, emotional volatility, or inappropriate euphoria.

Evidence concerning the first of these indications derives largely from the work of Folstein et al. (1977). They compared 10 patients disabled by stroke with 10 disabled from orthopedic causes, and found stroke to have a more depressive effect. A scale of activities of daily living was used to classify the groups according to degree of disability.

One possible explanation for Folstein et al.'s (1977) data is that, even if the degree of disability is matched, the subjective sensation of disability from a stroke is more unpleasant than that of disability from other causes. Robins (1976), however, presented evidence against this conclusion.

Starkstein et al. (1990) described two cases that they regarded as confirming the Folstein et al. hypothesis. Both patients had stroke disability from left-hemisphere lesions but suffered from anosognosia and did not know they were paralyzed. Despite being unaware of their disability, they were severely depressed.

Primeau (1988) felt that none of these studies fully proved that the depression was not a reaction to the stroke-caused disability. He concluded, after a comprehensive review of the literature, that "it remains unproven that depression is more common in patients after stroke than among the elderly with other physical illnesses" (p. 762).

Site of Infarct

The problem of comparability of groups also arises when the emotional effects of the site of a brain infarct are considered. Infarcts in some locations cause more physical disability than those in other locations, and an infarct causing more disability might also cause more depression.

Two main bodies of evidence exist concerning the effect the site of an infarct has on mood: a series of recent papers on the role of left anterior lesions (Lipsey et al. 1986; Robinson et al. 1984; Starkstein et al. 1987), and the older work on the frontal lobe syndrome (Lishman 1968).

Left Anterior Hypothesis

One group of researchers (Lipsey et al. 1986; Starkstein et al. 1987) has presented evidence for an entity of "poststroke depression," which possesses certain specific features and is not merely a reaction to a depressing situation. When compared with a group of patients hospitalized for "functional depression," the poststroke depression patients were found to be less likely to have a history of psychiatric disorder and more likely to have cognitive and functional impairment; in addition, these patients were less physically active and had slower speech. These researchers have associated poststroke depression with left anterior brain infarction. The conflicting evidence concerning this proposed link is summarized in Table 14–1. No true meta-analysis has been done.

Lipsey et al. (1983) studied 15 patients with bilateral brain injury due to stroke or trauma. Nine of these patients had left anterior lesions, and these 9 were also found to be significantly more depressed—according to Zung and Hamilton scale measurements—than the rest.

Robinson et al. (1984), working with young black stroke patients in Baltimore, Maryland, found that the infarcts most associated with depression were those in the left frontal lobe, and that the farther forward in the left hemisphere and the farther backward in the right hemisphere the infarct was, the more likely depression was. Thus, a far-back infarct in the right hemisphere did not cause depression as severe as that from a far-back left-hemisphere infarct. Robinson and colleagues (1985) found this to be true for both left-handed and right-handed patients.

Several possible objections have emerged to the hypothesis that left anterior lesions specifically cause depression. One is that major depression may be overdiagnosed in stroke patients because of changes in appetite, sleep, or sexual interest caused by their medical illness. The Baltimore group (Fedoroff et al. 1991) addressed this issue in a study in which they surveyed the incidence of "autonomic" symptoms of depression among depressed stroke patients. The autonomic, or "vegetative," symptoms of depression are more or less physical in nature and can be associated with physical illness. The autonomic symptoms studied by Fedoroff and colleagues included anxiety, anxious foreboding, morning depression, weight loss, delayed sleep, subjective anergia, early awakening, and loss of libido. They found that these symptoms were strongly associated with depressed mood in patients with acute stroke. Autonomic symptoms were not common among acutely ill stroke patients unless they also had depressed mood. Fedoroff et al. claimed that the rate of autonomic symptoms in nondepressed acute stroke patients was low and that these symptoms were not likely to cause an erroneous diagnosis of major depression.

An objection made by House et al. (1991) was that the Baltimore group classified all negative moods as depression, failing to differentiate conditions such as anxiety, irritability, and emotional lability. In the Oxfordshire Stroke Project, House and colleagues studied a random community sample of 128 British stroke patients with a mean age of 71, using a control group. Symptoms of mood disorder were more common in the stroke patients than in the control subjects, but the differences were not substantial and had largely disappeared after 12 months. Psychiatric prob-

Table 14–1. Localization of brain infarcts and depression

Authors	Description of study	Support for left anterior hypothesis
Lipsey et al. 1986	Compared "poststroke depression" with "functional depression" patients	++
Starkstein et al. 1987	Compared "poststroke depression" with "functional depression" patients	++
Lipsey et al. 1983	Studied patients with bilateral lesions and compared Hamilton and Zung scores in those with and without left anterior lesions	++
Robinson et al. 1984	Studied young black patients; found that the farther forward in the left hemisphere and the farther backward in the right hemisphere the infarct was, the more likely depression was	+++
Robinson et al. 1985	Found above results true for left-handed patients as well as right-handed ones	++
Fedoroff et al. 1991	Found vegetative symptoms of depression more common among depressed than among non-depressed stroke patients	++
House et al. 1991	Random community sample of elderly British stroke patients	–
Bolla-Wilson et al. 1989	Excluded patients with any language disorder	–
Ebrahim et al. 1987	Elderly British patients	–
Eastwood et al. 1989	Patients were predominantly male, white, nondemented, and nonaphasic (mean age = 65.5); found more depression among those with right-hemisphere lesions	–
Signer et al. 1989	Aphasic and behaviorally disturbed inpatients (mean age = 58)	++

(continued)

Table 14–1.   Localization of brain infarcts and depression *(continued)*

Authors	Description of study	Support for left anterior hypothesis
Åström et al. 1993b	Population-based cohort of elderly Swedish stroke patients	?
Jeste et al. 1988	Literature review	++
Delvenne et al. 1990	SPECT and PET scan studies	–
Lishman 1968	345 brain-injured soldiers	–

Note. Hamilton = Hamilton Rating Scale for Depression (Hamilton 1960); PET = positron-emission tomography; SPECT = single photon emission computed tomography; Zung = Zung Self-Rating Depression Scale (Zung 1965); – = no support for the hypothesis; + = slight support; ++ = moderate support; +++ = strong support; ? = questionable support.

lems encountered included agoraphobia, social withdrawal, apathy, self-neglect, irritability, and pathological emotionalism. Only two cases of major depression persisted for the entire 12 months. There was a trend toward improvement of psychiatric disturbances over the year.

Bolla-Wilson et al. (1989) found no relationship between left anterior lesions and depression. They attributed this discrepancy with other studies to the fact that their study excluded patients with any language disorder, whereas previous studies had excluded only those with severe language disorders.

Ebrahim et al. (1987), in studying 150 elderly British patients, did not find any difference between right-hemisphere and left-hemisphere lesions in tendency to cause depression. Feibel and Springer (1982) found no relationship between side of stroke and depression, a finding duplicated by Sharpe et al. (1990, 1994), who studied patients from the Oxford Stroke Project.

De Haan et al. (1995) studied a cohort of 760 consecutively admitted Dutch stroke patients (mean age 73 years). They found no association between emotional dysfunction and the side of the infarct.

Herrmann et al. (1995) studied a group of German stroke patients (median age 62 years) selected as having a single demarcated unilateral infarct. They found no significant difference in depression rating scores between patients with right- and left-hemisphere infarcts, and no correlation between severity of depression and how far forward the infarct was.

Herrmann and colleagues found that a DSM-III-R (American Psychiatric Association 1987) diagnosis of major depressive disorder was most commonly associated with left basal ganglia infarcts.

Eastwood et al. (1989) in Toronto studied a predominantly male population of relatively young (mean age 65.5 years) patients without dementia or aphasia who had been hospitalized for stroke and were in rehabilitation. These researchers used the Geriatric Depression Scale (Brink et al. 1982) and the Hamilton Rating Scale for Depression (Hamilton 1960) and measured disability with the Barthel Index (Mahoney and Barthel 1965). They compared patients in the study population who were depressed with those who were not. The depressed patients were more likely to have had either a previous psychiatric illness or a previous stroke, were more severely disabled, and had suffered their stroke less recently. The results varied with the depression scale used. Regarding the site of the lesion, Eastwood and colleagues found more depression among the patients with right-hemisphere lesions than among those with left-hemisphere lesions. In the left hemisphere, frontal lesions caused more depression than posterior lesions. In the right-hemisphere patients, there was no relation between the site of the lesion and depression.

Stern and Bachman (1991) found a significant but complex association between the site of the infarct and various depressive symptoms. Their study population was predominantly white, with a mean age of 65.8 years. No difference was found with regard to eating disturbance. The infarct locations most closely related to dysphoric mood and sleep disturbance were the left parietal, left occipital, left inferior frontal, right superior frontal, and right temporal regions.

Signer et al. (1989) supported the theory that right anterior lesions are more likely than right posterior lesions to cause depression. They found elation to be more common with right posterior lesions. Their study subjects consisted of 61 aphasic and behaviorally disturbed inpatients (mean age of 58), of whom 16 had vascular lesions.

Åström et al. (1993b), in a population-based cohort of elderly Swedish stroke patients, found that those with left-hemisphere infarcts initially had significantly more depression than those with right-hemisphere infarcts, but that at the end of 3 years, those with right-hemisphere infarcts had more depression.

Jeste et al. (1988) reviewed the literature from the preceding 55 years about the effects of brain damage on mood and found much inconsistency. The consensus was that damage to the front of the left hemisphere and to the back of the right hemisphere was associated with depression. These authors noted that the association between left frontal damage and depression was more marked for stroke than for brain injury.

Results of single photon emission computed tomography (SPECT) and positron-emission tomography (PET) studies of depression in patients without strokes have not been conclusive regarding lateralization. Delvenne et al. (1990), using SPECT, found no significant difference between right- and left-hemisphere blood flow when they compared control subjects and different subgroups of depressed patients defined by either biological markers or clinical characteristics.

Frontal Lobe Syndrome

The disinhibited type of frontal lobe syndrome (Chapter 12) is, in some respects, the reverse of depression. Victims are described as uncaring, cheerful, and facetious.

Lishman (1968) examined 345 soldiers with brain injuries. Although computed tomography (CT) scans were not available, the localization of the damage in each case was well defined because the injuries had penetrated the dura mater and required surgery. Lishman found a higher-than-expected incidence of depression among those with right frontal lobe injury, but some of those with right frontal injury showed the disinhibited type of frontal lobe syndrome. The disinhibited frontal lobe syndrome was characteristic, but it was relatively rare, occurring in only 32 of 114 patients with right frontal lobe injury. In contrast, 58 of the 114 patients had marked and persistent depression.

Emotional Incontinence

Although emotional incontinence is a cause of such symptoms as weeping and looking sad, it may not be strictly correct to consider it as a cause of depression, because there is doubt about whether these symptoms truly constitute a manifestation of depression. ICD-10 (World Health Organization 1992) describes a "right hemispheric affective disorder" (p. 68) in which the patient superficially appears to be depressed, but depression is not present. First-person narratives describe an emotion of social embarrassment associated with the weeping, but no particular severity of depression (Josephs 1992; Pintoff 1992).

Ross (1981; Ross and Rush 1981) included spontaneous weeping in his category of "aprosodias" (Chapter 6), which are said to constitute a specific set of disturbances in the ability to express emotion, analogous to the inability to express thought in aphasia. This spectrum of disorders also includes a "motor aprosodia" in which there is inability to adequately express a deeply felt sadness. Ross described a patient with a right inferior frontoparietal infarct who was suffering from a major depression that subsequently responded to antidepressant medication. The patient would say he was depressed and that he thought of suicide, but spoke these words in a flat, monotonous voice.

Endocrine Imbalance

The dexamethasone suppression test measures the reduction of plasma levels of cortisol following a dose of dexamethasone. Abnormalities of the test results have been found in research studies of depression, but the abnormalities are not consistent.

Finklestein et al. (1982) found abnormalities of dexamethasone suppression associated with mood disturbance after stroke. Lipsey et al. (1985) found that large cerebral infarcts were associated with abnormal dexamethasone suppression test results independently of depression. Persistent abnormalities 3 years after a stroke correlate better with depression than do early abnormalities (Åström et al. 1993a). Josephs (1992) and Wender (1986) both felt that the corticosteroid drugs given as part of their treatment caused depression.

Relationship of Depression to Dementia

Awareness of impending dementia could hypothetically cause depression. On the other hand, dementia could reduce depression resulting from disabilities by reducing awareness of the disabilities. Fischer et al. (1990), using the Hamilton Rating Scale for Depression (Hamilton 1960) and global rating scales, compared dementia patients who had Alzheimer's disease with those who had brain infarcts. In general, the patients in the brain infarct group were less depressed, but when the dementia in Alzheimer's disease was very severe, there was less depression in the Alzheimer's disease group. Very severe dementia thus anesthetized against depression in the case of Alzheimer's disease but not in the case of brain infarction.

Neurotransmitter Depletion

The neurotransmitters most probably involved in depression are serotonin and the catecholamines (epinephrine, norepinephrine, and dopamine). Infarcts that destroy localized sites of production, such as the locus coeruleus and substantia nigra or the tracts leading from these, might specifically affect mood.

A suggestion based on animal experiments is that right-hemisphere damage is more likely than left-hemisphere damage to block the cortical input of catecholamines from the locus coeruleus (Robinson and Coyle 1980).

Damage closer to the frontal lobes may be more likely to affect catecholamine-mediated brain activity than is damage closer to the locus coeruleus. An infarct at the locus coeruleus would destroy a source of catecholamines that might be replaced from several other brain sources. The frontal cortex nerve cells that use catecholamines in neurotransmission could use their intact neural processes to access these alternative supplies (Robinson and Szetela 1981).

Antihypertensive Medication

Another hypothetical link between stroke and depression is the medications used to treat hypertension. Thiessen et al. (1990) have confirmed that beta-blocking drugs can be associated with depression, but there is no published evidence linking stroke-related depression to the use of these drugs.

First-Person Narratives

The dispute remains unresolved between those who suggest that poststroke depression is a psychologically determined reaction to the illness and those who say it is a direct consequences of organic brain changes caused by the illness. One group that might be able to provide some enlightenment on this topic is the patients themselves. The first-person stroke narratives might be the best sources for learning about what a stroke feels like. Some of the best known of these have been reports of famous people such as Agnes de Mille, Patricia Neal, and May Sarton.

These accounts all suggest that poststroke depression is reactive rather than endogenous. They do not describe delusions or pervasive guilt and self-blame; rather, they relate how dreadful it is to suffer a stroke, and describe the frustrations of being unable to talk and the humiliation of disfigurement. From these narratives, one might conclude that depression is a natural reaction to the situation, not a chemical imbalance. On the other hand, although these authors are firsthand witnesses, they may not be representative ones. Survivors of strokes who are well enough to be able to write about their strokes may not be typical.

Wender (1986) reported, "The first six months after I got home were in many ways the worst of all. Now, for the first time ever for me, I felt totally, desperately depressed. If it hadn't been for my daughters, I might have seriously considered killing myself" (p. 62). She attributed her depression partly to having been given corticosteroids, but primarily to the disabilities and deprivations caused by the stroke.

According to Josephs (1992), "For each person a time of mourning is not only proper but necessary. Each must grieve for that part of him which has died. The day will come when you will bury the fact that you aren't the person you once were. For most, the mourning lasts at least a year. During those funereal months it takes a stout heart not to remain depressed" (p. 36).

Prognosis

Depressive illness in general is usually self-limited for those who survive the risk of suicide, although advanced age and concurrent medical illness worsen the prognosis (Caine et al. 1993).

Robinson et al. (1984) found that, in a group of young black men with neurologically evident stroke, the incidence of depression increased with time after the stroke, and the depression was of long duration. Some of the authors' data suggest that the depression occurring in the period directly after the stroke was more likely to be biochemically based, whereas that in the later stages resulted from unhappiness over stroke-caused impairments.

Ebrahim et al. (1987) followed 150 elderly British patients for 6 months after a stroke. One-quarter of these patients were found to be severely depressed at the end of that time, and there was no tendency toward spontaneous recovery from depression.

Management of Depression

Psychotherapy

There are obvious obstacles to individual psychotherapy when, as so often happens, the stroke patient cannot talk coherently and cannot take part in a conversation.

The psychotherapeutic approach varies, depending on whether a patient's depression is believed to be endogenous or a reaction to adverse circumstances. In the latter case, most psychotherapists concentrate on the patient's low self-esteem and sense of guilt.

Freud (1917/1957), while propounding possible origins in anger directed inwardly toward an introjected love object, also felt that melancholia accompanied by weight loss, sleep disturbance, diurnal variation, and delusions of guilt might well be organic in origin, and he did not recommend psychoanalytic treatment. This does not mean that he eschewed all treatment of dysphoric moods—and, indeed, many subsequent psychoanalysts treated psychosis and organic conditions—but a trend developed of reserving psychodynamically oriented psychotherapy for young and verbally articulate patients who did not have organic brain disease.

Various psychotherapies for depression, while overtly based on behaviorist rather than psychoanalytic doctrines, owe something to the concept that a weakened ego has become the victim of a punishing superego. In the rational-emotive therapy of Ellis (Dryden 1991) and the cognitive therapy of Beck (Williams 1992), a direct attempt is made to identify and combat the unreasonable self-denigrating beliefs. Although these therapies demand less verbal fluency on the part of the patient than does psychodynamically oriented psychotherapy, they are contingent on some ability to communicate.

Psychotherapists who believe that the stroke patient's depression is a reaction to adverse circumstances will adopt a different approach than that used with depression thought to be endogenous, because the component of guilt and self-blame for one's misfortunes is lacking in reactive depressions. (The patient's sense of worth, however, may be diminished.) In this kind of depression, direct advice, counseling, education, and social or medical interventions are therefore more likely to be used. Group therapy is likely to take the form of a support group (see Chapter 17) consisting of other patients with similar disabilities.

Antidepressant medications and electroconvulsive therapy (ECT), like psychotherapeutic methods, also pose problems when the patient cannot communicate, because such treatments for depression are precise instruments. Applying them properly is not a simple matter. The psychiatrist treating depression by these methods will first of all want to establish a diagnosis, and to elicit the features known to predict a good response to such treatments. This is done primarily by talking to the patient. If the patient cannot talk, determining the right psychopharmacological treatment is almost as difficult as conducting psychotherapy.

Antidepressant Medication

Because stroke patients are often elderly individuals with concurrent medical illness, the administration of antidepressant drugs requires prudence. Many such patients are already taking five or six different drugs, which increases the possibility of adverse reactions, drug interactions, and side effects. Cardiovascular actions and seizure precipitation are antidepressant drug effects that warrant special consideration in stroke.

The side effects of the older generation of tricyclic antidepressants—amitriptyline (Elavil), nortriptyline (Pamelor, Aventyl), imipramine (Tofranil), trimipramine (Surmontil), and desipramine (Norpramin, Pertofrane)—are anticholinergic. Such effects include dryness of the mouth, blurring of vision, constipation, retention of urine, acute closed-angle glaucoma, and delirium. All of these are particularly likely to be problems for elderly patients. The cardiovascular effects are quinidine-like, with varying effects on cardiac impulse conduction.

Despite these side effects, the tricyclics have advantages and are frequently used, especially when a patient has previously responded to them or one of the newer drugs has not been successful. Their advantages include the extensive experience that has been gained with them and the ready availability of blood levels for help in regulating dosage. Many practitioners favor nortriptyline for the elderly (Salzman et al. 1993). Lofepramine and dothiepin are the most popular choices of psychiatrists working with elderly patients in Great Britain (Wattis et al. 1994).

Problems with side effects have led to the introduction of newer antidepressants that have fewer anticholinergic properties and are more precisely targeted at serotonin or norepinephrine reuptake. These include trazodone (Desyrel), bupropion (Wellbutrin), sertraline (Zoloft), paroxetine (Paxil), fluoxetine (Prozac), and venlafaxine (Effexor). This newer group of drugs is now used more commonly than the tricyclics in initial treatment of depression, but literature concerning their use in stroke is limited (Berthier and Kulisevsky 1993). A variety of other drugs are also used in the treatment of refractory depression, but are less likely to find a place in the treatment of the elderly stroke patient with multiple medical problems.

Some psychiatrists insist that most apparent failures of antidepressant drugs are due to inadequate trials. They recommend high dosages, with blood tests to ensure adequate serum levels, and emphasize that the drugs may take several weeks to show benefit.

Although the effectiveness of the medications in certain types of depression is no longer widely doubted, the results in double-blind trials in poststroke patients have been equivocal. Reding et al. (1986) used trazodone, and Lipsey et al. (1984) used nortriptyline. Six out of the 17 patients given the nortriptyline had to stop treatment because of side effects. Reding suggested that, in retrospect, there was a group of patients with abnormal dexamethasone suppression tests who benefited from trazodone. In Åström et al.'s series (1993b), most of those treated with antidepressant medications discontinued the drugs after short periods because of side effects or were eliminated from the trials because of poor compliance.

The most unequivocal justification for use of organic treatments is in a patient who previously had a depression that responded well to such medications and is now experiencing a depression with similar features. Stroke and depression are two very common conditions, so that some overlap may occur by chance. Patients with circular manic-depressive disorder, for example, may continue to have spells of elation and depression after a stroke. In such cases, two independent illnesses overlap.

Electroconvulsive Therapy

ECT is sometimes described as being controversial. In fact, this treatment's place in modern psychiatry, in certain limited circumstances, is well established, and it is somewhat safer than most drugs. Nevertheless, ECT is regarded as an extreme and dangerous remedy by the general public. This opprobrium, however unmerited, realistically limits its use to cases of severe and life-endangering depression. Positive indications for the use of ECT in depression include the presence of delusions, the presence of the vegetative signs of endogenous depression, and previous good response to ECT (Vanelle 1991).

The medical risks of modern ECT are lower than those of the anesthesia that is administered before ECT treatment. If the anesthesiologist can safely put the patient to sleep, then the psychiatrist can safely administer the ECT. Stroke patients tend to have a high risk of heart disease, and this condition must be monitored during anesthesia for ECT, just as it must be with any other anesthesia. A transient rise in blood pressure of about 20 mm Hg occurs during the treatment (Mulgaokar et al. 1985). Theoretically, such a rise in pressure could be dangerous in the presence of a berry aneurysm, but no cases have been reported of subarachnoid hemorrhage precipitated by ECT. It is important in patients with evidence of cerebrovascular disease to assess cognitive function prior to and throughout a course of ECT (Benbow and Slade 1995). Murray et al. (1986) described ECT treatment of 14 patients with poststroke depression and reviewed the possible risks. One of their patients had a transitory cardiac arrhythmia. No patient experienced a worsening of neurological status as a result of the treatment.

Eclectic Approaches

In practice, the treatment of poststroke depression is usually eclectic. A fairly typical example is the following consultation done for an internist, who had asked for a psychiatric consultation after having consulted with a neurologist.

> Mrs. R was a 70-year-old patient with a left hemiparesis who was seen in the hospital because of failure to rehabilitate and antagonistic attitudes toward the staff. The only psychiatric history prior to the stroke was that, on some occasions, she had had chlordiazepoxide (Librium) prescribed by her family physician. On these occasions, she might have been nervous. She had been going to work until the day before her stroke. She knitted, sewed, and gardened. Her husband had recently had open-heart surgery. He said that she had been looking after him prior to the stroke. It was not clear why he needed looking after, and he was so upset that he could not explain. They had one daughter and one son, both of whom were involved and concerned. On examination, Mrs. R was in bed and in a hospital gown at 2:00 in the afternoon. Her right limbs were paretic, but her speech was not obviously impaired. The nursing staff reported that she was incontinent of urine, and she was diapered. Her mood was negative, with statements that she was depressed and complaints of difficulty sleeping. There was a great deal of anger and resentment. She was querulous and demanding and an unpopular patient. Her daughter said that this was contrary to her previous personality. Mrs. R complained that she was not getting enough therapy, but the physical therapists complained that she was uncooperative and used the word "depressed" to describe how she felt.
>
> It was recommended that Mrs. R not spend too much time in bed, that she wear day clothes in the daytime, and that she have visits outside the hospital. The physical therapists, occupational therapists, and nurses agreed that she should be involved in a program of recreational group activities. A program of bladder training was suggested. Although she did not have all the classic symptoms of a medication-responsive depression, trazodone (Desyrel) was suggested, starting at 100 mg each night. This particular antidepressant was chosen because of her complaint of insomnia, and because her electrocardiogram (ECG) showed a left bundle branch block, which is a relative contraindication to the older tricyclics. Discussion with the utilization

review committee regarding insurance coverage for this regimen on a medical floor was suggested, with possible transfer to a psychiatric or stroke unit.

The Human Touch

Accurate and precise diagnosis of depression is important, because the specific treatments for its pathological forms and organic treatments of major mood disorders are among the most effective in modern medicine. In addition, failure to use them, when properly indicated, can be grounds for a malpractice suit (Kingsley 1991). Nevertheless, both organic treatments and psychotherapy have limitations in stroke, and a third kind of treatment may be more important.

When stroke patients describe what helped them feel better, it is usually some touch of human sympathy or ray of optimism rather than any antidepressant medication. However, these warm and helpful human touches are not usually a part of formal psychotherapy. They do not occur during sessions in the office of a psychiatrist or psychologist. The therapists to whom gratitude is expressed do not think of themselves as psychotherapists, and may be chagrined to find that they are so regarded by these patients.

When the first-person narrators say good things about their neurologists, internists, speech therapists, occupational therapists, and physical therapists, they are usually referring to those people's warm and caring personalities rather than to any technical marvels they accomplished. Josephs (1992) said that "doctors forget the healing quality from just a few words of encouragement. Words which may turn nightmare into hope, and hope into health" (p. 33).

Common humanity and cheerful and considerate care will go a long way toward elevating mood. Isaacs (1976), in Scotland, found that patients often did not receive physical therapy and rehabilitation services recommended by their physicians and that social work services to ensure patient rights in finances and housing were needed. Dealing with social isolation by participating in activities such as a stroke club was helpful. (See Appendix B for the address of the National Stroke Association.)

Perhaps the last word regarding this topic should belong to a proponent of a psychological approach:

I had my first stroke April 82 and second one July 84. Both on my right side. I have learned to do everything with my left side as you [can] tell from this writing. Had my gas pedal put on left side so I could drive my car. I am 62 years old and live alone. Do everything for myself.

It has been awful and still is at times. I had to fight this alone, my family just seem to turn from me. Oh, how that hurt. Then two years ago I was walking out to my car at Madison Hospital after therapy. Steve, a boy that was in the hospital for cure from drugs, ask me what would make me happy. I said, talk to my son. He ask his number. Called him that night and my son called me. Now my son and his family so good to me. I don't know what that boy said to my son, but thank God for Steve.

I have been taking therapy until two months ago at Madison Hospital. They call me when they have a stroke patient and I go talk to them, or cry, laugh, pray or whatever they need. I have learned so much by fighting this alone.

The main thing is don't give up, and trust. What hurts most is people stare at my walk, cane and brace.

I wish I could have pretty shoes for the brace. Then I thank God I can walk. (V.G. 1987)

Summary

There is evidence for an entity of poststroke depression that has certain specific features and that is not merely a reaction to a depressing situation. This entity may depend on the location of the infarct, and there is evidence that it is especially associated with left anterior infarcts. Other negative moods, such as anxiety and irritability, may mimic depression in stroke. Spontaneous weeping in stroke may cause distress but is not due to major depression. Psychotherapy with depressed stroke patients is often impeded by dementia or aphasia. Antidepressant drugs may have cardiovascular or neurological side effects. Some cases of depression respond better to electroconvulsive therapy (ECT) than to drugs or psychotherapy. ECT causes a slight transient rise in blood pressure but has been used safely in stroke patients, the main risks being those of anesthesia. Social work services to help patients with finances, housing, and isolation are often needed. Stroke patients who are depressed attach more importance to friendly and encouraging attitudes than to specific antidepressant treatments.

References

American Psychiatric Association: Diagnostic and Statistical Manual of Mental Disorders, 3rd Edition, Revised. Washington, DC, American Psychiatric Association, 1987

American Psychiatric Association: Diagnostic and Statistical Manual of Mental Disorders, 4th Edition. Washington, DC, American Psychiatric Association, 1994

Åström M, Olsen T, Asplund K: Different linkage of depression to hypercorticolism early versus late after stroke. Stroke 24:52–57, 1993a

Åström M, Adolfsson R, Asplund K: Major depression in stroke patients: a 3-year longitudinal study. Stroke 24:976–982, 1993b

Benbow SM, Slade R: ECT for patients with cerebrovascular disease (letter). International Journal of Geriatric Psychiatry 10:419, 1995

Berthier ML, Kulisevsky J: Fluoxetine-induced mania in a patient with poststroke depression (letter). Br J Psychiatry 163:698–699, 1993

Bolla-Wilson K, Robinson RG, Starkstein SE, et al: Lateralization of dementia of depression in stroke patients. Am J Psychiatry 146:627–634, 1989

Brink TL, Yesavage JA, Lum O: Screening tests for geriatric depression. Clinical Gerontologist 1:37–43, 1982

Caine ED, Lyness JM, King DA: Reconsidering depression in the elderly. American Journal of Geriatric Psychiatry 1:4–20, 1993

de Haan RJ, Limburg M, van der Meulen JHP, et al: Quality of life after stroke: impact of stroke type and lesion location. Stroke 26:402–408, 1995

Delvenne V, Delecluse F, Hubain PP, et al: Regional cerebral blood flow in patients with affective disorders. Br J Psychiatry 157:359–365, 1990

Dryden W: Reason and Therapeutic Change. London, Whurr Publishers, 1991

Eastwood MR, Rifat SL, Nobbs H, et al: Mood disorders following cerebrovascular accident. Br J Psychiatry 154:195–200, 1989

Ebrahim S, Barer D, Nouri F: Affective illness after stroke. Br J Psychiatry 151:52–56, 1987

Elon R, Pawlson IG: The impact of OBRA on medical practice within nursing facilities. J Am Geriatr Soc 40:958–963, 1992

Fedoroff JP, Starkstein SE, Parikh RM, et al: Are depressive symptoms nonspecific in patients with acute stroke? Am J Psychiatry 148:1172–1176, 1991

Feibel JH, Springer CJ: Depression and failure to resume social activities after stroke. Arch Phys Med Rehabil 63:276–278, 1982

Finklestein S, Benowitz LI, Baldessarini RJ, et al: Mood, vegetative disturbance, and dexamethasone suppression test after stroke. Ann Neurol 12:463–468, 1982

Fischer P, Simanyi M, Danielczyk W: Depression in dementia of the Alzheimer type and in multi-infarct dementia. Am J Psychiatry 147:1484–1487, 1990

Folstein MF, Maiberger R, McHugh PR: Mood disorder as a specific complication of stroke. J Neurol Neurosurg Psychiatry 40:1018–1020, 1977

Freud S: Mourning and melancholia (1917 [1915]), in The Standard Edition of the Complete Psychological Works of Sigmund Freud, Vol 14. Translated and edited by Strachey J. London, Hogarth Press, 1957, pp 237–260

Goodstein RK: Overview: cerebrovascular accident and the hospitalized elderly—a multidimensional clinical problem. Am J Psychiatry 140:141–148, 1983

Hamilton MA: A rating scale for depression. J Neurol Neurosurg Psychiatry 23:56–62, 1960

Herrmann M, Bartels C, Schumacher M, et al: Poststroke depression. Stroke 26:850–856, 1995

House A, Dennis M, Hawton K, et al: Methods of identifying mood disorders in stroke patients: experience in the Oxfordshire community stroke project. Age Ageing 18:371–379, 1989

House A, Dennis M, Mogridge L, et al: Mood disorders in the year after first stroke. Br J Psychiatry 158:83–92, 1991

Isaacs B, Neville Y, Rushford I: The stricken: the social consequences of stroke. Age Ageing 5:188–192, 1976

Jeste DV, Lohr JB, Goodwin FK: Neuroanatomical studies of major affective disorders: a review and suggestions for further research. BMJ 153:444–460, 1988

Josephs A: Stroke: An Owner's Manual. Long Beach, CA, Amadeus Press, 1992

Kingsley PL: Comments on the Klerman-Stone debate on *Osheroff v. Chestnut Lodge* (letter). Am J Psychiatry 148:139, 1991

Lipsey JR, Robinson RG, Pearlson GD, et al: Mood change following bilateral hemisphere brain injury. Br J Psychiatry 143:266–273, 1983

Lipsey JR, Robinson RG, Pearlson GD: Nortriptyline treatment of poststroke depression: a double blind study. Lancet 1:297–300, 1984

Lipsey JR, Robinson RG, Pearlson GD, et al: The dexamethasone suppression test and mood following stroke. Am J Psychiatry 143:318–323, 1985

Lipsey JR, Spencer WC, Rabins PV, et al: Phenomenological comparison of post-stroke depression and functional depression. Am J Psychiatry 143:527–529, 1986

Lishman WA: Brain damage in relation to psychiatric disability after head injury. Br J Psychiatry 114:373–410, 1968

Mahoney FI, Barthel D: Functional evaluations: the Barthel index. Maryland State Medical Journal 14:61–65, 1965

Mulgaokar GD, Dauchot PJ, Duffy JP, et al: Non-invasive assessment of electroconvulsive-induced changes in cardiac function. J Clin Psychiatry 46:479–488, 1985

Murray GB, Shea V, Conn DK: Electroconvulsive therapy for post-stroke depression. J Clin Psychiatry 47:258–260, 1986

Parmelee PA, Katz IR, Lawton MP: Depression among institutionalized aged. J Gerontol 1:M22–M29, 1989

Pintoff E: Bolt From the Blue. Salt Lake City, UT, Northwest, 1992

Primeau F: Post-stroke depression: a critical review of the literature. Can J Psychiatry 33:757–765, 1988

Radloff LS: The CES-D scale: a self-report depression scale for research in the general population. Applied Psychological Measurement 1:385–401, 1977

Reding MJ, Orto LA, Winter SW, et al: Antidepressant therapy after stroke: a double blind trial. Arch Neurol 43:763–765, 1986

Robins A: Are stroke patients more depressed than other disabled subjects? Journal of Chronic Disease 29:479–482, 1976

Robinson RG, Coyle JT: The differential effect of right versus left hemisphere cerebral infarction on catecholamines and behavior in the rat. Brain Res 188:63–78, 1980

Robinson RG, Szetela B: Mood change following left hemispheric brain injury. Ann Neurol 9:447–453, 1981

Robinson RG, Kubos KL, Starr LB, et al: Mood disorder in stroke patients: importance of location of lesion. Brain 107:81–93, 1984

Robinson RG, Lipsey JR, Bolla-Wilson K, et al: Mood disorders in left-handed stroke patients. Am J Psychiatry 142:1424–1429, 1985

Ross ED: The aprosodias: functional-anatomical organization of the affective components of language in the right hemisphere. Arch Neurol 38:561–569, 1981

Ross ED, Rush JA: Diagnosis and neuroanatomical correlates of depression in brain-damaged patients. Arch Gen Psychiatry 38:1344–1354, 1981

Salzman C, Schneider LS, Lebowitz BD: Antidepressant treatment of very old patients. American Journal of Geriatric Psychiatry 1:21–29, 1993

Sharpe M, Hawton K, House A, et al: Mood disorders in long-term survivors of stroke. Psychol Med 20:815–828, 1990

Sharpe M, Hawton K, Seagroatt V, et al: Depressive disorders in long-term survivors of stroke. Br J Psychiatry 164:380–386, 1994

Shinar D, Gross CR, Price TR, et al: Screening for depression in stroke patients. Stroke 17:241–245, 1986

Signer S, Cummings JL, Benson DF: Delusions and mood disorders in patients with chronic aphasia. Journal of Neuropsychiatry 1:40–45, 1989

Starkstein SE, Robinson RG, Price TR: Comparison of cortical and subcortical lesions in the production of poststroke mood disorders. Brain 110:1045–1059, 1987

Starkstein SE, Berthier ML, Fedoroff JP, et al: Anosognosia and major depression in two patients with cerebrovascular lesions. Neurology 40:1380–1382, 1990

Stern RA, Bachman DL: Depressive symptoms following stroke. Am J Psychiatry 148:351–356, 1991

Stern RA, Hooper SC, Morey CE: Development of visual analogue scales to measure mood in aphasia (abstract). Clinical Neuropsychologist 4:300, 1990

Sunderland T, Hill HL, Lawlor BA, et al: NIMH dementia mood assessment scale. Psychopharmacol Bull 24:747–753, 1988

Thiessen BQ, Wallace SM, Blackburn JL, et al: Increased prescribing of antidepressants subsequent to beta-blocker therapy. Arch Intern Med 150:2286–2290, 1990

Vanelle JM: Facteurs prédictifs de la réponse aux Électronarcoses. Encéphale 17 (Spec No 3):399–404, 1991

"V. G.": Readers' reflections. Open Channels (a publication of the National Stroke Association) 4:unpaged, 1987

Wattis J, Bentham P, Bestley J: Choice of antidepressants by psychiatrists working with old people. Psychiatric Bulletin 18:148–151, 1994

Wender D: At the edge of silence. Family Circle (March 26):62–69, 1986

Williams MG: The Psychological Treatment of Depression: A Guide to the Theory and Practice of Cognitive Behavior Therapy, 2nd Edition. London, Routledge, 1992

World Health Organization: International Statistical Classification of Diseases and Related Health Problems, 10th Revision. Geneva, Switzerland, World Health Organization, 1992

Zung WWK: A self-rating depression scale. Arch Gen Psychiatry 12:63, 1965

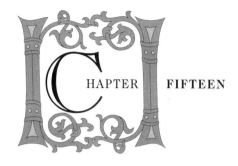

CHAPTER FIFTEEN

Anxiety

S troke is one of the dread illnesses whose name arouses fear. This evocation in itself constitutes a plausible link between stroke and anxiety, but there are other, more complex relationships.

The connection between stroke and anxiety differs from that between stroke and depression in that there is no body of evidence establishing that localized infarcts are a biological cause of anxiety. There are, however, possible biological associations between stroke and anxiety and between high blood pressure and anxiety. Some forms of anxiety produce symptoms of a physical nature that can mimic those of stroke, and the ubiquitous symptom of dizziness includes both stroke and anxiety in its differential diagnosis.

Diagnostic Aspects of Stroke and Anxiety

Anxiety is so universal a human experience that some feel that psychiatric attempts to label its varieties are misbegotten. Anxiety parallels depression in having an intuitively obvious dichotomy: one kind of anxiety is intrinsic to the individual, and another kind is caused externally. The former is sometimes called *trait anxiety* and the latter, *state anxiety*.

The varieties of anxiety disorder recognized in DSM-IV (American Psychiatric Press 1994) are generalized anxiety disorder, panic disorder, and anxiety disorder due to a general medical condition. (This last diagnosis applies only to cases in which the anxiety is biologically rather than psychologically due to the medical condition.)

The group of disorders in which anxiety is provoked to an abnormal degree by a situation that would be manageable for most people includes obsessive-compulsive disorder, simple phobia, social phobia, agoraphobia, and perhaps posttraumatic stress disorder.

If the anxiety is an understandable result of the stress imposed by a medical illness, DSM-IV would classify it as *adjustment disorder with anxiety*. ICD-10 (World Health Organization 1992) apparently does not find it feasible to separate the emotions under these circumstances, allowing only for *adjustment disorder with mixed anxiety and depressive reaction*.

Differentiation of Stroke From Anxiety

Panic Attacks and Agoraphobia

An acute panic attack is a devastating experience that can puzzle and alarm patients and health care workers alike. Such attacks constitute a very convincing simulacrum of physical illness. Because of the intensely felt physical symptoms, patients with panic attacks and agoraphobia often seek treatment from a general practitioner, internist, or neurologist, rather than a psychiatrist.

A panic attack involves shaking, sweating, rapid pulse, tingling of the hands and feet, chest pain, and difficulty breathing; there is dizziness, a sense of unreality, and an urgent fear that if the attack is prolonged 1 second more, something dreadful will happen. The feared "something dreadful" varies—it may be completely unnameable or it may be losing control, passing out, going insane, dying, or having a heart attack. Very often it is having a stroke. The person having a panic attack suffers social embarrassment and often tries to conceal the attack. This disproportionate concern for public opinion is a useful diagnostic point.

Agoraphobia is closely related to panic attacks. The individual with agoraphobia (who is usually female) does not say that she is frightened of supermarkets or elevators, but comes to the physician complaining of panic attack symptoms. On questioning, it is found that these symptoms are more likely to occur when the patient is far from home, or in situations from which there is no easy escape, and that the presence of a "safety person"—usually a close relative—can provide some measure of protection against them.

Psychogenic Syncope

Simple phobias are more specific and more easily recognized than is agoraphobia. They are also more akin to straightforward fear and do not produce the same range of physically felt symptoms. Sometimes the cardiovascular symptoms experienced in simple phobia are opposite in kind from those in panic and agoraphobia, and a vasovagal syncope is produced in which the pulse becomes slow rather than fast, the skin becomes pale, and blood pressure drops. The patient often loses consciousness (something the agoraphobic person fears will happen, although it seldom does in that disorder). This kind of reaction is produced especially by the sight of blood or medical procedures.

Vasovagal syncope enters into the differential diagnosis of attacks of unconsciousness. It can usually easily be distinguished clinically from stroke if the patient is seen during the acute attack, or if the psychological precipitants are known.

Dizziness

Both stroke and anxiety enter into the differential diagnosis of dizziness. This symptom is the most common reason for a patient over 72 years of age to visit a physician (National Center for Health Statistics 1984), and about one-fifth of elderly people occasionally experience dizziness (Sloane et al. 1989). Most dizziness seems to be psychological in origin, with patients characteristically describing themselves as nervous or depressed. A distinction can sometimes be made between true vertigo—the world spinning around—and a sensation of unsteadiness, but making this distinction requires good communication, fluent verbalization, and patience. The patient should ideally have time to give a spontaneous account of the symptom, but in doing so may introduce elements that seem irrelevant to the health practitioner, who may then respond by posing questions in a way that can seem brusque and overbearing. If, as the interview develops, it becomes apparent that the kind of dizziness being described is unlikely to be easily treatable, the practitioner can be tempted to rush to terminate the patient's session.

Slight abnormalities of the semicircular canals in the ear can produce an alarming vertigo that may convince people who experience such abnormalities that they are severely ill. Recurrent attacks of vertigo occur in Ménière's disease. Convincing people who have this disorder that they have not had strokes is not easy. Even after a careful and accurate diagnosis of Ménière's disease, the patient may remain convinced of having had a stroke and reexperience this conviction upon subsequent attacks.

The patient who presents with reports of dizziness but who has no stroke history or other neurological signs is unlikely to have had a stroke; however, an association of true vertigo with vascular disease can occur in disease of the vertebral and basilar arteries. Some cases of positional vertigo may be caused by brief kinking of the vertebral arteries. *Lateral medullary syndrome* (Wallenberg's syndrome), which is caused by infarction in the area supplied by the posterior inferior cerebellar artery, results in vertigo, disturbance of sensation on one side of the face and body, and various cranial nerve signs and symptoms—a cluster of phenomena that enables clinical diagnosis of the fully developed syndrome.

Although complaints of dizziness may increase after a diagnosed stroke (Åström et al. 1992), the presence of dizziness does not in itself predict a subsequent stroke (Boult et al. 1991; Sloane et al. 1989).

Transient Ischemic Attack

Transient ischemic attack (TIA) is one of the differential diagnoses that may be considered in panic disorder or agoraphobia, although the official consensus report on the diagnosis of TIA (National Institute of Neurological Disorders and Stroke [NINDS] 1990) does not specifically mention these conditions. The report states that dizziness is not to be regarded as a manifestation of TIA and that an attack that does not include motor defects, visual loss, or aphasia should be reviewed carefully before accepting TIA as the diagnosis (NINDS 1990).

Causes of Anxiety in Stroke

Stroke as a Cause of Anxiety

Anxiety typically does not precede the first stroke. The initial attack of unconsciousness is not ushered in by fear and does not come at the culmination of anything subjectively resembling a panic attack. Stocklin (1989) refers to herself as having felt "tired and deliciously sleepy." The emotional experience on return to consciousness includes bewildered

and dreamlike sensations but, according to the self-reports, is not typically dominated by fear.

Subsequent to recovery, fear of a second stroke becomes prominent
(Singler 1975). This fear is not so apparent in those with very severe
disability or those with no disability at all. It is greatest among those who
retain and cherish a capacity for independence in the face of an incapacity
that constantly reminds them of their vulnerability. Åström (1996) found
that stroke patients with anxiety were more likely to live alone and to
have fewer social contacts. She observed that the stress of sustaining a
stroke rendered those patients who lacked the support of a live-in family
particularly vulnerable to developing both anxiety disorder and depression. Anxiety is not universal, and it has been suggested that in some
patients with right-hemisphere infarcts there is a pathological lack of
anxiety. Such patients show an indifference that hampers rehabilitation
and social relationships (Williams 1992).

Anxiety and nervousness are most frequently experienced during the
first year after a stroke (Åström et al. 1992). Sharpe et al. (1990) found
that 20% of 60 surviving patients from a community-based stroke register,
when interviewed 3–5 years after their first stroke, suffered from anxiety
disorders, and that anxiety was more common than depression.

Anxiety as a Cause of Stroke

Patients commonly come to health practitioners to have their blood
pressure checked because they "can feel that it is high." It is unlikely
that high blood pressure can be subjectively felt in this way, although
some evidence exists that anxiety does predict hypertension in middle-
aged men (Markowitz et al. 1993).

The blood pressure rises when taken by a physician—especially if that
individual is a man who is not well known to the patient—by about 25 mm
Hg systolic and 15 mm Hg diastolic above the normal level as measured
by ambulatory blood pressure monitoring (Holverson 1991). This "white-
coat hypertension" is not independently associated with increased risk
of heart problems or stroke, although it is more common in obese and
hypercholesterolemic patients. The pulse rate also rises, which is consistent with an anxiety response. The white-coat effect persists in certain
individuals over many years, and no measure of general anxiety or any
other psychological trait is predisposing.

The white-coat effect may play a part in some of the fluctuations in blood
pressure immediately after stroke. There is a rise in blood pressure in the

acute phase, a fall after the patient has been in the hospital for a while, and then a rise after discharge from the hospital (Fotherby et al. 1993).

The direct effects of a panic attack on blood pressure are less dramatic than patients usually suppose. Patients need reassurance on this point; they are often convinced that during an attack their pressure rises almost to the point where a "blood vessel bursts" or some other cardiovascular catastrophe occurs. One way to reassure patients is to point out the excellent cardiac health enjoyed by marathon runners, who routinely raise their pulses to 200 beats per minute or more.

An occasional cause of an association between hypertension and anxiety is the abrupt withdrawal of sympatholytic drugs, especially those acting on the central nervous system (e.g., clonidine [Catapres]). Such a withdrawal can result in sympathetic overactivity with nervousness, agitation, and headache. Further psychological aspects of stroke risk factors are discussed in Chapter 3.

Surveys

Surveys that depend on self-report to diagnose stroke may exaggerate the association between stroke and anxiety. The larger the sample studied and the more representative it is of the general population, the more likely a survey is to rely on self-report rather than physical examination to detect stroke. Weissman et al. (1990) studied 60 subjects with panic disorder and found that they were twice as likely as control subjects with other psychiatric conditions to say that they had suffered a stroke.

A higher-than-expected rate of cardiovascular mortality in panic disorder was found by Coryell (1986) in a 12-year follow-up of 155 men with anxiety neurosis. According to death certificate information, three of these patients died from cardiovascular causes—one from "ruptured congenital aneurysm," one from "massive myocardial infarction," and one from "pulmonary embolism." There were no cardiovascular deaths in the control group.

Management of Anxiety in Stroke

The development of psychodynamic psychotherapy has been closely bound up with the treatment of anxiety. The limitations of such therapy for the elderly patient with both brain damage and impaired communication have been discussed in Chapter 14. The comments here pertain primarily to the anxiety that is an adjustment reaction to the situation of having a stroke, for which condition the emphasis is on supportive counseling and advice rather than on in-depth probing of unreasonable self-denigrating beliefs.

Reassurance and verbalization are cornerstones of supportive therapy in stroke. Information sought by the patient should be given in full. Some practitioners think that more knowledge will create more anxiety if the reality is that the prognosis is bad. However, more doom and gloom can be picked up from misinformation than from accurate facts. Brutally frank statements of poor prognosis have no place, and such statements are, in any case, seldom valid in stroke. The only patients with inevitably poor prognoses are those unable to take part in a verbal exchange, such as a patient in a coma or with dementia.

Following a stroke, so much of the reassurance needed is about the medical condition itself that psychotherapy cannot be handed over to a non-medical psychotherapist outside the treatment team. Not having a psychotherapist on the team places constraints on the time of the primary treating physician, who tends to be regarded as the sole authoritative source for information. Group therapy is more economical of time, but stroke groups have some drawbacks for the highly anxious patient. If a group contains severely impaired stroke patients or if a group member has a second stroke, an anxious patient's fear of getting worse again may increase.

Another source of reassurance for patients is information pamphlets available from the National Stroke Association and from private organizations. *The Road Ahead: A Stroke Recovery Guide,* issued by the National Stroke Association (1989), is a useful general handbook for stroke patients and their families that contains a great deal of practical advice about dealing with disabilities and getting help. Foley and Pizer's *The Stroke Fact Book* (1985) is even more comprehensive. An additional informational resource is the University of Virginia Medical Center's stroke hotline (1-804-295-9557).

Antianxiety Medications

Most drugs that can cause drowsiness have an antianxiety effect. They also commonly cause addiction and can result in seizures if abruptly withdrawn after prolonged use. This side-effect profile probably reflects a common site of action at the gamma-aminobutyric acid ($GABA_A$) receptors, as described in Chapter 5. The earliest drugs effective specifically in anxiety were phenobarbital and meprobamate; these have largely been replaced by benzodiazepines.

Benzodiazepines. The adverse benzodiazepine effects particularly relevant to stroke—especially in elderly patients—are drowsiness, liability to falls, and impairment of memory (Greenblatt et al. 1991). If these medications are stopped abruptly after being used for extended periods at high dosages, withdrawal effects may include seizures (Schneider et al. 1987). Such effects may occur upon hospitalization in stroke patients who are confused or comatose and whose previous intake is unknown.

A number of benzodiazepines are available, and it is possible that adverse responses can be minimized by judicious choice and dosage. Long-acting benzodiazepines include chlordiazepoxide (Librium), diazepam (Valium), clorazepate (Tranxene), flurazepam (Dalmane), clonazepam (Klonopin), and prazepam (Centrax). Short-acting ones include triazolam (Halcion), alprazolam (Xanax), oxazepam (Serax), and lorazepam (Ativan). The short-acting benzodiazepines are less likely to adversely affect rehabilitation in stroke, probably because the drowsiness and cognitive impairment they produce are less prolonged (Woo et al. 1991). It is governmentally recommended that the long-acting benzodiazepines be avoided in nursing homes (Health Care Financing Administration 1992).

Most practitioners endorse the temporary use of these drugs in anxiety-provoking medical situations, such as before frightening procedures. The benzodiazepines are much used in coronary care units, but their potential to produce drowsiness limits their use in the acute stage of stroke.

The long-term use of benzodiazepines to treat anxiety is controversial (Fernando 1989; Rickels et al. 1991). Some of the objection to such use comes from those who oppose *any* chemical treatment of emotional disorders, and some comes from concern about this class's potentials for addiction and tolerance (Tyrer and Murphy 1987). Given the evidence (Åström et al. 1992) that anxiety following stroke diminishes after the first year, a case can be made for using benzodiazepines during this limited period.

Buspirone.   Buspirone (BuSpar) is a recently introduced antianxiety drug which, unlike most other medications used for this purpose, does not cause drowsiness or addiction, presumably because it does not act—as most hypnotic-anxiolytic drugs do—on the $GABA_A$ receptors. The exact mechanism by which buspirone exerts its anxiolytic effects is not fully understood. However, anxiety disorders are believed to be associated with excessive amounts of serotonin in the synaptic cleft (Eison 1990), and buspirone appears to alter serotonergic transmission through its activity at serotonin receptor sites (Jann 1988).

The obverse side of buspirone's failure to cause drowsiness or addiction is that patients do not experience an immediate sensation of anxiety relief, which may be why this drug has not achieved the popularity of the benzodiazepines. So far, there have been no reports of buspirone's use specifically in stroke.

Treatment of Panic Attacks

Patients who present with panic attacks mimicking a stroke can be referred to mental health practitioners and can be effectively treated by modern methods. The psychological methods commonly used for treatment of agoraphobia and panic attacks are now usually based on behavioral rather than psychodynamic theories. However, the patient's relationship with the "safety person," the embarrassment experienced during the attack, and the restriction of activities produced by fear of subsequent attacks can often be fruitfully explored in psychodynamic therapy.

Many psychiatrists favor the use of medication for anxiety, including tricyclic antidepressants, monoamine oxidase inhibitors, or benzodiazepines. The benzodiazepine most commonly used is alprazolam (Xanax), a relatively short-acting drug with a half-life of 12–15 hours; the tricyclic antidepressant and monoamine oxidase inhibitor most often used are imipramine (Tofranil) and phenelzine (Nardil), respectively. Improvement is more rapid with the benzodiazepines than with antidepressants (Cross-National Collaborative Panic Study 1992).

Because panic disorder is a chronic condition, antianxiety drugs may need to be administered for long periods, and patients tend to relapse when their prescriptions are stopped. Relapse may be accompanied, in the case of benzodiazepines, by actual withdrawal symptoms (Noyes et al. 1991). Notwithstanding these drawbacks, drug treatment is usually effective, inexpensive, and convenient.

Some patients refuse medication, find behavioral remedies worse than the disorder, or are unable to afford office psychotherapy. Even those who respond to treatment sometimes need further reassurance that their symptoms are not due to an impending stroke, and they return to their primary care physician or neurologist for this purpose.

Management of Dizziness

A quandary for the practitioner managing a patient with dizziness is how far to investigate this very common symptom. There is general agreement on the desirability of a good history and physical examination. Investigation for stroke risk factors also seems reasonable. Baloh (1992) concluded that it is inappropriate to dismiss dizziness in elderly patients by attributing it to nonspecific entities, such as multiple sensory defects or presbyastasia, and that the great majority of elderly patients who present to a physician complaining of dizziness have an identifiable cause. He presented a vigorous schema for establishing the cause of dizziness.

Dizziness in the patient who has had a stroke is probably organic in origin, but patients with this symptom seem to respond better to reassurance and encouragement than to medication, although there are no controlled trials of treatment.

Summary

Panic attacks and agoraphobia may be self-diagnosed as stroke. Dizziness is the most common reason for a patient over 72 years of age to see a physician. Complaints of dizziness increase after a previously diagnosed stroke, but the presence of dizziness as a complaint does not in itself predict a subsequent stroke. Anxiety does not typically precede stroke, and stroke does not come at the culmination of anything subjectively resembling a panic attack."White-coat hypertension" is a rise in blood pressure that occurs when the measurement is taken in a formal medical setting. Syncope due to some phobias is vasovagal, with bradycardia and hypotension. The experience of returning to consciousness after stroke includes bewildered and dreamlike sensations but is not typically dominated by fear. After recovery, fear of a second stroke becomes prominent. Anxiety and nervousness are more frequent in the first year after a stroke but tend to diminish thereafter. Treatments for anxiety include medication and psychotherapy. Benzodiazepines are the most commonly used antianxiety medications. Most drugs that reduce anxiety can cause drowsiness, which is probably because they have a common site of action at the $GABA_A$ receptors. Drugs that alter serotonergic transmission can relieve anxiety without causing drowsiness. Explanation and reassurance about the illness are especially important in alleviating patients' anxiety in the aftermath of stroke. Groups may be helpful for stroke patients, but patients' anxiety may increase if a group member's condition worsens.

References

American Psychiatric Association: Diagnostic and Statistical Manual of Mental Disorders, 4th Edition. Washington, DC, American Psychiatric Association, 1994

Åström M: Generalized anxiety disorder in stroke patients. Stroke 27:270–275, 1996

Åström M, Asplund K, Åström T: Psychosocial function and life satisfaction after stroke. Stroke 23:527–531, 1992

Baloh RW: Dizziness in older people. J Am Geriatr Soc 40:713–721, 1992

Boult C, Murphy J, Sloane P, et al: The relation of dizziness to functional decline. J Am Geriatr Soc 39:858–861, 1991

Coryell W: Mortality among outpatients with anxiety disorders. Am J Psychiatry 143:508–510, 1986

Cross-National Collaborative Panic Study: Drug treatment of panic disorder: comparative efficacy of alprazolam, imipramine, and placebo. Br J Psychiatry 160:191–202, 1992

Eison MS: Serotonin: a common neurobiologic substrate in anxiety and depression. J Clin Psychopharmacol 10:26S–30S, 1990

Fernando L: Benzodiazepines unabashed (letter). Br J Psychiatry 155:717, 1989

Foley C, Pizer HF: The Stroke Fact Book. New York, Bantam Books, 1985

Fotherby MD, Potter JF, Panayiotu B, et al: Blood pressure changes after stroke (letter). Stroke 24:1422, 1993

Greenblatt DJ, Harmatz JS, Shapiro L, et al: Sensitivity to triazolam in the elderly. N Engl J Med 324:1691–1698, 1991

Health Care Financing Administration: Transmittal 250, Interpretive Guidelines, 483.25(1)(1). Washington, DC, Department of Health and Human Services, April 1992

Holverson HE: The "white coat" response to blood pressure measurement. Intern Med 12:24–32, 1991

Jann MW: Buspirone: an update on a unique anxiolytic agent. Pharmacotherapy 8:100–116, 1988

Markowitz JH, Matthews KA, Kannel WB, et al: Psychological predictors of hypertension in the Framingham study: is there tension in hypertension? JAMA 270:2439–2443, 1993

National Center for Health Statistics: Patterns of ambulatory care in internal medicine: the National Ambulatory Care Survey—United States, January 1980–December 1981 (Vital and Health Statistics Series 13, No 80; DHSS Publ No PHS-84-1741). Washington, DC, U.S. Government Printing Office, September 1984

National Institute of Neurological Disorders and Stroke: Classification of cerebrovascular diseases, III. Stroke 21:637–676, 1990

National Stroke Association: The Road Ahead: A Stroke Recovery Guide. Englewood, CO, National Stroke Association, 1989

Noyes R, Garvey MJ, Cook B, et al: Controlled discontinuation of benzodiazepine treatment for patients with panic disorders. Am J Psychiatry 148:517–523, 1991

Rickels K, Case WG, Schweizer E, et al: Long-term benzodiazepine users 3 years after participation in a discontinuation program. Am J Psychiatry 148:757–761, 1991

Schneider LS, Syapin PJ, Pawluczyk S: Seizures following triazolam withdrawal despite benzodiazepine treatment. J Clin Psychiatry 48:418–419, 1987

Sharpe M, Hawton K, House A, et al: Mood disorders in long-term survivors of stroke. Psychol Med 20:815–828, 1990

Singler JR: Group work with hospitalized stroke patients. Social Casework 56:348–354, 1975

Sloane P, Blazer D, George LK: Dizziness in a community elderly population. J Am Geriatr Soc 37:101–108, 1989

Stocklin A: My Stroke, My Blessing. Aurora, CO, Charles Delperdang, 1989

Tyrer P, Murphy S: The place of benzodiazepines in psychiatric practice. Br J Psychiatry 151:719–723, 1987

Weissman MM, Markowitz JS, Ouellette R, et al: Panic disorder and cardiovascular problems. Am J Psychiatry 147:1504–1508, 1990

Williams AM: Self-report of indifference and anxiety among persons with right hemisphere stroke. Res Nurs Health 15:343–347, 1992

Woo E, Proulx SM, Greenblatt DJ: Differential side effect profile of triazolam versus flurazepam in elderly patients undergoing rehabilitation therapy. J Clin Pharmacol 31:168–173, 1991

World Health Organization: International Statistical Classification of Diseases and Related Health Problems, 10th Revision. Geneva, Switzerland, World Health Organization, 1992

CHAPTER SIXTEEN

Dementia

In 1894, Alzheimer presented to the annual meeting of the Society of German Psychiatrists in Dresden his observations on 12 cases of arteriosclerotic atrophy of the brain (reprinted in translation by Foerstl and Levy 1991). The early stages of this disease were marked by headache, dizziness, fatigue, and weakness of thinking. In some cases, the illness began with an apoplectic attack in a person previously in normal mental health. Thereafter, there was increasing weakness of thought and judgment, although definite delusions were usually absent.

Alzheimer found that in this condition, as well as in the condition now called Alzheimer's disease and in syphilis of the brain, there were clinical features not found in melancholia or dementia praecox (schizophrenia). This observation led other psychiatrists, such as Kraepelin and Bonhoeffer, to establish a major division between *functional* and *organic* psychoses.

In illnesses such as schizophrenia and manic-depressive disorder, Alzheimer and his contemporaries saw no obvious diagnostic abnormalities on brain examination at autopsy. They noted that in these conditions, memory and certain intellectual abilities—those that are often loosely called *cognitive functions* by neurologists and psychiatrists—remained intact. (The definitions of cognitive function in the psychological literature are more precise).

Some kinds of brain damage impair memory and the kind of reasoning involved in playing chess or doing mathematics. Older books and older physicians will sometimes use *organic brain syndrome* for conditions of this type, but in some organically induced psychoses, such as the paranoid psychosis produced by chronic amphetamine use, memory is not affected. There is also increasing evidence of a biochemical disorder in schizophrenia and affective illnesses. The term *organic mental disorder* was therefore dropped from DSM-IV (American Psychiatric Association 1994). It was replaced by a category of "cognitive disorders" that comprises three entities: dementia, delirium, and amnestic disorders (American Psychiatric Association 1991).

The *organic mental disorder* of ICD-10 (World Health Organization 1992) includes several entities, three of which involve impaired memory and cognitive function: dementia, delirium, and amnestic disorder.

Diagnosis

Definition of Dementia

Although dementia is a useful working concept, debate and confusion continue regarding its exact definition. This definitional debate impinges especially on stroke, because vascular disease produces several entities that closely resemble dementia. These entities include disorders of language and memory, the separation of which from dementia may also be a matter of definition.

Attempts to define dementia precisely are relatively recent, and the development of the concept was gradual. The word *dementia* first appeared in English as a translation of the word *démence* in French psychiatric texts, which referred to a generalized loss of mental functions, as opposed to mania or melancholia. The forms occurring in elderly and syphilitic patients were later designated *dementia senilis* and *dementia paralytica,* and that in the young was termed *dementia praecox.* It was recognized that in dementia praecox, primary disturbances of memory and orientation were absent.

ICD-10 defines dementia as "a syndrome due to disease of the brain, usually of a chronic or progressive nature, in which there is a disturbance of multiple higher cortical functions, including memory, thinking, orientation, comprehension, calculation, learning capacity, language, and judgment" (World Health Organization 1992, p. 312).

The definition of dementia in DSM-III-R (American Psychiatric Association 1987) was more complex, with five criteria, designated A, B, C, D, and E. (Criteria B and E each contained alternative criteria.) Criterion A was the presence of impairment in long- and short-term memory. The four alternatives in B were impaired abstract thinking; impaired judgment; other disturbances of higher cortical function, such as aphasia, apraxia, agnosia, and "constructional difficulty"; or personality change (American Psychiatric Association 1987, p. 107). Criterion C was that the disturbance in A and B significantly interfered with work, usual social activities, or relationships with others. Criterion D stated that delirium must be absent. Criterion E contained two alternatives: evidence of a causative organic factor or absence of a nonorganic factor that could account for the illness.

This DSM-III-R definition was criticized in the *DSM-IV Options Book* (American Psychiatric Association 1991) because "the central construct of Dementia (i.e., the development of multiple cognitive deficits) was not clearly stated; and the inclusion of criterion B(4) (personality change) allowed individuals with memory loss and some mild personality change to be diagnosed as having Dementia instead of the more appropriate Amnestic Disorder" (p. D:6).

In conclusion, a succinct and generally accepted definition of dementia is elusive. For purposes of discussion, dementia will be considered here as an entity distinct from circumscribed neurological disabilities such as aphasia, apraxia, agnosia, and limited memory deficits. Table 16–1 presents working criteria for dementia and other cognitive disorders based on a synthesis of traditional usage and the official definitions.

Delirium.   There is even more disagreement about the definition of delirium than about that of dementia (Liptzin 1991; Spitzer 1991). *Delirium* was originally a term used in general medicine to describe confusion and other mental changes manifested in the course of fevers and toxic states. Almost one-half of hospitalized elderly patients experience delirium, according to some authorities and definitions (Lipowski 1992).

In traditional medical usage, delirium was a temporary state. According to ICD-10, the condition may last with fluctuations for up to 6 months. Some clinicians regard delirium as a form of dementia distinguished only by acute onset and fluctuations. Specific features such as illusions, hallucinations, rapid fragmented speech, and restlessness are recognized; some authorities insist that these must be present to make the diagnosis and that these features differentiate delirium from dementia. The term is also used synonymously with *acute brain syndrome, acute exogenous reaction type, acute confusional state, toxic psychosis,* and *metabolic encephalopathy.*

The DSM definitions have undergone many modifications and are not always accepted by nonpsychiatrists. The DSM-IV definition is very broad,

Table 16–1.   Symptoms in cognitive disorders

	Dementia	Delirium	Aphasia	Amnestic syndromes of vascular origin	
				Hippo-campal ischemia	Transient global amnesia
Long-term memory	Impaired	Impaired	Intact	Intact	Impaired
Ability to learn new material	Impaired	Impaired	Intact	Impaired	Impaired
Visual memory	Impaired	Impaired	Intact	Intact	Impaired
Performance on multiple-item tests for dementia	Impaired	Impaired	Impaired	Impaired	Impaired
ADL skills	Impaired	Impaired	Intact	Intact	Intact
Arithmetic skills	Impaired	Impaired	Intact	Intact	Intact
Medical illness outside the central nervous system	Absent	Present	Absent	Absent	Absent
Brain findings	Variable damage	Anatomically normal in most cases	Left brain damage	Damage to hippocampus	Not known
Aphasia	May be present by DSM-IV definition	Absent	Present by definition	Absent	Absent

Note.   ADL = activities of daily living. DSM-IV (American Psychiatric Association 1994).

requiring a rapid onset of mental disturbance due to a nonpsychiatric medical condition, with impairment of consciousness and changes in cognition. Such changes may include memory deficit, disorientation, language disturbance, or perceptual disturbance.

Stroke is not usually considered a cause of delirium, but there are stroke patients who meet the DSM definition. Such patients present with acute confusion and are found on computed tomography (CT) scan or full neurological examination to have evidence of a cerebral infarct. This presentation is more common with right-sided vascular disease (Dunne et al. 1986).

Mehler (1989) found that most patients with obstruction of the upper (rostral) basilar artery *(top-of-the-basilar syndrome)* present with acute confusion but rapidly recover. Martin et al. (1992) reported that electroconvulsive therapy (ECT)–induced interictal delirium was associated with recent infarcts involving the caudate nucleus.

Amnestic syndromes.   Although intellectual functioning and memory are closely linked, current nomenclature separates memory disorders from dementia. Memory loss can apparently occur without dementia if only certain kinds of memory are affected. Retention of intellectual capacity in the face of memory loss is demonstrated in *confabulation,* an exercise by which the patient attempts to conceal his or her memory loss by manufacturing plausible details to fill in the gaps. Confabulation suggesting a high degree of retention of verbal intellect is common with alcoholic brain damage but rare in stroke.

The nomenclature of the various kinds of memory loss is not completely standardized, and definitions vary (Shimamura and Gershberg 1992). Loss of memory for the events immediately preceding a stroke or other condition is termed *retrograde amnesia. Anterograde amnesia* refers to the inability to form new memories for subsequent events (Kopelman 1987).

Anterograde amnesia is classically associated with hippocampal damage. Although victims of this condition cannot learn new information or recall events of the preceding few hours or days, they remain able to take part in a conversation, a skill that requires the ability to remember what has just been said to one. This implies that some type of memory is still intact—specifically, that termed *primary memory* (also called *immediate* or *short-term memory).*

Some authors have described an amnestic syndrome of posterior cerebral artery occlusion due to infarction affecting the hippocampus (Benson et al. 1974). This syndrome is characterized by an inability to acquire new knowledge and some degree of retrograde amnesia without intellectual impairment or clouding of consciousness. Visual field defects accompany the memory loss because the posterior cerebral arteries supply the occipital cortex. In DSM-IV, this condition would be classified as an "amnestic disorder due to a general medical condition."

Von Cramon et al. (1988) studied 30 patients with unilateral posterior cerebral infarction demonstrated by CT scan. All had normal performance on the Wechsler Adult Intelligence Scale (WAIS; Wechsler 1955) and almost all had severe visual field defects. Most did not have memory loss. In 12 of the 30, there was a defect in the ability to learn new verbal information. These 12 patients all had left-hemisphere lesions.

Ott and Saver (1993) described six patients in which acute amnesia was the sole or primary manifestation of stroke. Four of these patients had hippocampal lesions and two had thalamic lesions.

Transient global amnesia.   Transient global amnesia is a temporary, severe memory loss that remits completely. Although individuals who have undergone this state can remember not having been able to remember, there have been few opportunities to measure the exact type of memory loss experienced during the episode. It is more common in elderly men, and is liable to follow stress such as swimming in cold water or sexual intercourse. Stern (1992) noted that "the nature of these disturbances has received a fascinating diversity of psychiatric interpretations which have not been unreservedly received by organically determined neurologists" (p. 435).

Bogousslavsky and Regli (1988) described cases in which isolated transient global amnesia was associated with stroke, and concluded that this symptom had no localizing value apart from a tendency for the lesions to be in the general area of the temporal lobes and basal nuclei. Lin et al. (1993), however, found that perfusion defects revealed by single photon emission computed tomography (SPECT) during a transient global amnesia attack indicated ischemia in the region of the posterior cerebral arteries.

Classifications of Dementia

The classification of dementia in DSM has varied from edition to edition, and differs from that in ICD-10 and also from popular usage.

In DSM-III-R, dementia in which the histological changes seen in the brain under the microscope were those of Alzheimer's disease was called *primary degenerative dementia of the Alzheimer type* (PDAT); in DSM-IV, this entity is named *dementia of the Alzheimer's type*. ICD-10 uses *demen-*

tia in Alzheimer's disease. Alzheimer's disease and *senile dementia* are the terms in common use.

Dementia due to cerebrovascular disease was called *multi-infarct dementia* in DSM-III-R and is called *vascular dementia* in DSM-IV. This condition was termed *arteriosclerotic dementia* in ICD-9 (World Health Organization 1975) as well as in most of the older literature. ICD-10 uses the term *vascular dementia,* specifying that it includes arteriosclerotic dementia and subdividing it in into *vascular dementia of acute onset* (which corresponds to *dementia post-apoplexiam,* or *poststroke dementia*), *multi-infarct dementia, subcortical vascular dementia* (which includes Binswanger's disease), *mixed cortical* and *subcortical vascular dementia,* and "other and unspecified" (see Table 16–2).

DSM-IV (American Psychiatric Association 1994, p. 146) specifies that criteria labeled A, B, C, and D must be present for the diagnosis of vascular dementia. Criterion A calls for the presence both of memory loss and of aphasia, apraxia, agnosia or "disturbance in executive functioning (i.e., planning, organizing, sequencing, abstracting)." Criterion B requires the presence of either focal neurological signs or "laboratory evidence indicative of cerebral vascular disease"—presumably a CT or magnetic resonance imaging (MRI) scan showing an infarct. Criterion C notes that the cognitive deficits must be seriously handicapping and of recent onset. Criterion D stipulates that the condition not be delirium.

Including aphasia, apraxia, and agnosia as evidence of dementia makes it easier to assign disabled patients to a category but limits the usefulness of the DSM-IV criteria in certain contexts, because, as mentioned earlier, one of the most common problems in stroke practice is that of deciding whether a disability is physical or mental. The concept of "disturbance in executive functioning" is not an easy one to pin down.

The diagnostic criteria listed in Table 16–3 are therefore idiosyncratic, mingling simplified DSM-IV criteria with the guidelines of ICD-10. They also largely correspond to the criteria of the state of California Alzheimer's Disease Diagnostic and Treatment Centers (ADDTC) and of the National Institute of Neurological Disorders and Stroke (NINDS)–Association Internationale pour la Récherche et l'Enseignement en Neuroscience (AIREN) group (Amar et al. 1996).

Pseudodementia

Pseudodementia is usually said to exist when patients perform poorly on tests of memory and cognitive function but are not demented. Most of the reported cases of this condition have been in depressed individuals, and the term is often restricted to depressed patients rather than including other causes of poor response such as psychosis or language impairment. Patients with pseudodementia have been found to exhibit a rapid—as opposed to gradual—onset of cognitive function loss that follows rather than precedes depression. They show relative preservation of activities of daily living (ADL) in contrast to their very low psychometric scores (McNeil 1993).

Table 16–2.   Classifications of vascular dementia

Source/type	Brain changes	Comments
Alzheimer		
Dementia post-apoplexiam	Infarct	Follows paralyzing stroke
Binswanger's disease	Arteriosclerosis without infarct	
Mental disorder due to arteriosclerosis	Infarct or arteriosclerosis	Includes entities without dementia
DSM-III-R		
Multi-infarct dementia	Infarct	
ICD-9 and most of the older literature		
Arteriosclerotic dementia	Infarct or arteriosclerosis	
ICD-10		
Vascular dementia		
Vascular dementia of acute onset	Infarct	Same as dementia post-apoplexiam
Multi-infarct dementia	Infarct	
Subcortical dementia	Infarct or arteriosclerosis	Includes Binswanger's disease
Mixed cortical and subcortical dementia	Infarct or arteriosclerosis	
Other and unspecified	Infarct or arteriosclerosis	
DSM-IV		
Vascular dementia	Infarct or arteriosclerosis	

Note.   Alzheimer (1895, 1898, 1902); DSM-III-R (American Psychiatric Association 1987); DSM-IV (American Psychiatric Association 1994); ICD-9 (World Health Organization 1975); ICD-10 (World Health Organization 1992).

Table 16–3. Suggested clinical diagnostic criteria for vascular dementia

Must have both	Must have one	Must not have
Memory loss	Hemiplegia not due to head injury or tumor	Delirium
Cognitive defects that are seriously handicapping and of recent origin	History of stroke or transient ischemic attacks	
	Infarct on CT scan	

Note. CT = computed tomography.

The distinction between pseudodementia and true dementia is not always absolute. Reding et al. (1985) studied patients who had been referred to a dementia clinic with a presumed diagnosis of dementia, but who were found to be depressed rather than demented. Most of them did go on to develop true dementia. The presence of "cerebrovascular disease with focal neurological signs" was found to be a factor that predicted this progression from pseudodementia to true dementia.

It has been suggested that pseudodementia may develop after a stroke because of a combination of aphasia and depression (Robinson et al. 1986; Starkstein and Robinson 1991). Diagnosis in such cases may depend on careful assessment of social behavior and emotional responsiveness, and perhaps may involve some degree of intuition.

Dementia Versus Aphasia

Those who do poorly on tests of memory and cognitive function include nondemented aphasic patients, dementia patients with or without aphasia, noncommunicating psychotic patients, severely depressed patients, and severely physically ill patients.

Among the first three groups, nondemented aphasic patients can be identified with the best degree of certainty. The nondemented aphasic patient stands out by doing well on tests of visual memory and on picture-recognition tests, such as are included in several aphasia test batteries. If visual acuity is intact and allowance is made for visual field defects, then such tests are reliable and valid. Nonspeaking patients who do well on tests for visual memory are unlikely to be demented.

The retention of ADL skills in some nondemented patients with aphasia helps identify them; however, other nondemented aphasic patients will have lost these skills because of right hemiplegia.

Scales of Severity of Dementia

Numerous scales have been devised to measure dementia (see Table 16–4). All include asking subjects questions to determine whether they know where they are, what the date is, what the name of the president is, and so forth. These measures rely heavily on testing memory, which limits their ability to distinguish between amnestic syndromes and dementia and results in score deflation among patients with less formal education.

Table 16–4.   Tests of severity of dementia

Test	Comments
Short Portable Mental Status Questionnaire (Pfeiffer 1975)	Short; as reliable as longer tests
Abbreviated Mental Test (AMT; Qureshi and Hodkinson 1974)	British; short; purely verbal; validated against autopsy findings
Maudsley Tests of the Sensorium (Withers and Hinton 1971)	Forms the basis of several later tests
Mental State Questionnaire (MSQ; Kahn et al. 1960)	Short; purely verbal; longest in use in U.S.
Memory for Designs Test (Kendall 1969)	Needs pencil and paper; affected by visual and motor impairment
Grober Tests of Nonlinguistic Memory (Grober 1984)	Needs special test material; validated in aphasic subjects
Mini-Mental State Examination (MMSE; Folstein et al. 1975)	Needs pencil and paper; affected by visual and motor impairment and literacy; most widely used in U.S.
Dementia Rating Scale (Hasegawa et al. 1986)	Most widely used in Japan
HAWIE Deterioration Index (Baxa and Pakesch 1972)	German; measures discrepancy between educationally acquired information and performance ability
Global Deterioration Scale (Riesberg et al. 1982)	Staging of dementia based on behavioral observations
Glasgow Coma Scale (Teasdale and Jennett 1974)	Measures level of consciousness of nonambulant patient

A particular drawback of these scales in stroke patients is their dependence on performance items that might be affected by specific neurological defects. Some scales assume that a patient is physically capable of seeing, hearing, writing, and drawing. They may include items in which the subject must copy a design, write a sentence, or read a written command. Such tests are very sensitive, which is useful in some situations, such as population surveys, but they are not selective or specific enough in other situations, such as when the patient is already known to have a neurological defect and the purpose of the test is to decide whether dementia is also present.

Scales that are vulnerable to bias on the basis of subjects' education are less useful in surveys, but may be useful clinically. Eastwood et al. (1983) compared, and provided references for, several of the older tests.

Tests that are very short and do not require any props are useful but can be influenced by a subject's deafness, receptive aphasia, education level, familiarity with the local area, and knowledge of English. Examples of very short tests are the Short Portable Mental Status Questionnaire, the Mental State Questionnaire, the Abbreviated Mental Test, and the Maudsley Tests of the Sensorium.

Pfeiffer's Short Portable Mental Status Questionnaire (Pfeiffer 1975) contains only 10 items yet seems as valid, reliable, sensitive, and selective as some of the more elaborate scales (Erkinjuntti et al. 1987). The Mental State Questionnaire (MSQ) of Kahn et al. (1960) has the advantages of great simplicity and the longest record of standardized use in the United States. It consists of simple spoken questions about memory and orientation such as have long been part of the standard neurological examination. The Abbreviated Mental Test (AMT; Flicker 1988; Qureshi and Hodkinson 1974) is similar to the MSQ in content and has been validated against autopsy criteria. The shortened forms of the Maudsley Tests of the Sensorium (Withers and Hinton 1971) are also substantially comparable to the MSQ.

The Memory for Designs Test (Kendall 1969) measures the subject's ability to reproduce geometric drawing; it is influenced by visual impairment and by paralysis, but is less likely to be affected by aphasia or deafness. The Maudsley tests and the Memory for Designs Test have been found equally successful in differentiating structural brain damage from schizophrenia (Birkett and Boltuch 1977).

The Mini-Mental State Exam (MMSE) of Folstein et al. (1975) is the most widely used test of general cognitive status in the United States. It requires a setup for writing and drawing and is very vulnerable to language barriers, illiteracy, deafness, blindness, and paralysis. Hasegawa's Dementia Rating Scale (Hasegawa et al. 1986) is the most widely used in Japan.

The HAWIE Deterioration Index of Baxa and Pakesch (1972) is designed to measure the discrepancy between educationally acquired information and performance ability; it also can detect a falling off from a previous level of achievement.

Several authors (e.g., Riesberg et al. 1982) have described schemes for staging the degree of severity of dementia based on behavioral observations. Criteria for defining mild, moderate, and severe levels of dementia are also provided in DSM-IV. When the patient is not paralyzed, an assessment of his or her capacity for independent ADL is often the most useful practical way of deciding between dementia and other diagnoses. There are several ADL scales in use (see Chapter 17).

Many of the most severely ill patients are unable to respond to any test questions. Such patients drop off the bottom of verbally administered scales. For the bedridden, a measure such as the Glasgow Coma Scale (Teasdale and Jennett 1974) can be useful because it measures responsiveness in those incapable of speech or movement.

A clinician dealing with stroke patients should be familiar with one of these scales, and should use it to assess each patient. There is much overlap between rating scales (Gurland et al. 1995). Clinician choice can therefore be based on convenience and familiarity. In terms of specificity and selectivity when used to screen for dementia, the longer scales such as the MMSE are not as good as short, simple scales such as the MSQ (Gurland et al. 1995; Wilder et al. 1995). Our own practice is to use the MSQ for patients who can talk, and to supplement it with a short test of visual memory (Birkett 1995) for patients with left-brain infarcts.

In conclusion, these rating scales are useful in documenting both the progress of dementia and the efficacy of treatment. They can be helpful as a screening device in allocating patients to appropriate care settings, such as rehabilitation facilities, dementia units, or nursing homes. An attempt should be made to assess for the presence and degree of dementia in every case of stroke.

Causes

How Much Dementia Is Vascular?

The title of a 1983 paper by Brust is "Vascular Dementia Is Overdiagnosed" and that of a 1988 paper by O'Brien is "Vascular Dementia Is

Underdiagnosed." As these titles suggest, no general agreement exists on the matter.

Among fully ambulant patients who come to psychiatrists' offices with complaints suggesting dementia, or who are seen in memory disorder clinics, only a minority will be found to have infarcts on CT scan. If patients who present with dementia but who do not have infarcts on CT scan are followed to autopsy, the majority will have Alzheimer's disease. However, attempts to more precisely determine how much of dementia is vascular have not resolved the disagreement between Brust and O'Brien.

Alzheimer's disease, artery disease, stroke, and dementia are all age-related disorders that can overlap and interact. The overlap between Alzheimer's disease and arteriosclerosis is probably no more or less than that due to chance, but there is one kind of vascular change, *congophil arteriopathy*, that does correlate with Alzheimer's disease.

Occasionally, congophil arteriopathy may itself produce enough damage to cause dementia (Scully 1991). The brain damage in this condition is caused by hemorrhages rather than infarcts. Although congophil arteriopathy is very rare in the United States, a hereditary form (hereditary cystatin C amyloid angiopathy) has caused many cases of dementia in young people in Iceland (Blondal et al. 1989) and Holland (Blumenthal and Premachandra 1990).

The consensus in the literature is that vascular dementia is less common than Alzheimer's disease; however, there have been few true population studies. The "ideal" experiment would be to take a random sample of Americans, test them by all our tests, and perform autopsy examinations immediately afterward. Since such an experiment is obviously out of the question, various surveys have been conducted. These generally conclude that less than one-half of dementia cases are of vascular origin, although results vary according to the population studied and the criteria used for vascular dementia (Brayne et al. 1995; Hershey 1990; Jorm 1991; Kase 1991; Rocca et al. 1991). Surveys of ambulant patients who present with symptoms of dementia find more Alzheimer's disease; community surveys and mental hospital and nursing-home surveys find more vascular disease.

Both prevalence and incidence must be considered. The figures for brain infarcts and neurologically evident stroke are relatively well known. For 20 years, Ueda et al. (1987) followed a population sample of 1,600 persons over 40 years of age. During the two decades, 255 strokes occurred, resulting in an annual incidence of 9.8 per thousand. In 1977, the National Health Survey estimated that there were 2.7 million adults in the United

States with a history of stroke, of whom about two-thirds had been hospitalized (Baum 1982). In addition to these are patients with brain infarcts in whom stroke has not been clinically diagnosed. Among patients in the Framingham cohort with autopsy-confirmed brain infarcts, only 40% had stroke mentioned on their death certificates (Baum and Manton 1987).

The prevalence of vascular dementia may be reduced by the tendency of patients to die sooner than those with Alzheimer's disease. Thirty percent of stroke patients die within 30 days of their stroke, and 70% are dead at the end of 5 years (Posner et al. 1984), whereas life expectancy after the onset of clinically detectable Alzheimer's disease is about 6 years.

A source of error in determining prevalence is that, in many patients, medical complications override the dementia. Such patients may not be included in the dementia statistics because they are obviously physically ill. General-hospital medical records often fail to document dementia in stroke patients (Harris et al. 1992). Nearly 2 million Americans are in nursing homes, which contain relatively large numbers of untestable and medically ill patients with dementia.

Fischer et al. (1990) in Vienna found that one-half of the chronic patients with dementia in the neurology department of a geriatric hospital had vascular dementia, but this proportion was a result of the organization of the department and was counterbalanced by higher rates of Alzheimer's disease in patients in the internal medicine and psychiatric departments. Livingston et al. (1990), in a survey of noninstitutionalized subjects over age 65 in London, found that 6% (48 of the sample) had dementia, and diagnosed vascular dementia in only 6 of the 48.

Swedish investigators conducted a population survey of all 85-year-olds living in Gothenburg (Skoog et al. 1993), using structured interviews, neurological examinations, and CT scans. They found that most cases of dementia were vascular rather than due to Alzheimer's disease.

Several reports have suggested that vascular dementia is relatively more common among East Asians (Ishino et al. 1990; Liu et al. 1991; Serby et al. 1987). Ueda et al. (1992), in a survey of all the elderly residents in a Japanese rural community, found that 59 (out of 887) had dementia. Among these, 32 died and came to autopsy during a 5-year follow-up, at which 13 were found to have the brain changes of Alzheimer's disease. In addition, 18 had CT scans of the head. Of the 59 persons with dementia, 13 had small multiple infarcts, 3 had large infarcts, 2 had small solitary infarcts; 7 had cerebral embolisms; 2 had Binswanger's disease; and 1 had intracerebral hemorrhage. Thus, 28 of the 59 demented residents had vascular lesions. Of these 28, 8 also were found to have the brain changes of Alzheimer's disease at autopsy. No comparable study has been done outside Japan.

Are Infarcts Necessary for Vascular Dementia?

Many authorities believe that artery disease does not cause mental changes unless it produces brain infarcts (Hachinski et al. 1974). This assumption was made by DSM-III-R, which replaced *psychosis with arteriosclerosis* with the term *multi-infarct dementia*. Proponents of the infarct theory point out that most patients with dementia who do not have severe Alzheimer's disease are found at autopsy or on CT scan to have brain infarcts. They also argue that it is physiologically unlikely for the brain to suffer a slow partial strangulation, because nerve cells are very sensitive to oxygen deprivation. A nerve cell with its arterial oxygen supply cut off for 3 minutes dies, and a localized area of dead cells, by definition, constitutes an infarct.

Evidence against the infarct theory has been reviewed by Birkett and Raskin (1982), Parnetti et al. (1990), Sulkava and Erkinjuntti (1987), and Wallin and Blennow (1991).

Sulkava and Erkinjuntti (1987) adduced evidence that cerebral hypoperfusion may cause dementia without producing infarcts. Wallin and Blennow (1991) describes a group of dementia patients without Alzheimer's disease or infarcts, but with evidence of vascular disease, who were found at autopsy to have changes in the myelin of the centrum ovale, which they considered may have been caused by hypoxia that stopped short of producing infarction. Kumar et al. (1992) found that leukoareiosis correlated with dementia among patients with stroke risk factors—a finding that also suggests a vascular contribution to dementia without definite infarcts. Langlois et al. (1989) found that memory disorder precedes infarction in vasculitis. Positron-emission tomography (PET) scans in acute stroke have revealed a zone, called the *penumbra*, beyond the area of irreversible nerve cell death, which suggests the possibility of partial damage in areas not infarcted (Hakim 1989).

Although the controversy is partly semantic, there are some practical implications. If patients with vascular dementia can be diagnosed before nerve cells have been killed, they might be more likely to respond to treatment. It may be that "both hypotheses, namely loss of brain volume and chronic hypoperfusion as factors responsible for cognitive impairment in MID [multi-infarct dementia], appear to be correct. They are not mutually exclusive, but depend on the stage and severity of MID" (Kawamura et al. 1991, p. 37).

Relationship Between Infarct Characteristics and Dementia

Some infarcts may be more likely to be associated with dementia than others. The association could depend on whether the infarcts are single or multiple, on the total volume of brain infarcted, or on the location of the infarcts.

Infarct Volume and Dementia

Multiplicity of infarcts.   The presence of more than one infarct is commonly regarded as a factor in causing dementia. Evidence from earlier autopsy studies, as well as from recent studies mostly based on CT scans rather than autopsy, is presented in the following paragraphs.

Mahendra et al. (1985) compared dementia patients with infarcts with nondementia patients with infarcts. They found that large infarcts confined to one hemisphere were unlikely to be associated with dementia, and suggested that dementia is associated with bilateral lacunar infarcts. The ages of their subjects were not mentioned, and the dementia was not quantified. It is not certain whether they were using the term *lacunar* in the strict sense defined by Fisher (1982; see Chapter 2) or applying it to small lesions anywhere in the brain.

Loeb et al. (1987) compared dementia patients with multiple infarcts with age-matched nondementia patients with multiple infarcts. They found that the presence of dementia was related to the presence of infarcts in both the thalamus and the cortex, to the total amount of cerebral substance lost, and to the presence of cerebral atrophy.

Ladurner et al. (1982a, 1982b) found that, although bilateral infarcts were more likely to be associated with dementia, there was no other association between dementia and multiple infarcts. Only one-half of their stroke patients with dementia had multiple infarcts. Thus, they proposed that the dementia was related to the presence of infarcts on both sides rather than to the multiplicity of the infarcts.

Volume infarcted.   It seems reasonable to assume that the volume of brain infarcted must have something to do with the presence of dementia, but few experimental studies of the relationship have been done. The findings of Tomlinson and colleagues (1968, 1970) have been interpreted to mean that brain infarctions below a certain threshold volume are not associated with dementia.

Tomlinson et al. (1968) described the brains of 28 nondemented patients aged 65–92 who had been active until shortly before their deaths. In 8 of the 28 patients, no ischemic foci were found. Seven had very small areas of softening. The remaining 13 all had softenings varying in volume from 2 mL to 91 mL. The authors summarized their findings as follows: "Multiple small bilateral basal ganglion softenings were prominent in this group, frequently accompanied by small softenings elsewhere" (Tomlinson et al. 1968, p. 341).

Tomlinson et al. (1970) also studied 50 elderly patients with dementia by similar methods. These 50 dementia patients served as a control group for the 28 patients without dementia previously described. In 10 of the 50 patients with dementia, no ischemic foci were found. Very small areas of softening were found in 9 others. The remaining 31 all had softenings varying in volume from 2 mL to 412 mL.

Tomlinson and Henderson (1976), summarizing the results of the 1968 and 1970 investigations as well as those of subsequent cases studied by the same methods, stated that "90% of well-preserved old people have less than 50 mL of cerebral softening and no nondemented old subjects have been found with more than 100 mL destroyed by ischemia. Against this, about 20% of demented old subjects have more than 100 mL of cerebral softening. The great majority of normal old people will be found to have less than 50 mL of cerebral softening and more than 90% of people with more than 50 mL of softening will be demented; from our present experience, old subjects with more than 100 mL of cerebral softening always show some dementia" (p. 191). Thus, few cases of dementia occur at volumes of softening less than 50 mL, and all patients with more than 100 mL of softening have dementia.

Del Ser et al. (1990), however, were not able to confirm this sharp division. They compared the brains of demented patients without Alzheimer's disease with those of nondemented control subjects, and found that the volume of infarcts was greater in the demented patients than in the nondemented subjects, even when the volume infarcted was less than 100 mL.

Mielke et al. (1992) considered their findings, based on PET scan, to contradict those of Tomlinson with regard to the threshold effect. They found that even very small infarcts could be associated with dementia, and that the determining factor was the volume of brain with impaired function as determined by PET scan rather than the volume infarcted as determined by CT. Mielke and colleagues suggested that there are areas of "incompletely infarcted" brain tissue—areas that are intact but deprived of afferent connections needed in order to function.

Infarct Location and Dementia

The possibility of a localized infarct's causing an amnestic syndrome was discussed earlier in this chapter in "Amnestic syndromes." Few studies have compared the locations of cerebral infarcts in patients with and without dementia.

Tomlinson et al. (1970) reported that infarcts in the frontal lobes, of the hippocampus and adjacent limbic structures, and in the corpus callosum were more frequent in demented patients than in nondemented control subjects with infarcts.

Del Ser et al. (1990) found that bilateral infarcts, and possibly infarcts in the front part of the brain, were more common in patients with dementia than in nondemented patients with infarcts. Tatemichi et al. (1992a) described cases in which dementia was associated with infarction involving the inferior genu of the left internal capsule; they suggested that this condition may represent "strategic-infarct dementia" due to loss of connections between the thalamus and frontal cortex.

Kitagawa et al. (1984) found, in 15 dementia patients with infarcts, that left midtemporal ischemia correlated with dyscalculia and memory disturbance, whereas ischemia of both frontal lobes correlated with disorientation to time and place.

Mahler and Cummings (1991) described several separate "syndromes of vascular dementia" associated with particular localized lesions. The diagnostic criteria for these syndromes include lateralized motor and sensory changes, and the definitions are based on the associated sets of localizing neurological signs. For example, these authors' *carotid artery syndrome* includes hemiplegia, and their *posterior cerebral artery syndrome* includes hemianopsia.

In summary, it has not been proven that an infarct's localization makes a substantial difference to its likelihood of causing dementia. This lack of association may be because dementia-associated infarcts are related to widespread intracranial cerebral arteriosclerosis (Birkett and Raskin 1982) or because infarcts big enough to cause dementia are so big that they produce widespread damage and are thus not truly localized.

Dementia Following Paralytic Stroke

In some cases, neurologically evident stroke is followed by dementia, a condition referred to in some of the older literature as "dementia post-apoplexiam." One way to find out which strokes are followed by dementia is to study patients known to have had strokes and see which ones develop dementia. It is, however, not easy to be sure that patients did not have dementia before their stroke. Alzheimer (1902) noted that even in dementia post-apoplexiam, the dementia had sometimes preceded the hemiplegia. This sequence is more common in older patients.

Kotila et al. (1986) found a very low incidence of dementia in 52 young (mean age 49) stroke patients, initially without dementia, followed for more than 4 years after a first stroke. Their patients tended to show improvement in mental function, with only 3 patients (ages 40, 43, and 49) developing loss of intellectual abilities severe enough to cause them to give up work. One of these 3 patients had small lacunar infarcts, another had bilateral multiple infarcts, and the third had a single left-hemisphere infarct.

Tatemichi et al. (1990) studied patients who had suffered strokes as defined by the National Stroke Data Bank Registry (which essentially means paralytic strokes; see Table 2–1). They found that 10% of the younger patients (ages 60–64) and 25% of the older patients (ages 80–84) developed dementia 10 days after their stroke. As time went on, the younger patients' dementia decreased and the elderly patients' dementia increased. A year after the stroke, 10% of the patients under 79 years of age and 75% of the patients over 85 had dementia. Hijdra et al. (1991) have criticized this study because the criterion used for diagnosis of dementia was the opinion of a neurologist. In another study, Tatemichi et al. (1992b) found that 3 months after hospitalization for stroke, 26% of the elderly patients had dementia according to DSM-III-R criteria, compared with only 9% of age-matched, nonstroke control subjects living in the community. Advanced age, lack of education, and nonwhite racial status increased the risk of dementia.

Gustafson et al. (1991) studied the incidence of acute confusional states in 155 elderly patients with acute cerebrovascular disorder. The independent predictors of acute confusional state were extensive paresis, previous acute confusional state, left-hemisphere brain lesions, old age, and treatment with drugs that had anticholinergic effects.

Ladurner et al. (1982a, 1982b) also studied dementia in 71 stroke patients. Admission criteria for stroke were not fully detailed. The authors reported that "in 67 patients there was a history of at least one ischemic episode with focal neurological signs in 66 cases" (Ladurner et al. 1982b, p. 97). Included in the 71 were 4 patients with no focal neurological signs, in whom "the diagnosis of ischemic stroke was based only on the CT which showed an infarct" (1982b, p. 97). In 9 of the 71, no infarct was found on CT scan. The HAWIE Deterioration Index of Baxa and Pakesch (1972) was used to assess the presence of dementia. The strokes had occurred, on average, about 2 years before the time of the investigations. Ladurner and colleagues found that, compared with nondementia patients, the dementia patients were significantly more likely to have bilateral infarcts, to have infarcts of the left side, to have general brain atrophy in combination with infarcts, to have hypertension (> 165/95 mm Hg), to have thalamic infarcts, and to have cerebral atrophy. The nondementia patients were more likely to have a CT scan without infarcts. Bilateral infarcts were more likely to be associated with dementia, but otherwise there was no association between multiplicity of infarcts and dementia.

Terayama et al. (1992) compared cerebral blood flow (CBF) in stroke patients both with and without dementia. The dementia group showed more hypoperfusion in the frontal, temporal, and occipital areas.

A measure called the *contingent negative variation* was found by Kofler et al. (1988) to differentiate stroke patients with dementia from those without dementia; however, this electroencephalographic factor may actually be a nonspecific measure of the severity of mental disorder.

Depression

As previously mentioned, depression can produce "pseudodementia" that adversely affects performance on tests of cognitive function. Authors who believe in the specific effect of left frontal lesions in causing dementia have therefore suggested that such lesions are also specifically associated with impaired performance on tests of cognitive function. Such an association was not found in the study of Bolla-Wilson et al. (1989), although lower test performance by depressed patients was confirmed.

Lacunar Strokes

The definition of the term *lacune* was discussed in Chapter 2. *Lacunes,* as described by Fisher, are located in the area of the basal ganglia and internal capsule, and Fisher himself, in his original description of the clinical entities (Fisher 1982), specified that confusion is rarely a lacunar manifestation, although he described an entity of "thalamic dementia" with abulia and impairment of memory. Del Ser et al. (1990) found that lacunes confined to the basal ganglia and internal capsule—that is to say, strictly Fisherian lacunes—were associated with dementia.

Some authors who recognize lacunar stroke as a clinicopathological entity describe it as being associated with dementia, emotional lability, abulia, and mood changes (Mahler and Cummings 1991); this condition has also been called *lacunar dementia* (Roman 1985).

Subcortical Dementia

Subcortical dementia refers to dementia due to disease below the cortex. The term is used in two ways. First, it is sometimes used in a broad sense for any dementia in which there is no disease of the cerebral cortex. The term can thus be used for dementia with infarcts of the white matter of the centrum ovale and for Binswanger's disease. (ICD-10 has a category of "subcortical vascular dementia" for vascular disease affecting the white matter only, including Binswanger's disease.) Second, the term is also used for dementia with disease of basal nuclei or other gray matter in the lower parts of the brain.

Erkinjuntti (1987, 1990) used the term in the broad sense. He compared two groups of dementia patients: one with cortical infarcts and the other with subcortical infarcts. Those with subcortical infarcts were less severely demented, had a less-abrupt onset of confusion, and had more depression and emotional lability. They also had less heart disease and less-severe stroke disability. In Erkinjuntti's original description, the dementia itself was not unusual but was distinguished by an accompanying neurological feature such as hemiparesis, bulbar signs, and dysarthria.

Some authors use the term in a narrower sense than Erkinjuntti did, employing it to describe the dementia seen in conditions such as Parkinson's disease, Huntington's chorea, and progressive supranuclear palsy. Defined in this context, subcortical dementia is conceptualized as being less likely to show speech disturbance as an early symptom; in addition, it is thought to be marked by a slowing down of thought processes—a condition called *bradyphrenia*. Patients with bradyphrenia can give correct answers to questions, but only after a long pause. A difficulty in using this feature to distinguish subcortical dementia has been that Parkinson's disease is marked by a slowing down of physical mobility (*bradykinesia*), and it is difficult to determine whether the cause of a patient's slowness in response is physical or mental. Most of the studies on this kind of subcortical dementia have been concerned with the effects of degenerative neurological disease rather than of infarction (Cummings 1986).

Mahler and Cummings (1991) described a "thalamic dementia" that is accompanied by apathy and slowing of the thought processes (features they regard as characteristic of subcortical dementia). They included in this entity the syndrome in which there is reduced spontaneous speech and reduced volume of speech, which is classified by others as an aphasia (Bruyn 1989) and associated by some with left thalamic lesions.

Katz et al. (1987) described six patients who had infarcts restricted to the thalamus and midbrain. These patients with paramedian mesencephalic-diencephalic infarcts (PMDIs) had what the authors claimed to be a distinctive syndrome of dementia, comprising two distinct phases. In the early stages, all patients had depressed levels of consciousness that gradually improved over days to weeks. They then became fully alert but showed dramatic slowness of response, either verbal or motor. Apathetic and unmotivated, they would lie fully awake, doing nothing for long periods. Only one patient had shown improvement at 15-month follow-up.

Does the Kind of Artery Blockage Make a Difference?

The artery disease most often associated with stroke is *arteriosclerosis*. Outside the brain, two kinds of arteriosclerosis can be distinguished: *atherosclerosis* and *arteriolosclerosis*. In atherosclerosis, plaques of cholesterol form under the endothelium. In arteriolosclerosis, the artery walls are thickened. This distinction is less evident inside the brain. Microscopically, other vascular changes in the arterioles and capillaries are also now recognized (Munoz 1991).

Blockage of an artery may be due to thrombosis, but there are several other possible mechanisms by which artery disease may cause brain infarcts: the artery may go into spasm; the lumen may be narrowed by plaque; or emboli may travel and block a brain artery.

Emboli may arise from several sources, and opinions differ regarding which is most important in causing brain infarction. Some kinds of emboli have long been known to arise from heart disease; these can cause *cardioembolic* stroke. "Artery to artery" embolism is caused by artery disease outside the skull. In this condition, a plaque of atheroma forms in an artery supplying the brain, such as the carotid, and subsequently ruptures. Blood clots form on the ruptured plaque, and these clots, or debris from the plaque itself, then travel into the brain as embolisms.

Carotid arteries and dementia.   It used to be thought that a brain infarct was always caused by a thrombus or plaque of atheroma that blocked the small artery immediately supplying the infarcted area. Strokes not due to hemorrhage were called *cerebral thrombosis*. However, autopsies have shown that the small arteries immediately supplying infarcted areas are usually patent (Hutchinson 1972), and this finding has focused attention on the importance of artery disease outside the skull in causing strokes, especially disease of the carotid artery, blockage of which is quite common and is found in 11% of people over age 50 at autopsy ("New Studies of Strokes," *BMJ* 1971). Most of the work on the clinical significance of carotid artery disease has been concerned with neurologically evident stroke, but there may be differences between the artery disease causing neurologically evident stroke and that causing dementia.

There have been a few studies of the relationship between dementia and measures of carotid artery flow. Carotid murmurs are found in about one-tenth of the general population (Hammond and Eisinger 1962). Naugle et al. (1986) studied six patients in whom carotid murmurs had been found on routine physical examination at a Veterans Administration center, and in whom subsequent ultrasound studies had shown 70% or greater stenosis in the right, left, or both carotid arteries. They compared these patients with age- and education-matched volunteer control subjects. Although none of the patients with stenosis had a clinical diagnosis of dementia, they did less well than the control subjects on several psychometric tests of memory, intelligence, and motor skills.

Müller et al. (1989) used sonography (direct/indirect Doppler and real-time techniques) to examine the carotid arteries of 18 institutionalized patients with severe dementia who had CT scan–proven infarcts, and found only 6 with pathological lesions in the extracranial blood supply.

Knowledge of the role of intracranial cerebral arteriosclerosis in dementia has been limited by the need for autopsy to study the smallest vessels. The small intracranial arteries may be more important in dementia than they are in neurologically evident stroke.

Corsellis and Evans (1965) and Birkett (1972) found that extracranial artery disease was relatively absent, but that intracranial arteriosclerosis was severe, in autopsied mental-hospital patients with infarcts. Del Ser et al. (1990) also found an absence of carotid and basilar atheromatosis in dementia patients with brain infarcts. Garcia et al. (1984) showed that the incidence of cognitive impairment in peripheral vascular disease and coronary artery disease was high, even in the absence of stroke, and that among patients with stroke, those with emboli were least likely to have dementia. This finding suggests that the pervasiveness of the vascular disease, rather than embolism, is what causes the dementia.

Judd et al. (1986), using ^{133}Xe blood-flow measurement techniques, found evidence of generalized intracerebral artery disease in patients with multi-infarct dementia. The intracranial arteries of these patients were less responsive to increases or decreases of inhaled oxygen than were those of nondemented control subjects or of control subjects with Alzheimer's disease. The degree of this loss of vasomotor responsiveness correlated with the severity of cognitive impairment, a finding that suggests a general rigidity or loss of reactivity in the intracranial arteries. The importance of such rigidity is supported by the work of Ries et al. (1993), who found that Alzheimer patients could be differentiated from vascular dementia patients, using transcranial Doppler examination, by the value of *pulsatility*—a measure of flow resistance in small blood vessels.

Alzheimer's Disease and Vascular Dementia

To what extent does the presence of concurrent Alzheimer changes determine whether artery disease will cause dementia? Is there an additive or potentiating effect? The question remains open, but there is probably a threshold effect rather than an additive or potentiating one. It takes definite Alzheimer-type histological brain changes to produce dementia, and the combination of an infarct with slight Alzheimer histological changes is not especially liable to cause dementia.

Among the 50 elderly dementia patients and 28 nondementia control subjects studied by Tomlinson et al. (1970), the presence of mild to moderate degrees of Alzheimer changes did not enhance the tendency for infarcts of any given size to be associated with dementia.

Clinical Differences Between Vascular Dementia and Alzheimer's Disease

The clinical differentiation of vascular disease and Alzheimer's disease depends on definitions. What exactly is it that we are predicting when we say a patient has vascular dementia? Are we predicting that autopsy would show more than 50 mL of brain tissue infarcted? Are we predicting that a consensus of experts would agree on a diagnosis of vascular dementia? Are we predicting that less than a certain amount of Alzheimer brain changes would be found at autopsy? Are we predicting that a CT scan would show an infarct? None of these questions has an unequivocal answer, and different studies have used different criteria.

In elderly patients with mental disorder (Birkett and Raskin 1982) and some other populations studied (Leung et al. 1993), the presence of any infarct is a strong predictor of generalized intracranial cerebral arteriosclerosis. Since infarcts can now be detected by CT, the presence of an infarct on CT in a dementia patient can be used as evidence of vascular dementia. However, some authors insist that infarcts above a certain size, or multiple infarcts, should be present.

Psychiatric features.   The possibility of purely mental differences between two kinds of organic brain disease is of theoretical interest, even if not of immediate practical importance.

In his original description of arteriosclerotic dementia, Alzheimer (1895; Foerstl and Levy 1991) emphasized that insight may continue to be present and that patients may be distressed by their disability, but he underscored these features to contrast arteriosclerotic dementia with general paralysis of the insane rather than with (subsequently to be described) Alzheimer's disease. In 1898, Alzheimer presented further work on the brain disorder caused by dementia senilis and atheromatous vascular disease and again mentioned that extensive parts of the original personality are preserved in the vascular cases (Förstl and Howard 1991). Relative preservation of personality was also noted by Mayer-Gross et al. (1960) as a feature of vascular—as opposed to Alzheimer-type—dementia, and has been confirmed in some recent studies (Birkett 1972; Erkinjuntti 1990).

This relative preservation of personality may be due to features extrinsic to the mental disease process itself. The Alzheimer patient is more likely to be healthy apart from the brain and may survive until the severity of the dementia leads to death, whereas second strokes or heart attacks may kill the stroke patient before the dementia has had as much chance to progress. Thirty percent of stroke patients die within 30 days of their stroke (Posner et al. 1984). The presence of concurrent neurological disability may cause institutionalization of patients with only mild dementia. A survey of institutionalized patients may therefore find that dementia is less severe in the vascular cases.

Birkett (1972) found that in mental-hospital patients followed to autopsy, preservation of personality and suddenness of illness onset distinguished those with infarcts, and that agitation was more characteristic of the Alzheimer cases; however, the presence of a stroke history was such a strong indicator of infarction that purely psychiatric features not secondary to a neurological disability were difficult to elucidate.

Bucht et al. (1984) reported that multi-infarct dementia patients were more likely to have a history of depression, whereas Alzheimer patients were more likely to be depressed at the time of examination.

Cummings et al. (1987) compared psychiatric symptoms in two groups of dementia patients, one group clinically diagnosed with Alzheimer's disease, and the other with multi-infarct dementia. The multi-infarct dementia patients had a history of at least one definite stroke or at least one visible lesion on CT. The Alzheimer patients had more dementia, whereas the multi-infarct patients were more depressed and more likely to have hallucinations, especially visual hallucinations. Two of the three multi-infarct patients with visual hallucinations had visual field defects, and one was almost blind from eye disease.

In general, then, there is support for the hypothesis that preservation of personality is a feature of vascular dementia, but attempts to isolate purely mental differentiating points are confounded by concomitant stroke-related physical disability. This confounding also applies to suddenness of onset.

It is often suggested that an abrupt onset and stepwise progression distinguish vascular dementia, whereas Alzheimer's disease is characterized by insidious onset and gradual progression (Erkinjuntti 1990). This dichotomization sounds plausible but is not easy to test experimentally. In retrospective histories, the onset of illness may be reported to be more sudden in vascular dementia, and there may be more episodes of sudden deterioration, but these features cannot clearly distinguish vascular dementia from neurologically evident stroke. The more steps the researcher takes to exclude neurologically evident stroke, the more vascular dementia cases are excluded. There are certainly many cases of vascular dementia with insidious onset (Birkett 1972; Fischer et al. 1990).

Hachinski Ischemic Score.   This measure was derived from a paper by Hachinski et al. (1975), who classified dementia patients with a score containing 13 items derived from the textbook of psychiatry by Mayer-Gross et al. (1960). Five of the items were physical (history of hypertension, history of strokes, "evidence of arteriosclerosis," focal neurological symptoms, and focal neurological signs); four were mental (nocturnal confusion, relative preservation of personality, depression, and emotional incontinence); and another four were equivocally mental or physical (abrupt onset, stepwise deterioration, fluctuating course, and depression). These authors found that patients with high scores had reduced CBF as measured by the intracarotid ^{133}Xe method.

Rosen et al. (1979) applied the Hachinski Ischemic Score to 14 dementia patients who were followed to autopsy. Four of these patients were found to have cerebral infarcts without great numbers of Alzheimer changes, 5 had Alzheimer changes without infarcts, and 5 had both infarcts and Alzheimer changes. The groups could not be differentiated by fluctuating course, by "evidence of arteriosclerosis," or by any of the mental items. Abrupt onset (not defined), stepwise deterioration, history of stroke, focal neurological signs, and focal neurological symptoms characterized those with infarcts. However, 3 of the 5 patients with abrupt onset, and all 3 cases with stepwise deterioration, had a history of stroke.

The Hachinski score is effectively equivalent to asking whether or not the patient has had a neurologically evident stroke. This information, although very useful in certain contexts, has only limited usefulness for purposes such as assessing the amount of dementia that is due to vascular disease among patients attending a dementia clinic. If patients with stroke are not sent to the clinic, then, as O'Brien (1988) points out, the number of patients with dementia attributed to vascular disease will be vanishingly small.

Radiological techniques.   The use of CT and MRI is limited in dementia by the nature of the illness. The justification for performing a CT scan is less to diagnose cerebral infarction than to exclude certain other treatable forms of dementia, although finding such treatable forms in very elderly patients is a great rarity.

An impetus to precise diagnosis of dementia has been provided by recent legislation in the United States, which mandates that mentally ill patients may not be put into nursing homes unless they have dementia, and sets up standards for documenting that the illness *is* dementia. Even this incentive, however, may not be enough to justify subjecting a patient to the trouble and expense of CT if he or she is at an age where dementia is very common. Most New Yorkers and Londoners over 90 years of age have some evidence of dementia (Gurland et al. 1983).

In some cases, the behavioral disturbance associated with the dementia may make the investigation difficult to carry out. CT scans with contrast involve injecting a dye intravenously, which can cause complications in those with high blood sugar or urea (blood urea nitrogen [BUN]). Clinical judgment and a good rapport with the patient's family are needed to make the decision of whether to perform radiological examination.

The CT scan will show most areas of softening but can be negative in patients with clinical stroke. At present, the significance of many MRI-detected brain changes in elderly patients and in dementia patients is under investigation (see Chapter 2).

Other research procedures.   PET, SPECT, and regional cerebral blood flow (rCBF) show a pattern in Alzheimer's disease patients of reduced metabolic activity and blood flow in both parietal and temporal areas, referred to as "bilateral temporoparietal defects." The pattern in patients diagnosed with multi-infarct dementia is less consistent and varies from asymmetrical focal defects to normality (Geaney and Abou-Saleh 1990). McKeith et al. (1993) found that multi-infarct dementia patients showed higher activity in the anterior parietal areas than did those with Alzheimer's disease.

Kuwabara et al. (1992) found that PET could differentiate Alzheimer's disease patients from those with vascular dementia by the patient's response to breathing carbon dioxide. The carbon dioxide increased rCBF and oxygen consumption in the Alzheimer cases, but not in the vascular dementia cases.

Electroencephalographic recording.   Dementia of any kind tends to cause diffuse slowing of the electroencephalogram (EEG) (Leuchter et al. 1993). The normally dominant alpha (8–13 Hz) and beta (faster than 13 Hz) waves are replaced by a preponderance of slow theta (4–8 Hz) or even slower delta (slower than 4 Hz) waves. A normal EEG or one that is asymmetrical is indicative of multi-infarct dementia rather than Alzheimer's disease (Erkinjuntti 1990).

Koshino et al. (1990) found that slow and sharp activity in temporal leads was frequent in vascular dementia, rare in primary degenerative dementias, and absent in stroke patients without dementia. A computer-derived measure of coherence between the parietal and temporal areas has been shown to be significantly different in vascular and senile dementia (Leuchter et al. 1992; O'Connor et al. 1979). Bucht et al. (1984) found that generalized slowing was more common in Alzheimer cases and localized slowing was more common in multi-infarct cases.

Stroke risk factors.   The presence of stroke risk factors predicts the presence of infarction on CT or at autopsy; it also predicts that the clinician will make a diagnosis of multi-infarct dementia (Tresch et al. 1985).

St. Clair and Whalley (1983) compared infarct patients with dementia with Alzheimer's disease patients with dementia. The evidence of infarcts and Alzheimer's was obtained at autopsy, and the dementia diagnosis and blood pressure measurements were obtained from retrospective record review. None of the Alzheimer patients had received antihypertensive medication. The systolic and diastolic blood pressures of the infarct group were significantly higher than those of the Alzheimer group. In a stroke-free community sample of elderly people in New York, diabetes and hypercholesterolemia—but not hypertension, heart attack history, or smoking—correlated with cognitive impairment (Desmond et al. 1993).

Treatment

Drugs for Vascular Dementia

There is no medication of proven benefit for vascular dementia. Research follows two main lines. The first has been to look for drugs specific to vascular disease of the brain. The second line of research has been to seek drugs that are hoped to improve dementia regardless of etiology, sometimes called *nootropic agents.*

Several special difficulties arise in trials of the efficacy of drugs for vascular dementia. These include ambiguity in diagnosis of the condition, the frequent presence of concomitant illness, and problems in defining useful improvement.

Vascular drugs.   Drugs that can dilate arteries seem a rational approach, but if dementia is caused by infarcts, then it may be futile to use a drug that improves brain blood supply but merely brings more oxygen to dead nerve cells. The response of blood vessels in different parts of the body to drugs varies. For example, drugs that dilate coronary arteries may cause peripheral vasoconstriction and therefore be useful in coronary artery disease but harmful in peripheral artery disease of the legs.

Pentoxifylline (Trental) has an approved use for peripheral vascular disease of the legs. Black et al. (1992) were not able to show that this drug improved vascular dementia, although they noticed a slowing in the decline of cognitive function, which was more marked for patients who had neurologically evident strokes. Cyclandelate (Cyclospasmol) and other drugs have been shown to increase CBF and cortical perfusion rates but have not proved clinically useful in dementia, even in cases identified as caused by cerebral artery disease (Birkett 1971).

Vinpocetine is claimed to increase CBF. In an open trial, Tamaki et al. (1985a, 1985b) showed that increases in CBF followed the use of vinpocetine in patients with cerebrovascular disorders. Subhan and Hindmarsh (1985) found that it improved memory in healthy volunteers.

Balestreri et al. (1987) carried out a double-blind placebo-controlled trial of vinpocetine. The criteria for subject selection were not clearly stated; subjects were "patients with chronic cerebral dysfunction of variable duration, of vascular origin, with consequent impaired cognitive function" (Balestreri et al. 1987, p. 425). They apparently were institutionalized during the time of the study. Statistically significant improvements were claimed on several measures of cognitive capacity.

Otomo et al. (1985), using global ratings in an open-label trial, found that vinpocetine produced improvement in patients with "sequelae of cerebral infarction and cerebral hemorrhage, cerebral arteriosclerosis and transient ischemic attacks" (p. 811). Thal et al. (1989) reported that vinpocetine was not effective in Alzheimer's disease.

Nootropic drugs.   The assessment of mental improvement in response to a drug presents special difficulties in vascular disease. Measurement may be hampered by defects in patients' motor functioning, perception, or speech, which can impair performance on certain scales. In some reported drug trials, it is not clear whether the investigators intended the drug to be specific for vascular dementia or to be a treatment for dementia in general. There have been several trials of medications in which the subjects were said to have had vascular dementia without the criteria being clearly defined.

The literature on Hydergine (a mixture of ergot derivatives variously known as co-dergocrine, co-dergocrine mesylate, ergoloid mesylate [or mesylates], dihydroergotoxine, and dihydroergotoxine mesylate) is confusing. Hydergine was originally promoted as being likely to dilate brain arteries, but more recently as a nootropic (Schneider and Olin 1994; Wadworth and Chrisp 1992). It is approved and marketed in the United States as a treatment for dementia, and has very little in the way of adverse side effects (although single doses of more than 12 mg may cause headache and nausea). Some earlier studies, such as that of Yesavage et al. (1979), used dementia patients regardless of the cause of the dementia.

Yoshikawa et al. (1983) performed a double-blind comparison of the effects of dihydroergotoxine mesylate (Hydergine) at 6 mg daily versus 3 mg daily in 550 patients experiencing "sequelae of cerebral infarction" and "other cerebrovascular disturbances" (p. 2). The symptoms most benefited were "heavy-headedness," "difficulty in concentrating at work," and "loss of vigor" (p. 6). Arrigo et al. (1989) used intravenous infusions of 3 mg daily of co-dergocrine (Hydergine) in multi-infarct dementia, and claimed improvement in a controlled trial.

Oxiracetam was used in a double-blind placebo-controlled trial that included both multi-infarct patients and Alzheimer patients (Maina et al. 1989). The drug was given at a dose of 800 mg twice a day for 12 weeks and produced significant improvement in dementia-scale scores. Baumel et al. (1989) performed a single-blind trial in patients diagnosed as having multi-infarct dementia. Although the subjects in this trial showed improvement in global ratings, they failed to demonstrate improvement in psychometric measures of cognitive function. Oxirecetam is marketed in Italy as "Neuromet" but has not been found successful in Phase II drug trials in the United States (Cooper 1991), and is not marketed here.

Carotid Artery Surgery

There are several recent and ongoing trials of carotid endarterectomy (Gelabert and Moore 1991). The North American Symptomatic Carotid Endarterectomy Trial (Strandness 1995) ceased randomizing symptomatic patients with severe carotid artery stenosis because the benefits of the operation in this group were so definite. The definition of "symptomatic" used in this trial referred only to prior stroke, and patients with dementia were presumably considered asymptomatic.

So far, there is no definite report of any benefit in dementia, although the surgery caused an overall reduction in stroke, which presumably means there is some effect in preventing dementia.

Baird (1991) reviewed earlier studies, including trials of other surgical procedures for improving cerebral blood supply, and found no strong evidence of behavioral improvement after surgery.

In the cohort of 49 patients with presumed multi-infarct dementia studied by Meyer et al. (1986), there were 8 patients with bilateral occlusive carotid artery disease. Six of these were treated by superficial temporal artery grafting to the middle cerebral artery, and 5 of those 6 improved in cognitive function. Seven of the 8 patients improved after carotid endarterectomy. The eighth improved after stabilization of his blood pressure in the upper range of normal.

Treatment of Nonarteriosclerotic Artery Disease

Occasionally, the treatable condition of giant cell (or temporal) arteritis may cause dementia with infarcts (Caselli 1990). This illness should be possible to diagnose clinically, although it is often the presence of a very high erythrocyte sedimentation rate (ESR) on a routine blood test that alerts clinicians to the diagnosis.

Stroke Prevention Measures

An important question is whether dementia can be helped or prevented by measures intended to reduce the risk of a second stroke. This question becomes particularly difficult when the patient in question has dementia and the measures involve inconvenience or risk.

Some evidence exists that dementia may be reduced by controlling high blood pressure. Hypertension is itself a cause of cognitive impairment in elderly patients (Starr et al. 1993). Meyer et al. (1986) followed 49 patients with multi-infarct dementia for 2 years and compared their clinical course and cognitive performance with those of control groups of age-matched healthy volunteers and of Alzheimer patients. Thirty-five of the 49 patients with multi-infarct dementia were hypertensive. Cognition in the hypertensive multi-infarct cases improved or stabilized in those whose systolic blood pressure was controlled within a range of 135–150 mm Hg.

Several studies have indicated that it is important to avoid episodes of hypotension (Morley 1991). These investigations raise the possibility that hypotension may impair mental function, perhaps by reducing the blood supply to the brain. Such studies must be considered against the background of the evidence that treatment of hypertension is lifesaving and of crucial importance in stroke prevention. In Meyer et al.'s (1986) study, cognition deteriorated if systolic blood pressure fell below 135 mm Hg. Hamamoto et al. (1990) found that scores on a dementia rating scale diminished when the systolic blood pressure of elderly hypertensive patients was reduced below 140. They recommended that the target systolic blood pressure not be below 160.

In the investigation conducted by Meyer et al. (1986), giving up smoking reduced cognitive impairment among normotensive multi-infarct patients. However, most severely demented patients do not smoke anyway. Exercise may also help, but it is difficult for dementia patients to exercise at all vigorously. The role of exercise may be mainly to maintain mobility and daily activities and to prevent contractures and bedsores.

Meyer et al. (1989) published a report of the usefulness of aspirin in multi-infarct dementia. The subjects took one 325-mg aspirin tablet a day for 1 year. A matched control group was used but was not treated with placebo. Two measures of improvement were employed: one was a measure of CBF using ^{133}Xe, and the other was a measure of dementia. Significant improvement was found for the aspirin-treated group on both of these measures. The authors also stated in their discussion that "the aspirin treated group showed improvement in their ADL and became less dependent on others, which was not seen among the control patients" (Meyer et al. 1989, p. 553).

No studies have examined the usefulness of stroke-prevention measures such as diabetes treatment and cholesterol reduction. One investigator has claimed benefits from the use of anticoagulants in all kinds of dementia (Walsh 1993).

Antipsychotic Drugs

An extensive literature now exists on the use of antipsychotic drugs in dementia in general, although there is relatively little concerning vascular dementia in particular.

Barnes et al. (1982), in a controlled trial of antipsychotic medications in nursing-home patients with dementia, did not find that the cause of the dementia affected the response to medications. Anxiety, excitability, and emotional lability were the most likely types of symptoms to be helped.

In 1985, Helms reviewed the existing studies on the efficacy of antipsychotics in treating the behavioral complications of dementia, and found a paucity of well-controlled trials. Drugs that had shown significant advantages over placebo on standardized scales in double-blind trials included thiothixene (Navane), loxapine (Loxitane), haloperidol (Haldol), and thioridazine (Mellaril). None of these agents had been shown to produce any improvement in memory or cognitive function. Rating-scale factors reported to have shown significant improvement were "manifest psychosis," "global improvement," "total assets" (on the Nurses' Observation Scale for Inpatient Evaluation [NOSIE; Honigfeld et al. 1966]), "anxiety," "emotional lability," and "uncooperativeness."

The use of antipsychotic drugs in stroke and in paranoid disorders is further discussed in Chapters 5, 11, and 13.

Treatment of Concurrent Mental Disorder

Apart from the use of antipsychotic drugs to control symptoms of dementia, an improvement in the status of an apparently demented patient may sometimes result from treatment of a concurrent psychosis. The development of paranoid disorders as a result of vascular disease is discussed in Chapter 13. Patients already under treatment for a chronic psychosis, such as schizophrenia, may have their medication regimen interrupted when hospitalized for stroke. The psychotic symptomatology may then recur, especially if hospitalization is prolonged and the patient is transferred to a nursing home or rehabilitation facility. It is important to obtain an accurate history and to communicate with the patient's previous providers of psychiatric care.

The management of depression in general is discussed in Chapter 14. Pseudodementia will sometimes respond to appropriate antidepressant treatments, resulting in improvement of cognitive function.

Treatable Causes of Secondary Dementia

Clinical history and examination should prevent more-treatable conditions from being mistaken for vascular dementia in a new patient. Such conditions are more likely to be missed when they occur as complications causing deterioration of a patient already known to have mild dementia.

> A patient on thyroid medication had a stroke, was hospitalized, and was found to have mild dementia. A battery of blood tests, including thyroid function tests, was normal. Her history of thyroid medication was not recorded. The patient was transferred to a nursing home, where her mental capacity deteriorated until she was noticed to have classic myxedema.

Batteries of blood tests recommended in investigating dementia, and lists of drugs likely to impair cognitive function, are provided in several sources (Conn 1991). A careful review of all medication the patient is taking is an integral part of the assessment of any case of dementia. Iatrogenic cognitive impairment might more correctly be termed delirium than dementia, but regardless of nomenclature, the medication review is one of the most likely ways to improve the mental function of a patient with apparent dementia.

Treatment of debilitating or anoxia-producing conditions can result in improvement of cognitive function. Stroke patients are especially likely to suffer from concurrent cardiovascular disease.

Rehabilitation Modalities

The place of physical and occupational therapy in dementia is partly diagnostic. The physical therapist may be the first to detect that a patient's dementia is emerging as an obstacle to rehabilitation. The occupational therapist will be concerned with elucidating which of the patient's disabilities in ADL are due to specific neurological defects and which are due to dementia.

Even if the disabilities are due to dementia, the therapist may still play a role in optimizing the patient's independence and devising programs for recreation and reality orientation. Occupational therapists have also taken part in helping caregivers of a dementia patient to improve their strategies for dealing with the patient at home (Corcoran and Gitlin 1992).

The place of speech therapy in the treatment of dementia is still being explored. Any successes must raise the question of whether what is being treated is truly dementia or a primary language disorder. Methods such as that of Glickstein and Neustadt (1993; see Table 6–3) are directed at treating aphasia in the presence of dementia. Bourgeois (1992) has used a system of *memory wallets* to treat dementia. These memory wallets contain pictures and sentences about familiar things that the patient has difficulty remembering, and are used during prompted conversations with familiar partners.

Psychosocial Treatments

All of the hard work involved in caring for a patient with dementia constitutes treatment in some sense, although it may seem that not much is being achieved. When institutionalized, dementia patients consume a lot of nursing time, even though the beneficial results of this increased time are hard to measure (Stevens and Baldwin 1988). Sometimes programs such as *friendly visitors,* which seem to improve morale, fail when it comes to demonstrating any measurable effect on memory (Denney 1988). Little work has been done specifically on vascular dementia as opposed to Alzheimer's disease.

Reality orientation.   In institutions, one of the most frequently used treatments for dementia is called *reality orientation* (Holden and Woods 1988). The techniques used are close to what common sense might suggest as methods to improve patients' awareness. There are two kinds of reality orientation—informal and formal. Informal reality orientation goes on throughout the day, and the instructions assume that the patient is in a nursing home or day center. Staff caregivers keep reminding the patient of the date, the time of day, and what is going on around him or her. Staff members are encouraged to speak slowly and clearly, and to make use of aids such as large-print calendars, clocks, and pictures. Formal reality orientation involves small groups of patients meeting daily with a therapist for about 30 minutes, preferably in a special classroom equipped with clocks and calendars and so forth. A description of the original program can be obtained to serve as a basis for training (American Psychiatric Association 1969). There is also a useful general description in a paper by Powell-Proctor and Miller (1982), which critically reviews the evidence for this technique's effectiveness.

Measurements of the effectiveness of reality orientation have been obscured by the use of different techniques and by uncontrolled trials. In general, there is some immediate effect on a patient's ability to remember certain items but little generalization to overall behavior or useful improvement in ADL capacity (Powell-Proctor and Miller 1982). These gains are modest but compare favorably with the meager results of the experimental organic interventions. The effect is greatest on the interest and enthusiasm of the staff and family.

Home Versus Institutional Placement for Patients With Dementia

The placement of the stroke patient in the spectrum of care is discussed in Chapter 20. Most dementia patients are in their own homes, and they may remain there in quite severe states of dementia if the onset of the illness was insidious. When a patient is admitted to an acute-care general hospital following stroke, it will sometimes be found that he or she cannot be discharged home because of dementia. Because state psychiatric hospitals are usually reluctant to take patients with dementia and stroke rehabilitation units also avoid admitting them, such patients usually go to a nursing home.

An increasing number of nursing homes provide special care units for dementia patients (Leon 1994; Weiner and Reingold 1989), but it has been difficult to demonstrate any advantage for dementia care units by controlled trials (Buckwalter 1992; Teresi et al. 1994).

The Team Approach

The lack of effective drugs has sometimes led to the statement that dementia cannot be treated. It is true that in many trials of treatment of dementia, the best that can be done is to demonstrate a slowing down of the progress of the illness, and there are no successful recoveries. There is, however, certainly a great deal of work to be done by health care professionals in the management of dementia. The morale of the family can be considerably helped by a friendly and caring attitude, and even if the treatment of dementia tends to be a losing battle, it is all the more important to encourage and support the individuals involved in providing care. Professionals who care for stroke patients should be expert in dealing with the behavioral disturbances of dementia and the social and economic aspects of this common and tragic condition. Team leaders must demonstrate their knowledge of dementia and their interest in this fascinating challenge to medical science.

Summary

Most dementia patients who do not have severe Alzheimer's disease are found on computed tomography (CT) or at autopsy to have brain infarcts. The overlap between Alzheimer's disease and vascular dementia is probably no more or less than what would be expected by chance. The consensus in the literature is that vascular dementia is less common than Alzheimer's disease. A history of stroke or the presence of an infarct on CT is commonly used to distinguish vascular dementia from Alzheimer's disease. The onset of illness is often more sudden in vascular dementia, and there are more episodes of sharp deterioration.

Multiplicity of infarcts is commonly regarded as a factor in causing dementia. Dementia may also be related to the presence of infarcts in both the thalamus and the cortex, and to the existence of bilateral infarcts. Infarcts with a volume of less than 100 mL are unlikely to cause dementia. Infarcts of the frontal lobes and the hippocampus are more common in patients with dementia than in those without dementia.

Subcortical dementia is unlikely to show speech disturbance as an early symptom, and is marked by a slowing down of thought processes.

No drug has been proven to improve memory and cognitive function in dementia. Helping caregivers with social and economic problems is probably more important than any specific treatment yet available. Vascular dementia may be reduced by controlling high blood pressure, but it is also important to avoid episodes of hypotension. Exercise, aspirin, and giving up smoking have been claimed to help. Antipsychotic medications are used in treating the behavioral complications of dementia. The goal of reality orientation is to improve awareness in dementia patients, but its effectiveness has not been proven.

References

Alzheimer A: Die artiosklerotische Atrophie des Gehirns: Jahresversammlung des Vereins der deutschen Irrenärzte zu Dresden 1894. Allgemeine Zeitschrift für Psychiatrie 51:809–811, 1895

Alzheimer A: Neuere Arbeiten über die Dementia senilis und die auf athero-matoser Gefässerkrankung basierenden Gehirnkrankheiten. Monat-schrift für Psychiatrie und Neurologie 3:101–115, 1898

Alzheimer A: Die Seelenstörungen auf arteriosklerotisher Grundlage: Jahres-versammlung des Vereins der deutschen Irrenärzte. Allgemeine Zeit-schrift für Psychiatrie 59:695–711, 1902

Amar K, Wilcock GK, Scott M: The diagnosis of vascular dementia in the light of the new criteria. Age Ageing 25:51–55, 1996

American Psychiatric Association: Reality Orientation: A Technique to Re-habilitate Elderly and Brain Damaged Patients with a Moderate to Se-vere Degree of Disorientation. Washington, DC, American Psychiatric Association Hospital and Community Psychiatric Service, 1969

American Psychiatric Association: Diagnostic and Statistical Manual of Mental Disorders, 3rd Edition, Revised. Washington, DC, American Psy-chiatric Association, 1987

American Psychiatric Association: DSM-IV Options Book. Washington, DC, American Psychiatric Association, 1991

American Psychiatric Association: Diagnostic and Statistical Manual of Mental Disorders, 4th Edition. Washington, DC, American Psychiatric Association, 1994

Arrigo A, Casale R, Giorgi I, et al: Effects of intravenous high dose co-der-gocrine mesylate (Hydergine) in elderly patients with severe multi-in-farct dementia: a double-blind placebo-controlled trial. Curr Med Res Opin 11:491–500, 1989

Baird AD: Behavioral correlates of cerebral revascularization, in Neurobe-havioral Aspects of Cerebrovascular Disease. Edited by Bornstein RA, Brown GG. New York, Oxford University Press, 1991, pp 297–313

Balestreri R, Fontana L, Astengo F: A double-blind, placebo controlled evalu-ation of the safety and efficacy of vinpocetine in the treatment of pa-tients with chronic vascular senile cerebral dysfunction. J Am Geriatr Soc 35:425–430, 1987

Barnes R, Veith R, Okimoto J, et al: Efficacy of antipsychotic medications in behaviorally disturbed dementia patients. Am J Psychiatry 139:1170–1174, 1982

Baum HM: Stroke prevalence: an analysis of data from the 1977 National Health Interview Survey. Public Health Rep 97:24–30, 1982

Baum HM, Manton KG: National trends in stroke-related mortality: a com-parison of multiple cause mortality data with survey and other health data. Gerontologist 27:293–300, 1987

Baumel B, Eisner L, Karukin M, et al: Oxiracetam in the treatment of multi-infarct dementia. Prog Neuropsychopharmacol Biol Psychiatry 13:673–682, 1989

Baxa W, Pakesch E: Mitteilung über die Verwendung eines Index am HAWIE zur Bestimmung einer sekundaren Intelligenzreduzierung. Wiener Zeitschrift für Nervenheilkunde und deren Grenzgebiete 30:119–130, 1972

Benson DF, Marsden CD, Meadows JC: The amnesic syndrome of posterior cerebral artery occlusion. Acta Neurol Scand 50:133–145, 1974

Birkett DP: Vasodilators in geriatric psychiatry. Journal of the Medical Society of the State of New Jersey 68:619–625, 1971

Birkett DP: The psychiatric differentiation of senility and arteriosclerosis. Br J Psychiatry 120:321–324, 1972

Birkett DP: Diagnosis of dementia in the non-communicating patient (abstract). American Journal of Geriatric Psychiatry 3:261, 1995

Birkett DP, Boltuch B: Measuring dementia. J Am Geriatr Soc 25:153–156, 1977

Birkett DP, Raskin A: Arteriosclerosis infarcts and dementia. J Am Geriatr Soc 30:261–266, 1982

Black RS, Barclay LL, Nolan KA, et al: Pentoxyphylline in cerebrovascular dementia. J Am Geriatr Soc 40:237–244, 1992

Blondal H, Guomundssen G, Benedikz E, et al: Dementia in hereditary cystatin C amyloidosis. Prog Clin Biol Res 317:157–164, 1989

Blumenthal TH, Premachandra BN: The aging-disease dichotomy: cerebral amyloid angiopathy—an independent entity associated with dementia. J Am Geriatr Soc 38:475–482, 1990

Bogousslavsky J, Regli F: Transient global amnesia and stroke. Eur Neurol 28:106–110, 1988

Bolla-Wilson K, Robinson RG, Starkstein SE, et al: Lateralization of dementia of depression in stroke patients. Am J Psychiatry 146:627–634, 1989

Bourgeois MS: Evaluating memory wallets in conversations with persons with dementia. J Speech Hear Res 35:1344–1357, 1992

Brayne C, Gill C, Huppert FA, et al: Incidence of clinically diagnosed subtypes of dementia in an elderly population. Br J Psychiatry 167:255–262, 1995

Brust JCM: Vascular dementia is overdiagnosed. Stroke 14:298–300, 1983

Bruyn RPM: Thalamic aphasia. J Neurol 236:21–25, 1989

Bucht G, Adolfsson R, Winblad B: Dementia of the Alzheimer type and multi-infarct dementia. J Am Geriatr Soc 32:491–498, 1984

Buckwalter KC: Specialized dementia care units (review of book edited by DH Coons). J Am Geriatr Soc 40:305–306, 1992

Caselli RJ: Giant cell (temporal) arteritis, a treatable cause of multi-infarct dementia. Neurology 40:753–755, 1990

Conn DK: Delirium and other organic mental disorders, in Comprehensive Review of Geriatric Psychiatry. Edited by Sadavoy J, Lazarus LW, Jarvik LF. Washington, DC, American Psychiatric Press, 1991, pp 311–336

Cooper JK: Drug treatment of Alzheimer's disease. Arch Intern Med 151:245–249, 1991

Corcoran M, Gitlin LW: Dementia management: an occupational therapy home-based intervention for caregivers. Am J Occup Ther 46:801–808, 1992

Corsellis JAN, Evans PH: The relation of stenosis of the extracranial cerebral arteries to mental disorder and cerebral degeneration in old age. Proceedings of the Fifth International Congress on Neuropathology, 1965, pp 546–548

Cummings JL: Subcortical dementia. Br J Psychiatry 149:682–697, 1986

Cummings JL, Miller B, Hill MA, et al: Neuropsychiatric aspects of multiinfarct dementia and dementia of the Alzheimer type. Arch Neurol 44:389–393, 1987

Del Ser T, Bermejo F, Portera A, et al: Vascular dementia: clinico-pathological study. J Neurol Sci 96:1–17, 1990

Denney NW:. A reanalysis of the influence of a friendly visitor programme. Am J Community Psychol 16:409–433, 1988

Desmond DW, Tatemichi TK, Paik M, et al: Risk factors for cerebrovascular disease as correlates of cognitive function in a stroke-free cohort. Arch Neurol 50:162–166, 1993

Dunne JW, Leedman PJ, Edis RH: Inobvious stroke as a cause of delirium and dementia. Aust N Z J Med 16:771–778, 1986

Eastwood MR, Lautenschlaeger E, Corbin S: A comparison of clinical methods for assessing dementia. J Am Geriatr Soc 31:342–347, 1983

Erkinjuntti T: Types of multi-infarct dementia. Acta Neurol Scand 75:391–399, 1987

Erkinjuntti T: Multi-infarct dementia: clinical features and diagnosis. Geriatric Medicine Today 9:22–40, 1990

Erkinjuntti T, Sulkava R, Wikstrom J, et al: Short Portable Mental Status Questionnaire as a screening test for dementia and delirium among the elderly. J Am Geriatr Soc 35:412–416, 1987

Fischer P, Gatterer G, Marterer A, et al: Course characteristics in the differentiation of dementia of the Alzheimer type and multi-infarct dementia. Acta Psychiatr Scand 81:551–553, 1990

Fisher CM: Lacunar strokes and infarcts: a review. Neurology 32:871–876, 1982

Flicker J: Hodkinson scale and predicting performance (letter). J Am Geriatr Soc 36:1072, 1988

Foerstl H, Levy R: Arteriosclerotic brain atrophy (translation of Alzheimer A: Die artiosklerotische Atrophie des Gehirns: Jahresversammlung des Vereins der deutschen Irrenärzte 1894). International Journal of Geriatric Psychiatry 6:129–130, 1991

Folstein MF, Folstein SE, McHugh PR: Mini-mental state a practical method for grading the cognitive state of patients for the clinician. J Psychiatr Res 12:189–198, 1975

Förstl H, Howard R: Recent studies on dementia senilis and brain disorders caused by atheromatous vascular disease: by A. Alzheimer 1898. Alzheimer Dis Assoc Disord 5:257–265, 1991

Garcia CA, Tweedy JR, Blass JP: Underdiagnosis of cognitive impairment in a rehabilitation setting. J Am Geriatr Soc 32:339–342, 1984

Geaney DP, Abou-Saleh MT: Use and applications of single-photon emission computerised tomography in dementia. Br J Psychiatry 157 (suppl 9): 66–75, 1990

Gelabert HA, Moore WS: Reducing the risk of stroke: identifying patients to refer for carotid endarterectomy. Geriatrics 46:22–27, 1991

Glickstein JK, Neustadt GK: Speech-language interventions in Alzheimer's disease. Clinics in Communication Disorders 3:15–30, 1993

Grober E: Nonlinguistic memory in aphasia. Cortex 20:67–73, 1984

Gurland B, Copeland J, Kuriansky J, et al: The Mind and Mood of Aging. New York, Haworth Press, 1983

Gurland B, Wilder D, Cross P, et al: Relative rates of dementia by multiple case definitions over two prevalence periods in three sociocultural groups. American Journal of Geriatric Psychiatry 3:6–20, 1995

Gustafson Y, Olsson T, Ericksson S, et al: Acute confusional states (delirium) in stroke patients. Cerebrovascular Disease 1:257–264, 1991

Hachinski VC, Lassen NA, Marshall J: Multi-infarct dementia: a cause of mental deterioration in the elderly. Lancet 2:207–209, 1974

Hachinski VC, Iliff LD, Zilhka E, et al: Cerebral blood flow in dementia. Arch Neurol 32:632–637, 1975

Hakim AM: Hemodynamic and metabolic studies in stroke. Semin Neurol 9:286–292, 1989

Hamamoto M, Tsushima T, Miyazaki T, et al: The effects of antihypertensive therapy on the aged—an intervention study in a home for the aged. Nippon Ronen Igakkai Zasshi 27:559–563, 1990

Hammond JH, Eisinger RP: Carotid bruits in 1,000 normal subjects. Arch Intern Med 109:563–565, 1962

Harris Y, Miles HY, Bozzola F: Vascular dementia: a clinical and death certificate study. Neuroepidemiology 11:53–58, 1992

Hasegawa K, Homma A, Imai Y: An epidemiological study of age-related dementia in the community. International Journal of Geriatric Psychiatry 1:45–55, 1986

Helms PM: Efficacy of antipsychotics in the treatment of the behavioral complications of dementia. J Am Geriatr Soc 33:206–209, 1985

Hershey LA: Dementia associated with stroke. Stroke 21 (suppl 2):9–11, 1990

Hijdra A, Derix MMA, Tennisse S, et al: Dementia after stroke (letter). Stroke 22:416, 1991

Holden UP, Woods RT: Reality Orientation: Psychological Approaches to the Confused Elderly. Edinburgh, Churchill Livingstone, 1988

Honigfeld G, Roderic D, Klett JC: NOSIE-30: a treatment-sensitive ward behavior scale. Psychol Rep 19:180–182, 1966

Hutchinson EC: Lesions in cerebrovascular disease and their clinical implications. BMJ 1:89–91, 1972

Ishino H, Seno H, Inagaki T, et al: Relative frequencies of dementia of the Alzheimer type and vascular dementia in Japanese nursing homes. Jpn J Psychiatry Neurol 44:551–556, 1990

Jorm AF: Cross-national comparisons of the occurrence of Alzheimer's and vascular dementias. Eur Arch Psychiatry Clin Neurosci 240:218–222, 1991

Judd BW, Meyer JS, Rogers RL, et al: Cognitive performance correlates with cerebrovascular impairments in multi-infarct dementia. J Am Geriatr Soc 34:355–360, 1986

Kahn RL, Goldfarb AI, Pollack M, et al: Brief objective measures for the determination of mental status in the aged. Am J Psychiatry 117:326–328, 1960

Kase CS: Epidemiology of multi-infarct dementia. Alzheimer Dis Assoc Disord 5:71–76, 1991

Katz DL, Alexander MP, Mandell AM: Dementia following strokes in the mesencephalon and diencephalon. Arch Neurol 44:1127–1133, 1987

Kawamura J, Meyer JS, Terayama Y, et al: Cerebral hypoperfusion correlates with mild and parenchymal loss with severe multi-infarct dementia. J Neurol Sci 102:32–38, 1991

Kendall BS: Memory for designs performance in the seventh and eighth decades of life. Percept Mot Skills 14:399–404, 1969

Kitagawa Y, Meyer JS, Tachibana H, et al: CT-CBF correlations of cognitive deficits in multi-infarct dementia. Stroke 15:1000–1009, 1984

Kofler B, Harrer G, Ladurner G: Contingent negative variation (CNV) differences between cerebrovascular patients with and without dementia. Arch Gerontol Geriatr 7:311–318, 1988

Kopelman MD: Amnesia: organic and psychogenic. Br J Psychiatry 150:428–442, 1987

Koshino Y, Murata T, Oomori M, et al: Temporal minor slow and sharp activity in psychiatric patients. Clin Electroencephalogr 21:225–232, 1990

Kotila M, Waltimo O, Niemi M-L, et al: Dementia after stroke. Eur Neurol 25:134–140, 1986

Kumar A, Yousem D, Souder E, et al: High intensity signals in Alzheimer's disease without cerebrovascular risk factors: a magnetic resonance imaging evaluation. Am J Psychiatry 149:248–250, 1992

Kuwabara Y, Ichiya Y, Otsuka M, et al: Cerebrovascular responsiveness to hypercapnia in Alzheimer's dementia and vascular dementia of the Binswanger type. Stroke 23:594–598, 1992

Ladurner G, Iliff LD, Sager WD, et al: A clinical approach to vascular (multi-infarct) dementia. Exp Brain Res 5 (suppl):243–250, 1982a

Ladurner G, Iliff LD, Lechner H: Clinical factors associated with dementia in ischemic stroke. J Neurol Neurosurg Psychiatry 45:97–101, 1982b

Langlois PF, Sharon GE, Gawryl MS: Plasma concentrations of complement-activation complexes correlate with disease activity in patients diagnosed with isolated central nervous system vasculitis. J Allergy Clin Immunol 83:11–16, 1989

Leon J: The 1990/1991 national survey of special care units in nursing homes. Alzheimer Dis Assoc Disord 8 (suppl 1):S72–S86, 1994

Leuchter AF, Newton TF, Cook IA, et al: Changes in brain functional connectivity in Alzheimer-type and multi-infarct dementia. Brain 115:1543–1561, 1992

Leuchter AF, Daly KA, Rosenberg-Thompson S, et al: Prevalence and significance of electroencephalographic abnormalities in patients with suspected organic mental syndromes. J Am Geriatr Soc 41:605–611, 1993

Leung SY, Ng THK, Yuen ST, et al: Pattern of cerebral atherosclerosis in Hong-Kong Chinese. Stroke 24:779–786, 1993

Lin K-N, Liu R-S, Yeh T-P, et al: Posterior ischemia during an attack of transient global amnesia. Stroke 24:1093–1095, 1993

Lipowski ZJ: Update on delirium. Psychiatr Clin North Am 15:335–346, 1992

Liptzin B: Revising diagnostic criteria for delirium. Am J Psychiatry 148:1612, 1991

Liu HC, Tsou HK, Lin KN, et al: Evaluation of 110 consecutive patients with dementia: a consecutive study. Acta Neurol Scand 84:421–425, 1991

Livingston G, Sax K, Willison J, et al: The Gospel Oak study stage II: the diagnosis of dementia in the community. Psychol Med 20:881–891, 1990

Loeb C, Gandolfo C, Bino G. Intellectual impairment and cerebral lesions in multiple cerebral infarcts. Stroke 19:560–565, 1987

Mahendra B, Lumley JSP, Nimmon CC: Atheroma infarction and dementia (letter). Br J Psychiatry 146:211, 1985

Mahler ME, Cummings JL: Behavioral neurology of multi-infarct dementia. Alzheimer Dis Assoc Disord 5:123–130, 1991

Maina G, Fiori L, Torta R, et al: Oxiracetam in the treatment of primary degenerative and multi-infarct dementia: a double blind, placebo-controlled trial. Neuropsychobiology 21:141–145, 1989

Martin M, Figiel G, Mattingly G, et al: ECT-induced interictal delirium in patients with a history of CVA. J Geriatr Psychiatry Neurol 5:149–155, 1992

Mayer-Gross W, Slater E, Roth M: Clinical Psychiatry. Baltimore, MD, Williams & Wilkins, 1960, p 525

McKeith IG, Bartholomew PH, Irvine EM, et al: Single-photon computerized tomography in elderly patients with Alzheimer's disease and multi-infarct dementia. Br J Psychiatry 163:597–603, 1993

McNeil JK: False negative and false positive cases of pseudodementia. Clinical Gerontologist 13:67–70, 1993

Mehler MF: The rostral basilar artery syndrome. Neurology 39:9–16, 1989

Meyer JS, Judd BW, Tawakhina T, et al: Improved cognition after control of risk factors for multi-infarct dementia. JAMA 256:2203–2209, 1986

Meyer JS, Rogers RL, McClintic K, et al: Randomized clinical trial of daily aspirin therapy in multi-infarct dementia. J Am Geriatr Soc 37:549–555, 1989

Mielke R, Herholz K, Grond M, et al: Severity of vascular dementia is related to volume of metabolically impaired tissue. Ann Neurol 49:909–913, 1992

Morley JE: Is low blood pressure dangerous? J Am Geriatr Soc 39:1239–1240, 1991

Müller M, Schreiner R, Bayar B: Halsgefässonographie Stellenwort in der Differentialdiagnose dementieller Syndrome. Fortschr Med 107:733–735 (English abstract), 1989

Munoz DG: The pathological basis of multi-infarct dementia. Alzheimer Dis Assoc Disord 5:77–90, 1991

Naugle RI, Bridgers SL, Delaney RC: Neuropsychological signs of asymptomatic carotid stenosis. Archives of Clinical Neuropsychology 1:25–30, 1986

New studies of strokes (editorial). BMJ 2:723–724, 1971

O'Brien MD: Vascular dementia is underdiagnosed. Arch Neurol 45:797–798, 1988

O'Connor KP, Shaw JC, Ongley CO: The EEG and differential diagnosis in geriatrics. Br J Psychiatry 135:156–162, 1979

Otomo E, Atarashi J, Abaki G, et al: Comparison of vinpocetine with ifenprodil tartrate and dihyroergotoxine mesylate treatment and results of long-term treatment with vinpocetine. Current Therapeutic Research 37:811–821, 1985

Ott BR, Saver JL: Unilateral amnesic stroke: six new cases and a review of the literature. Stroke 24:1033–1042, 1993

Parnetti L, Mecocci P, Santucci C, et al: Is multi-infarct dementia representative of vascular dementia? A retrospective study. Acta Neurol Scand 81:484–487, 1990

Pfeiffer E: SPMSQ: short portable mental status questionnaire. J Am Geriatr Soc 23:433–441, 1975

Posner JD, Gorman KM, Woldow A: Stroke in the elderly, I: epidemiology. J Am Geriatr Soc 32:95–102, 1984

Powell-Proctor L, Miller W: Reality orientation: a critical appraisal. Br J Psychiatry 140:457–463, 1982

Qureshi KN, Hodkinson HM: Evaluation of a ten-question mental test in the institutionalized elderly. Age Ageing 3:152–157, 1974

Reding M, Haycox J, Blass J: Depression in patients referred to a dementia clinic. Arch Neurol 42:894–896, 1985

Ries F, Horn R, Hillekamp J, et al: Differentiation of multi-infarct and Alzheimer dementia by intracranial hemodynamic parameters. Stroke 24:228–235, 1993

Riesberg B, Ferris SH, De Leon MJ, et al: The global deterioration scale for assessment of primary degenerative dementia. Am J Psychiatry 139:1136–1139, 1982

Robinson RG, Bolla-Wilson K, Lipsey JR, et al: Depression influences intellectual impairment in stroke patients. Br J Psychiatry 148:541–547, 1986

Rocca WA, Hofman A, Brayne C, et al. for the EURODEM-Prevalence Research Group: The prevalence of vascular dementia in Europe: facts and fragments from 1980–1990 studies. Ann Neurol 30:817–824, 1991

Roman GC: The identity of lacunar dementia and Binswanger disease. Med Hypotheses 16:389–391, 1985

Rosen WG, Terry RD, Fuld PA, et al: Pathological verification of ischemic score in differentiation of dementias. Ann Neurol 7:486–488, 1979

Schneider LS, Olin JT: Overview of clinical trials of hydergine in dementia. Arch Neurol 51:787–798, 1994

Scully RE: Case records of the Massachusetts General Hospital. N Engl J Med 325:42–54, 1991

Serby M, Chou JC, Franssen EH: Dementia in an American-Chinese nursing home population. Am J Psychiatry 144:811–822, 1987

Shimamura AP, Gershberg FB: Neuropsychiatric aspects of memory and amnesia, in The American Psychiatric Press Textbook of Neuropsychiatry, 2nd Edition. Edited by Yudofsky SC, Hales RE. Washington, DC, American Psychiatric Press, 1992, pp 345–362

Skoog I, Nilsson L, Palmertz B, et al: A population-based study of dementia in 85-year-olds. N Engl J Med 328:153–158, 1993

Spitzer RL: Revising diagnostic criteria for delirium. Am J Psychiatry 148:1611–1612, 1991

Starkstein SE, Robinson RG: Dementia of depression in Parkinson's disease and stroke. J Nerv Ment Dis 179:593–601, 1991

Starr JM, Whalley LJ, Inch S, et al: Blood pressure and cognitive function in healthy old people. J Am Geriatr Soc 41:753–756, 1993

St. Clair D, Whalley LJ: Hypertension, multi-infarct dementia and Alzheimer's disease. Br J Psychiatry 143:274–276, 1983

Stern G: Book review of Transient Global Amnesia, by H. J. Markowitsch. Br J Psychiatry 160:435, 1992

Stevens GL, Baldwin GA: Optimizing mental health in the nursing home setting. J Psychosoc Nurs Ment Health Serv 26:27–31, 1988

Strandness DE: What you did not know about the North American Symptomatic Carotid Endarterectomy Trial. J Vasc Surg 21:163–165, 1995

Subhan Z, Hindmarsh J: Psychological effects of vinpocetine in normal healthy volunteers. Eur J Clin Pharmacol 28:567–571, 1985

Sulkava R, Erkinjuntti T: Vascular dementia due to cardiac arrhythmias and systemic hypotension. Acta Neurol Scand 76:123–127, 1987

Tamaki N, Kusunoki T, Matsumoto S: Effect of vinpocetine on cerebral blood flow in patients with cerebrovascular disorders. Advances in Therapy 2:53–59, 1985a

Tamaki N, Kusunoki T, Matsumoto S: The effect of vinpocetine on cerebral blood flow in patients with cerebrovascular disorders. Hungarian Medical Journal 33:13–21, 1985b

Tatemichi TK, Foulkes MA, Mohr JP, et al: Dementia in stroke survivors in the stroke data bank cohort. Stroke 21:858–866, 1990

Tatemichi TK, Desmond DW, Prohovnik I, et al: Confusion and memory loss from capsular genu infarction. Neurology 42:1966–1979, 1992a

Tatemichi TK, Desmond DW, Mayeux R, et al: Dementia after stroke: baseline, frequency, risks and clinical patterns in a hospitalized cohort. Neurology 42:1185–1193, 1992b

Teasdale G, Jennett B: Assessment of coma and impaired consciousness. Lancet 2:81–84, 1974

Terayama Y, Meyer JS, Kuwamara J, et al: Patterns of cerebral hypoperfusion compared among demented and non-demented patients with stroke. Stroke 23:686–692, 1992

Teresi J, Lawton MP, Ory M, et al: Measurement issues in special care populations: dementia special care. Alzheimer Dis Assoc Disord 8 (suppl 1): S144–S183, 1994

Thal LJ, Salmon DP, Lasker B, et al: The safety and lack of efficacy of vinpocetine in Alzheimer's disease. J Am Geriatr Soc 37:515–520, 1989

Tomlinson BE, Henderson G: Some quantitative cerebral findings in normal and demented old people, in Neurobiology of Aging. Edited by Terry RD, Gershon S. New York, Raven, 1976, pp 183–204

Tomlinson BE, Blessed G, Roth M: Observations on the brains of non-demented old people. J Neurol Sci 7:331–356, 1968

Tomlinson BE, Blessed G, Roth M: Observations on the brains of demented old people. J Neurol Sci 11:203–242, 1970

Tresch DD, Folstein MF, Rabins PV, et al: Prevalence and significance of cardiovascular disease and hypertension in elderly patients with dementia and depression. Am J Psychiatry 33:530–537, 1985

Ueda K, Fujii I, Kawano H, et al: Severe disability related to cerebral stroke: incidence and risk factors observed in a Japanese community, Hisayama. J Am Geriatr Soc 33:616–622, 1987

Ueda K, Kawano H, Hasuo Y, et al: Prevalence and etiology of dementia in a Japanese community. Stroke 23:798–803, 1992

Von Cramon DY, Hebel N, Schuri U: Verbal memory and learning in unilateral posterior cerebral infarction. Brain 111:1061–1077, 1988

Wadworth AM, Chrisp P: Co-dergocrine mesylate: a review of its pharmacological and pharmacokinetic properties and therapeutic use in age-related cognitive decline. Drugs and Aging 2:153–173, 1992

Wallin A, Blennow K: Pathogenetic basis of vascular dementia. Alzheimer Dis Assoc Disord 5:91–102, 1991

Walsh AC: Anticoagulant therapy and Alzheimer's disease (letter). Am J Psychiatry 150:530, 1993

Wechsler D: Manual for the Wechsler Adult Intelligence Scale. New York, Psychological Corporation, 1955

Weiner AS, Reingold J: Special care units for dementia. Journal of Long-Term Care Administration 17:14–19, 1989

Wilder D, Cross P, Chen J, et al: Operating characteristics of brief screens for dementia in a multicultural population. American Journal of Geriatric Psychiatry 3:96–107, 1995

Withers P, Hinton I: Three forms of the clinical tests of the sensorium and their reliability. Br J Psychiatry 119:1–8, 1971

World Health Organization: International Statistical Classification of Diseases, Injuries, and Causes of Death, 9th Revision. Geneva, Switzerland, World Health Organization, 1975

World Health Organization: International Statistical Classification of Diseases and Related Health Problems, 10th Revision. Geneva, Switzerland, World Health Organization, 1992

Yesavage JA, Hollister LE, Burian E: Dihydroergotoxine: 6 mg versus 3 mg in the treatment of senile dementia. J Am Geriatr Soc 27:80–82, 1979

Yoshikawa M, Shunsaku H, Aizawa T, et al: A dose-response study with dihydroergotamine mesylate in cerebrovascular disturbances. J Am Geriatr Soc 31:1–7, 1983

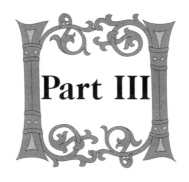

Part III

Outcome and Effects

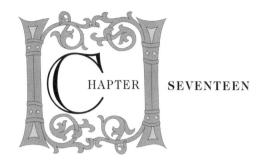

CHAPTER SEVENTEEN

The Stroke Recovery Process

The Neurological Process

Even after the most severe stroke, there is, in those who do not immediately die, some kind of recovery. The most common sequence of events is coma followed by recovery of consciousness. The reasons that brain damage causes coma are not entirely known. Strokes that affect the cerebral hemispheres alone *(supratentorial strokes)* may not produce coma unless they cause massive damage. These strokes may cause paralysis or speech impairment against a background of clear consciousness while the patient struggles to carry on with normal activities. The emotion usually described in retrospect is that of puzzlement or bewilderment. It is unusual for a patient to immediately realize that a stroke is what has caused the perplexing disability. Strokes that affect the pons and brain stem are more likely to produce coma, presumably by specifically affecting the reticular activating system (Frank and Biller 1992), but it is also possible, as in the top-of-the-basilar-syndrome, for such strokes to present as states of confusion. The recovery of consciousness is followed by the discovery of a neurological disability, such as paralysis or aphasia, which then makes a further recovery.

The neurological processes involved in recovery from acute stroke may be classified as *resolution of diaschisis, unmasking, compensation,* and *long-term potentiation* (Goldstein 1990; Meyer 1991).

Resolution of Diaschisis

When one part of the brain is acutely and severely damaged, the entire central nervous system may temporarily cease functioning. Such a generalized effect resulting from a local injury is sometimes called *diaschisis,* a term introduced by von Monakow in 1914 (1969).

One explanation of diaschisis is that, in the acute stage, no injury to the brain is truly localized. There are several possible mechanisms by which the effects of injury can spread. One of these is the production of *cerebral edema*. If one spot on the surface of the living brain is touched, the whole brain can become waterlogged. The condition of cerebral edema is a nonspecific response to any injury or acute disease, including infarction.

Cerebral edema is classified as either *cytotoxic* or *vasogenic*. Cytotoxic edema arises from the fact that the surface of each nerve cell is delicately primed to produce a controlled set of chemical and electrical changes when precisely stimulated. Any irritation can start an uncontrolled cascade of these changes, resulting in an influx of water into the cell. Vasogenic edema results from leakage of fluid from blood vessels into the spaces between the cells, and predominantly occurs in white matter rather than gray matter.

Diaschisis is also brought about by transmission along nerve fibers. As described earlier (see Chapter 5), damage passed along to one nerve cell from another nerve cell may be mediated by a surge of excitatory neurotransmitters.

One part of recovery from acute stroke is, therefore, the resolution of diaschisis. Mentally, this process corresponds to recovery from coma to consciousness; neurologically, it corresponds to recovery from complete flaccid paralysis of all limbs to partial spastic paralysis of some limbs.

Unmasking, Compensation, and Long-Term Potentiation

These three processes are more easily separated in neuroscientific theory than in clinical practice. *Unmasking* is the taking over of the function of a damaged part of the brain by another part that already had the ability to perform that function. *Compensation* is the replacement of one function by another function. *Long-term potentiation* is a neurological process whereby nerve cells learn new functions.

In long-term potentiation, the passage of a nerve impulse across a synapse is made easier by repetition. This facilitation occurs in some types of animal learning. Biochemically, it involves opening of N-methyl-D-aspartate (NMDA) receptors in the postsynaptic neuron, followed by influx of calcium, and then release of nitric oxide, which feeds back to the presynaptic neuron. Anatomically, such potentiation has been localized (although not entirely) to the hippocampus, where there are histologically identifiable neural circuits within which the process occurs. This anatomical location suggests that long-term potentiation is normally concerned with registering freshly learned information (see the discussion of posterior cerebral artery syndrome in Chapter 16). Experimentally, long-term potentiation can be blocked by trifluoperazine and possibly other antipsychotic drugs, but the clinical implications of this finding are not yet known.

The role of long-term potentiation in recovery from stroke is speculative (Goldstein 1990). It may be anatomically and functionally circumscribed, but it is also a possible mechanism for enabling parts of the nervous system to change and undertake new functions. Such changes of function apparently occur in children. Even in childhood there is no growth of fresh nerve cells, and yet children with sizable infarcts of one hemisphere may develop normally (Grotta and Hanson 1993), which suggests that they are able to regain function by developing the other hemisphere (Wehrmacher and Gonzalzles 1990).

Compensation is a process whereby a partially paralyzed patient learns techniques to compensate for the paralysis. For example, some well-muscled young patients with a flaccid hemiplegia are able to walk, carrying the bad side with their good side. Compensatory tricks may be taught by professionals, or patients may learn these themselves. The techniques may be acquired without the patient being aware that he or she is acquiring them. If the shoulder joint is frozen, for example, the patient can learn to move the arm by moving the scapula. In some cases, an unconsciously acquired compensatory trick may even be undesirable, and the therapist may want to make the patient unlearn it.

Unmasking and long-term potentiation are perhaps more physiological, and compensation more psychological, but they are not functionally separate. The three processes blend together as a patient recovers from coma, is left with a residual neurological disability such as hemiplegia, and then makes a slow further recovery from this impairment, with the whole process influenced by such psychological variables as the degree of dementia and extent of motivation.

The Psychosocial Process

The most obvious initial mental event after a stroke is that the patient enters a coma. As the patient begins to recover from the comatose state, he or she becomes progressively more aware of the surroundings. There may be a gradual improvement in cognitive function after the acute stroke. Continuation of the short-term improving trend is more likely in patients with intense subjective physical and emotional symptoms such as headache, vertigo, anxiety, and irritability. It is less likely in older patients and in those with severe motor weakness and impairment of activities of daily living (ADL) (Fujita et al. 1989); in these individuals, the confusion evident upon awakening from coma tends to continue and to become a chronic dementia. Patients who make a rapid and complete recovery from a severe stroke are usually unaware of the severity of their illness, and may even describe having had a pleasant experience (Grotta and Bratina 1995).

In other cases, the initial mental event is not coma but a period of confusion. Brief attacks of confusion or aphasia are not always easily identified. The initial reaction of observers to the acute onset of aphasia is often to assume that the sufferer has a mental disorder. Descriptions of the earliest stage of onset of stroke, from patients and observers alike, are often unclear because of difficulty in describing what was seen or felt. Sometimes the event is described in terms such as "She stopped talking and then her words came out jumbled," or "He stared into space and didn't answer us." Many of these episodes are so short that it is not possible to elicit an accurate account of what happened.

Socially, the period after the initial event is marked by helplessness, with the patient often in a hospital. During this phase, the patient may be unable to meet obligations and fulfill responsibilities. Work does not get done, bills are not paid, homes are neglected, deadlines unmet, and dependents uncared for. Realization of neglected duties comes with return to consciousness and frequently adds to the patient's agitation. The stigmatization of the stroke patient often begins at this point, so that the highly functioning professional may tend to want to conceal his or her diagnosis to avoid losing clients. Then there is slow further recovery, progressing to transfer to a rehabilitation setting or returning home.

Returning home involves further revelation of the extent of handicap, strains on family relationships, and economic adversity. Psychiatric disorders short of severe dementia often become more obvious at this point, because family members will notice emotional changes too subtle to be detected in the hospital. There is a trend for some stroke-associated emotional and personality disorders to improve over the course of about a year, if there is no second stroke or intercurrent illness. Attempts, if they are made, to return to work and to normal social activities involve further struggles until the patient reaches his or her permanent limitations.

The Prognosis of Stroke

The prognosis of stroke, especially regarding mental function, is variable and affected by many factors. Survival-length estimates (Posner et al. 1984) are strongly affected by death in the acute phase and death from concurrent cardiovascular disease. Psychosocially, stroke is a chronically disabling illness rather than a relentlessly progressive one, but one over which the threat of a second stroke or heart attack looms.

Although traditional teaching has been that recovery from stroke reaches its maximum after about 6 months, and that little change takes place after that, it has recently been shown that improvement continues over longer periods. This long-term improvement, especially in elderly patients, is often the result of learning compensatory strategies to cope with disability rather than being caused by purely neuromuscular factors (Ferrucci et al. 1993). According to some estimates, only about 10% of stroke survivors become severely disabled (Brandstater 1990), but such estimates are often based on samples that exclude patients with dementia and those with second strokes who are not rehospitalized. Bamford et al. (1991) also give a relatively optimistic overall prognosis based on a community sample.

Greveson et al. (1991) in England found that, at 3 years after admission to a hospital with a first stroke, 40% of the patients had survived. Of these, 71% were independent or only mildly disabled and 76% were living at home. The degree of physical disability had little to do with whether or not the patient was institutionalized. Reasons for institutionalization were advanced age, lack of a surviving spouse, and mental impairment.

Medical Factors Affecting Prognosis

The medical factors that predict that survival from the acute stroke is unlikely are the same ones that predict severe impairment in survivors. Prolonged deep unconsciousness, flaccid paralysis, advanced age, previous stroke, and the presence of concurrent illness are among these factors, although some patients overcome all of these. The persistence of stroke risk factors is a major determinant of a second stroke. Kalra and Crome (1993) describe several prognostic scoring instruments based on clinical features.

Psychosocial Factors Affecting Prognosis

Among those who survive the initial stroke, social circumstances and mental state (especially dementia) are stronger predictors of stroke recovery than is medical condition. Age is the most consistent predictor. However, the psychological and social cannot readily be disentangled from the physical and medical. The most recent and carefully controlled investigations have increased the importance that must be accorded to social factors, especially in the degree of functional recovery after hospitalization in survivors of a first stroke. Social isolation carries a high risk for poor outcome (Glass et al. 1993).

Kotila et al. (1984), studying Finnish stroke patients with a mean age of 61 years, found that old age, acute-stage hemiparesis, impairment of intelligence and memory, visuoperceptual deficits, "nonadequate emotional reactions," and living alone all had a major negative influence on outcome. More than one-half of the patients had returned to work by 12 months. There was no difference between left- and right-hemisphere strokes. Kotila and colleagues' category of "nonadequate emotional reactions" included emotional lability, indifference, euphoria, anosognosia, and depression. These emotional reactions correlated both with longer hospital stays and with dependence on others for assistance with ADL.

Åström et al. (1992) followed elderly stroke survivors for 3 years, excluding patients who died or who had second strokes. They found that ADL and neurological symptoms changed little after 3 months poststroke, whereas psychiatric symptoms showed changes later. Between 3 and 12 months poststroke, the prevalence of major depression decreased, but then it increased again. Leisure-time activities and social contacts were partially resumed at between 3 and 12 months, and life satisfaction improved. Once good life satisfaction was restored, it was maintained, and poor life satisfaction at 1 year remained poor for the entire 3 years. Patients who were disoriented at 3 months remained disoriented.

Labi et al. (1980) found that a significant proportion of survivors manifested social disability despite complete restoration of physical function, and that this disability could not be accounted for by age, physical impairment, or specific neurological defects. These researchers also found that women patients, better-educated patients, and those who lived with their families did worse, in the sense that they reduced their outside social activities. Some of these findings were unexpected, given that those with more education and those with family support do better in physical rehabilitation. Labi and colleagues suggested that women and highly educated patients may feel more stigmatized by disability and disfigurement, and that some families may be overprotective. Stroke survivors most likely to maintain outside social activities were those who lived alone but who had a close friend.

Measuring Recovery

The subjective element in recovery may defeat our attempts to measure it.

> A 73-year-old woman had made what seemed to be a remarkable recovery from a stroke. After days in a coma and months in a nursing home, she had returned to her own home. She walked into her physician's office and had no obvious disturbance of speech, movement, or memory. However, she said that she had lost her job as a result of her illness, could no longer drive a car to visit her friends or go shopping, and thought her life was miserable. She had been expressing this opinion so often and so vigorously that her children and grandchildren were beginning to avoid her company.

Various ways of assessing recovery exist; these include clinical impressions, global assessments, and rate of institutionalization. Several scales have been devised for this purpose. Apart from measurements of purely mental function, instruments have been formulated to test ADL, stroke-specific disability, and quality of life.

Several ADL scales were compared by Gresham et al. (1980), who found a high degree of agreement among them. The Barthel Index (Mahoney and Barthel 1965) had advantages in completeness, sensitivity to change, and amenability to statistical manipulation. Gresham and colleagues suggested that this scale also enjoyed greater familiarity due to its more widespread use, although the minimum data set (e.g., New York State Department of Health 1991), a comprehensive standardized assessment of functional capacity federally mandated for nursing-home patients in the United States by the Omnibus Budget Reconciliation Act of 1987 (OBRA '87), has probably now become the best-known instrument (Fanous 1993). Anderson (1992) found that the Barthel score underestimated the degree of handicap. For example, whereas the maximum distance scored for ability to walk is 50 yards or more, those who can walk only 50 yards can be severely limited. This underestimation may reflect the fact that the Barthel Index is adapted to U.S. conditions and assumes the availability of a private automobile.

Scales of physical disability measure such capacities as the range of movement of separate limbs and the strength of particular muscle groups. Gowland et al. (1993) has reviewed some of those scales specific to stroke.

Does Treatment Help Recovery?

It has been argued that "stroke recovery is a complex process, the bulk of which is spontaneous and cannot be accelerated by any known method" (Paris 1991, p. 8). If treatment is defined in narrow terms, and measures of improvement exclude effects on emotional well-being and morale, then it becomes doubtful whether treatment beyond the acute phase makes much difference to recovery from stroke. Apart from looking at the outcomes of objective measurements in controlled trials, it is necessary to consider whether treatment should be defined narrowly and whether emotional benefits should be excluded. The physical therapy of stroke patients consists of complex techniques to prevent contractures, encourage the exercise of paretic muscles, and prevent atrophy of non-paralyzed muscles. There is much individual variation and personal interaction in such therapy. The physical therapist applies anatomical and physiological knowledge, as well as following techniques such as those of Brunnstrom, Bobath, or Kabat (Foley and Pizer 1985, pp. 84–86).

From a comprehensive review of the literature up to 1988, Flicker (1989) concluded that no specific type of rehabilitation had been demonstrated to be superior to others, and in particular, that no benefit could be attributed to the newer neurofacilitation techniques. Wagenaar et al. (1990) were likewise unable to show any difference between methods of physical therapy.

Matyas and Ottenbacher (1993) pointed out that some of the faults of the reported trials are just as likely to result in false rejection of a beneficial treatment as in false claims for an ineffective one. A particular deficiency in this direction has been the small sample sizes used, resulting in a lack of statistical power.

Brocklehurst et al. (1978) contended that physical therapy is given to the wrong patients and is continued too long. They found that the most severely disabled patients received the most physical therapy yet had the worst prognosis. Their recommendation was that physical therapy be limited to the early months, and that alternative treatment by volunteers or by less-specialized personnel should be considered. Kalra and Crome

(1993) concluded that elderly stroke patients with either very good or very poor prognoses are those least likely to benefit from physical therapy, and suggested methods of targeting patients in the middle range for rehabilitation.

Many of the therapeutic methods used in rehabilitation may be simply morale builders, working on patients' psychology rather than their physiology. It could be argued that morale building is as important as anything else—that it does not matter if the benefits of the treatment are due to a placebo or Hawthorne effect. Although possibly true, such a statement may not meet with the agreement of an insurance company or managed care reviewer. If it is demonstrated that continuing physical therapy beyond the third month after the stroke does not improve muscle power, but that halting the physical therapy causes the patient to feel abandoned and plunges him or her into depression, what should be the decision about continuing the physical therapy?

Discussions among stroke treatment team members about treatment must include consideration of this issue. The team can feel impelled to recommend continuing the treatment on emotional grounds yet also consider that doing so is not scientific medicine and is wasteful of resources. Including the patient's emotional well-being in discussions of the care plan can ease this dilemma but will not always resolve it.

Although they may be intangible, the benefits of psychosocial interventions can also be definite. Situations exist in which a social work intervention can produce a very concrete benefit, such as obtaining additional funds or transport access for a patient who was entitled to but had not been receiving them. If common sense and intuition suggest that an intervention will make life more pleasant and comfortable for a stroke patient, that intervention is probably beneficial.

Psychotherapy and Stroke

If many of the benefits of rehabilitation are psychological, then the possibility arises of producing those benefits more directly by psychological methods. This hypothetical replacement of physical therapy by psychotherapy has not yet been accomplished. It may be that the morale-boosting effect requires a certain context of goal-directed organic treatment, a placebo effect that cannot be obtained by obviously psychiatric treatment. In the Headington study (Bucher et al. 1984), physical therapy was valued more highly than occupational therapy, even though it was not producing measurable results, because it could be seen to be goal directed.

Another obstacle is that psychotherapists themselves are not certain of their place in neuropsychiatry. Freud himself (1904/1953) did not consider brain-damaged patients to be legitimate subjects for psychoanalytic treatment. He gave various reasons for this assessment, such as that the quantity of libidinal energy was reduced and that "near or above the fifties, the elasticity of the mental processes, on which the treatment depends, is as a rule lacking—old people are no longer educable" (p. 264).

Psychotherapy with stroke patients places certain special strains on the therapist. Speech impediments, for example, can tax the listener as well as the talker. The listener may struggle sometimes to make sense of words, and may experience guilt when occasionally giving up trying to understand. It can also be difficult just to be around someone with a severe illness, even for professionals trained in dealing with distressing situations. Holland and Whalley (1981) said, "Faced with such concrete reasons for unhappiness it becomes hard to dissociate oneself from the patient's isolation and despair, and easy to become engulfed in the patient's unhappiness" (p. 227). The psychotherapist may join the band of those who shun people who have experienced misfortune.

Stroke patients with communication problems will often insist on bringing into the therapy sessions a family caregiver who acts as interpreter, and will want the therapist to direct questions through this person. There are several possible reasons that a patient may insist on having a translator present. The patient's demand may represent a wish to continue dependency or may simply be a way of demonstrating that the family member is indispensable to him or her. It may also represent resistance to insight or a refusal of therapy. How the therapist deals with such a situation will depends on his or her therapeutic orientation and intuitive understanding of what the patient's insistence represents. In my practice, I do not completely prohibit an interpreter, because the reality is that this caregiver is deeply in need of my help and understanding, and the relationship between the stroke patient and the caregiver is ultimately likely to be the most important aspect of therapy. Nevertheless, I always want some time spent alone with the stroke patient, regardless of the extent of his or her speech impairment. Having a private session allows the patient the opportunity to express feelings at leisure in any way he or she chooses. The caregiver is often glad to know that such an opportunity has been provided, regardless of how little advantage is taken of it.

When the patient is articulate and receptive, the therapist's communication might consist of direct advice and explanation of the medical and neurological condition and of matters such as how to obtain disability payments, as well as delving into deeper emotional concerns. Although therapy with stroke patients departs from conventional psychodynamic models by including practical help, friendly advice, and direct expressions of sympathy, the addition of such elements does not detract from the benefit of contact with an unhurried listener. Communicatively impaired patients have a special need for compassionate and understanding listening.

Group Therapy, Stroke Support Groups, and Stroke Clubs

Classical group therapy as described by Schilder, Slavson, Moreno, and others was based on psychodynamic principles. Early group work with stroke patients was based on these models. The pioneer in this field was Singler (1975), who worked in a rehabilitation hospital with stroke patients who had neither aphasia nor dementia. Although her valuable description of her work includes no mention of measurement of results or use of a control group, it contains acute insights and useful descriptions and deserves to be read by anyone concerned with the emotional reaction to stroke.

Singler found that modifications of classical group therapy were necessary with this population. Meetings were held for 1 hour a week. A departure from traditional group structure was that patients joined or left the group when they entered or left the hospital. New members were invited to begin by telling the group about their initial stroke experience.

Singler (1975) noted that discussion among members could be divided into three main areas: gathering information about stroke, sharing experiences and feelings, and identifying fears and problems. At first, patients got most satisfaction out of sharing stories of their frustrations and successes. Group support was useful for the symptom of inability to control emotions, with embarrassment from weeping. Group members gradually became better able to confront their fears. Singler found that head-injury patients did not fit in well with stroke patients in groups because, despite the similarity in the handicaps present, they did not have fear of a second injury, whereas a second stroke was a prominent concern of the stroke patients.

Bucher et al. (1984) ran groups in a rehabilitation hospital in England for young (average age 50) stroke patients whose language and comprehension were sufficient to allow such participation. Their account, like Singler's, is anecdotal and uncontrolled, but nonetheless useful and readable. The authors mentioned several practical points, such as the need to have central locations accessible to wheelchairs, the need to set aside adequate time to transport patients, and the fact that stroke patients are easily fatigued and do better if group sessions are not scheduled too late in the day.

Bucher and colleagues found that adequate preparation and briefing and a preliminary induction session were important. Some patients would express grievances about the institution and then become angry if the group leaders could not correct the problems. This anger might prevent expression of other concerns by the group. There were sharp sex differences, apparently related to the fact that the women in this population mostly did not work outside the home or drive. Women had different concerns from men—they were often forced to realize the extent of their disability sooner because they could not cope with housework when on leave from the hospital, whereas men postponed this realization by delaying their return to work.

Patients tended to measure their general progress by their walking ability, and this was consistently an emotive topic for the groups. They were also likely to overvalue physical aspects of treatment, which they could understand as directed toward a return to walking. Occupational therapy was sometimes found to be threatening if it revealed basic intellectual defects.

Bucher and co-workers found that the expectations of treatment results held by the patients in her groups were higher than those held by the neurological and rehabilitation specialists who worked with them. The patients were overoptimistic, often expecting full return to such activities as driving. This unrealistic optimism was a two-edged sword: although in some respects it improved morale, it also caused group members to become disappointed and upset if other patients were still severely disabled at the time of discharge.

Finally, Bucher and colleagues noticed that emotional lability was a problem for some patients, but that when a patient felt comfortable and confident in a group, he or she appeared able to exert more control and was notably less distressed.

Since these two papers were written, the number of stroke clubs and stroke support groups has grown. There is a slight difference between these modalities. Stroke clubs are run by patients and their families (although they may be sponsored by local chapters of the National Easter Seal Society, the American Heart Association, or local hospitals), whereas stroke support groups are professionally run by a hospital or clinic and concentrate on the concerns of the family members. The National Stroke Association (see Appendix B) maintains a file of all stroke clubs and support groups.

Summary

Small supratentorial infarcts may not produce a coma. Strokes that affect the pons and brain stem are more likely to cause a coma but can present as states of confusion. Younger patients and those with headache, vertigo, anxiety, and irritability are more likely to continue to improve in their awareness of the surroundings after recovery from coma. Descriptions of the earliest stage of onset of stroke are often unclear.

Emotional and personality disorders improve over the course of about a year. Physical recovery from stroke usually reaches its maximum after about 6 months. There is a high mortality rate during the first year after stroke. Although disability is not progressive, about 10% of stroke survivors become severely disabled. Most long-term stroke survivors live at home. Institutionalization occurs because of advanced age, lack of a surviving spouse, and mental impairment rather than because of physical disability. Prolonged deep unconsciousness, flaccid paralysis, advanced age, previous stroke, and the presence of concurrent illness predict that survival from the acute stroke is unlikely and that survivors will have severe impairment. Social circumstances and mental state (especially the presence of dementia) are stronger predictors of recovery of function than is medical condition. Age is the most consistent predictor. Social isolation carries a high risk for poor outcome.

Patients want to see a direct connection between rehabilitation methods and their expected goals. Medical and rehabilitation treatment beyond the acute phase may benefit patients' emotional well-being and morale, but often cannot be shown objectively to affect physical recovery.

Emotional well-being and morale may be helped by psychotherapy, but psychotherapists are not always prepared to deal with individuals who have sustained brain damage. The dynamic aspects of therapy often concern the relationship between the patient and caregivers. Frequently, direct advice and counseling are needed. Stroke clubs are run by patients and their families; stroke support groups are run by a hospital or clinic.

References

Anderson R: The Aftermath of Stroke. Cambridge, UK, Cambridge University Press, 1992

Åström M, Asplund K, Åström T: Psychosocial function and life satisfaction after stroke. Stroke 23:527–531, 1992

Bamford J, Sandercock P, Dennis M, et al: Classification and natural history of clinically identifiable subtypes of cerebral infarction. Lancet 337:1521–1526, 1991

Brandstater ME: An overview of stroke rehabilitation. Stroke 21 (suppl II): II-40–II-42, 1990

Brocklehurst JC, Andrews K, Richards B, et al: How much physical therapy for patients with stroke? BMJ 1:1307–1310, 1978

Bucher J, Smith E, Gillespie C: Short-term group therapy for stroke patients in a rehabilitation center. Br J Med Psychol 57:283–290, 1984

Fanous MH: New OBRA guidelines for nursing facilities (letter). J Am Geriatr Soc 41:194, 1993

Ferrucci L, Bandinelli S, Guralnik JM, et al: Recovery of functional status after stroke. Stroke 24:200–205, 1993

Flicker L: Rehabilitation for stroke survivors—a review. Aust N Z J Med 19:400–406, 1989

Foley C, Pizer HF: The Stroke Fact Book. New York, Bantam Books, 1985

Frank JI, Biller J: Coma in focal cerebrovascular disease: an overview. Stroke Clinical Updates 3:9–12, 1992

Freud S: On psychotherapy (1905 [1904]), in Standard Edition of the Complete Psychological Works of Sigmund Freud, Vol 7. Translated and edited by Strachey J. London, Hogarth Press, 1953, pp 257–268

Fujita T, Kurihara M, Hasegawa K: Short-term therapeutic prognosis of cognitive impairment with cerebrovascular diseases in chronic stages. Nippon Ronen Igakkai Zasshi 26:499–506, 1989

Glass TA, Matchar DS, Belyea M, et al: Impact of social support on outcome in first stroke. Stroke 24:64–70, 1993

Goldstein LB: Pharmacology of recovery after stroke. Stroke 21 (suppl 3): 139–142, 1990

Gowland C, Stratford P, Ward M, et al: Measuring physical impairment and disability with the Chedoke-McMaster stroke assessment. Stroke 24:58–61, 1993

Gresham GE, Phillips TF, Labi ML: ADL status in stroke: relative merits of three standard indexes. Arch Phys Med Rehabil 61:355–358, 1980

Greveson GC, Gray CS, French JM, et al: Long-term outcome for patients and carers following hospital admission for stroke. Age Ageing 20:337–344, 1991

Grotta JC, Bratina P: Subjective experiences of 24 patients dramatically recovering from stroke. Stroke 26:1285–1288, 1995

Grotta JC, Hanson S: Acute stroke management. Stroke Clinical Updates 4:13–16, 1993

Holland LK, Whalley MJ: The work of the psychiatrist in a rehabilitation hospital. Br J Psychiatry 138:222–229, 1981

Kalra L, Crome P: The role of prognostic scores in targeting stroke rehabilitation in elderly patients. J Am Geriatr Soc 41:396–400, 1993

Kotila M, Waltimo O, Niemi ML, et al: The profile of recovery from stroke and factors influencing outcome. Stroke 15:1039–1044, 1984

Labi MLC, Phillips TF, Gresham GE: Psycho-social disability in physically restored long-term stroke survivors. Arch Phys Med Rehabil 61:561–565, 1980

Mahoney FI, Barthel D: Functional evaluations: the Barthel index. Maryland State Medical Journal 14:61–65, 1965

Matyas TA, Ottenbacher KJ: Confounds of insensitivity and blind luck: statistical conclusion validity in stroke rehabilitation clinical trials. Arch Phys Med Rehabil 74:559–565, 1993

Meyer JS: Does diaschisis have clinical correlates? Mayo Clin Proc 66:430–432, 1991

New York State Department of Health: Minimum data set (Form DOH-2666). Albany, NY, New York State Department of Health, Division of Health Care Standards and Surveillance, October 1991

Omnibus Budget Reconciliation Act of 1987 (OBRA), Public Law 100-203

Paris JA: Comments on the case of Susan Bendor. Medical Malpractice Prevention 6:8, 1991

Posner JD, Gorman KM, Woldow A: Stroke in the elderly, I: epidemiology. J Am Geriatr Soc 32:95–102, 1984

Singler JR: Group work with hospitalized stroke patients. Social Casework 56:348–354, 1975

von Monakow C: Diaschisis (1914), in Brain and Behaviour, Vol 1: Mood States and Mind. Edited by Pribram KH. Baltimore, MD, Penguin Books, 1969, pp 27–36

Wagenaar RC, Meijer OG, Van Wieringen PC, et al: The functional recovery of stroke: a comparison between neurodevelopmental treatment and the Brunnstrom method. Scand J Rehabil Med 22:1–8, 1990

Wehrmacher WH, Gonzalzles A: Stroke in the young. Internal Medicine for the Specialist 11:88–93, 1990

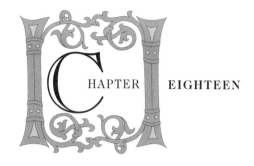

CHAPTER EIGHTEEN

The Family

The study of the family has become a vast field of its own. The work of practitioners such as Nathan Ackerman, Murray Bowen, and Robin Skynner possesses an interest that extends outside the medical area, but although such studies of family dynamics merit the attention of anyone involved with a stroke victim's family, they have seldom examined the effects on the family of having a member with neurological disease. Published studies about the effects of stroke on the family have mostly focused on socioeconomic rather than psychodynamic factors.

The perspective from which the practitioner sees the family varies with the location of practice. Hospital-based practitioners usually have little contact with members of a patient's family unless they deliberately decide to do so. In stroke, the patient is often brought unconscious to the hospital and given intensive care by specialists whom the family has not previously known, and who may be too busy to spend much time with the family. It is important to be aware of the potential for poor relationships and resentment in this situation.

In the initial stages of hospitalization, the decisions about care are mostly made by medical professionals, but as time goes on, more devolves upon the family. At this point, a reverse situation sometimes develops, with the discharge planners complaining that they cannot contact the family. Although difficulty in reaching family members is sometimes interpreted as evidence that the family wants to evade its responsibilities, such problems are more likely attributable to members' attempting to make up time missed at work, needing to travel long distances to visit, or having otherwise drained their emotional and financial resources during the acute stage.

In private office practice, on the other hand, the stroke patient seldom comes alone, and some aspects of the family structure are evident at the first visit. Much can be learned from observing who it is that comes with the patient. Some family members, especially sons, seem more adept at absolving themselves of responsibility than others. These absent sons are often favorites of the patient against whom not a word can be spoken.

Even more can be learned from a home visit. Although such visits are now more often made by nurses and social workers than by physicians, and are made with the object of assessing the level of assistance needed rather than the family dynamics, they are often more revealing of family emotional structure than is formal family therapy. Apparently loyal and dedicated families may not be able to give adequate care.

> The devoted elderly husband of an aphasic and hemiplegic patient insisted that he needed no outside help in caring for his wife. He would frequently call on their daughter for help but would turn away home aides and visiting nurses, telling them they were not needed. He himself was mildly demented and paranoid. The home was filthy and his wife was dirty and neglected.

Such denial in the face of a situation that is obviously out of hand can be an indication that the caregiving spouse has a psychiatric disorder. Behavior of this kind can also represent a method of imposing on a child for help.

The child elected to carry the greatest burden is often a daughter who is vulnerable to being manipulated by a guilt-inspiring parent—and susceptible to the depression associated with that guilt. A nonhelping child may vigorously point this out, and claim to be in better mental health than the martyr of the family. Each of these children in turn may have their own husbands and wives and children to cope with.

The overburdened daughter may need direct advice about asserting herself, and the practitioner can often provide both encouragement and concrete suggestions in this regard. One method is to tell her to announce to the other family members the dates when she is going on vacation.

Even when, as is often the case, such advice is not taken, it can be helpful in developing insight into the situation and relieving the burden of imposed guilt.

The effect of parental stroke on younger children has been little studied, in part because most strokes occur in older people. In the absence of clinical studies, the sensitive account by Colm Tóibín (1992) is worth reading.

Ethnicity

There are few areas of human behavior in which religious and ethnic background has as profound an effect as in family attitudes. Almost all of the literature about the effect of stroke on the family has come from English-speaking countries, and even that from the United States has focused little attention on ethnic factors. Practitioners who work with stroke patients must try to understand the considerable variation in family structure with nationality/race and religion. This variability is often particularly evident in decisions about managing a chronically disabled stroke patient at home versus putting him or her into a nursing home. The underrepresentation of African Americans as patients in nursing homes is striking, and is probably (although not certainly) related to the attitudes of this group toward family obligations.

Even within ethnic groups, the minor nuances of cultural variations in family custom can become important. For example, in some groups, such as Italian Americans, the family eats together at set times. This practice can cause tension if a stroke patient is unable to eat in a socially acceptable way. A messy eater may be easier to tolerate in a home where family members eat irregular snacks without sitting together at a table.

Family Influence on Prognosis

In stroke, the family may help or hinder recovery. Family members may undertake many tasks for the patient. Apart from the extra work this entails for the family, such catering is not always a good thing for the patient. Although social isolation is usually an adverse prognostic factor, stroke patients sometimes do better living alone, because an overprotective family can sabotage a patient's rehabilitation by doing too much for him or her (Isaacs 1977).

Evans et al. (1987b) found that prestroke family interaction was a better predictor of the length of hospital stay than were the typical forecasters of stroke outcome. They reported that patients whose families had more behavior problems spent less time in the hospital. It might seem counterintuitive that family behavior problems would result in shorter hospital stays, but Evans and colleagues suggested that the behavior problems were the result of vigorous and creative attempts to deal with the predicament caused to the family by the stroke. Families less emotionally involved would make less effort and give themselves fewer problems.

Stress on Family Caregivers

Family members may themselves experience adverse effects when a relative suffers a stroke. These adverse effects can be severe enough to require professional help. It seems to be the mental effects of stroke that cause the most stress for caregivers, although the methodology of attempts to prove this has been disputed (Daly and Fredman 1993). Intuition and clinical experience suggest that the stress produced by a family member's dementia varies with the closeness of the caregiver's relationship to the patient. Dementia is harder to deal with in a spouse than in a parent, and in the young than in the old. In living with a dementia patient, the cognitive deficits can sometimes be more easily tolerated than the accompanying behavioral disturbance.

Even successful rehabilitation can add to the burden of the caregivers, if it results in more responsibility being thrust upon them, as is illustrated in the following example:

> An elderly woman had dominated the life of her unmarried daughter, with whom she lived, by constant demands for attention, many physical complaints, and refusal to set foot outside the house. The daughter had become alcoholic. The mother suffered a stroke with left hemiplegia, was hospitalized, and was subsequently transferred to a nursing home. The daughter anticipated that placement would be permanent, and, as a result, her mental health improved. She stopped drinking and began to develop an independent social life. However, her mother progressed to being able to walk alone, and vociferously expressed her wish to return home. The daughter was very upset.
>
> With social work intervention and psychiatric consultation, it was established that much of the mother's previous illness had been due to agoraphobia. A program of treatment for this disorder was initiated, along with counseling for the daughter and recruitment of support from another daughter and son to share the burden.

A frequent research finding has been that the troubles of family caregivers are more severe than was formerly realized, and that these caregivers need more help. However, stress and mental illness cannot be equated, and although stressed caregivers may describe themselves as anxious or depressed, they seldom become mentally ill to the point of needing psychiatric treatment (Eagles et al. 1987).

Family caregivers lose sleep, restrict their social lives, and worry about whether the care they are providing is adequate. In the immediate aftermath of a stroke, fears that the patient may die result in concerns about the patient's physical health being dominant. These fears are subsequently replaced by concerns about psychosocial issues such as living arrangements and emotional relationships, and finally, concerns about physical dependency come to dominate (Anderson 1992).

Greveson et al. (1991), in England, using standardized rating scales, compared families of stroke patients with age- and sex-matched control subjects. They found that the family members were under generalized stress, with sleep problems, social isolation, and financial burdens. The financial burdens resulted not only from the direct cost of care but also from a family member's having given up work to attend to the patient. Whereas a patient's contact with friends and neighbors is reduced after stroke, that with his or her children remains high.

Silliman et al. (1986), in North Carolina, compared families who cared for stroke patients at home with those who had them institutionalized, and found no significant differences. The home caregivers suffered from loss of time for themselves and from financial burdens, but those with institutionalized family members also suffered from these difficulties. Wade et al. (1986) studied a community sample in England, using rating scales but not a control group. They found that increased anxiety was the most commonly reported change in family caregivers 6 months after a stroke. The degree of disability in the patient seemed unrelated to the amount of anxiety and depression seen in family caregivers at 2-year follow-up.

Carnwath and Johnson (1987), on the other hand, also in an English community sample but with a control group, found that depression increased among spouses of stroke patients over the 3 years after the stroke and was related to the stroke's severity. Regular contact with friends and neighbors was protective against depression. Although these spouses tended to resent being labeled as patients and to reject psychiatric help, they welcomed visits from a branch of the Association of Carers.

The differences between the findings of these two English groups may be attributable to the reality that it is more emotionally taxing to deal with disability in a spouse than in a parent, and the Carnwath and Johnson study was limited to spouses.

Management of Stress in the Family

Treatments recommended for stress have ranged from meditation and relaxation to medications and vacations, but it is always primary to examine and list the sources of stress and then to remove them if possible, and to discuss them if not. Discussion can be with others going through the same ordeal, with family and friends, or with professionals.

Families can be helped by some of the following publications: "What Every Family Should Know About Stroke," "Home and Work Adaptations," "Suggestions for Communication With an Aphasic Person," "Living at Home After a Stroke," "Stroke Questions and Answers," "Adaptive Resources Guide," "Family Care-Givers Guide," and *Disability Workbook for Social Security Applicants* (all from the National Stroke Association in the United States). Also useful are *When a Loved One Has a Stroke* (religiously oriented), from Abbey Press, and *Stroke: A Handbook for the Patient's Family,* from the Council of Health Service Agencies (CHSA) in Britain (addresses are provided in Appendix B).

A team approach can helpful in providing practical advice and factual information to family members. The family's goals for the patient should be defined early during the rehabilitation course and discussed in relationship to the treatment team's goals (Teroaka and Burgard 1992). Each member of the treatment team has a specific role. The physicians and nurses provide information about prognosis and medical aspects. The social worker may be especially involved in providing information regarding access to financial assistance, home care, and support groups. Rush (1992) provided a step-by-step account of such a team approach with a family involved in home care of a severely ill stroke patient.

Evans et al. (1987a, 1987b, 1988) reported on stroke patients' families in a series of articles, using rating scales and control groups. They assessed the usefulness of interventions and found that the addition of counseling, consisting of seven follow-up problem-solving sessions with a social worker, to classroom instruction for family caregivers was beneficial.

When we turn to the first-person narratives of caregivers to judge the efficacy of interventions such as support groups and counseling, we find that few caregiver-authors received any such interventions at all. In *The Matthew Tree,* by H. T. Wright (1975), what stands out is that psychological help provided for her by professionals was not just inadequate, but totally nonexistent.

Wright described a buildup of stress to the point where she typed a note saying, "If ever I am in a condition similar to my father's, please get a fast and final happy pill or shot from a reliable source and make certain I absorb it" (Wright 1975, p. 23). She subsequently killed her father, who had been paralyzed by a stroke for 7 years, by giving him an overdose of barbiturates. An especially alarming realization from reading this book is that, in many ways, the author faced fewer stresses than do many family caregivers. She had support from her own family, and no apparent financial problems.

A point sometimes made in connection with such tragic cases is that perhaps nothing can make the intolerable tolerable. Traditionally, grief was held to be outside the domain of medical treatment, but trained therapists now have a body of experience and skills that can be useful even in dealing with this extremity.

At the very least, practitioners must realize that caregivers endure a great deal of stress and that they have a responsibility to provide support and assistance. Often, medical and nursing staff regard this responsibility as less important than other aspects of care.

> Recently, at a nursing home, I admitted a stroke patient and wrote a series of orders for diet and medication. Having talked to the family, I also wrote an order for certain stroke informational literature and useful addresses to be given to them. Returning a week later, I found that every diet and medication order had been faithfully carried through, but nothing had been done about the orders to get information for the family, because no one had "gotten around to it."

Patient Advocates

In some cases, a patient advocate rather than a mental health professional is needed—for example, in situations where the basic needs of a patient or a patient's family have been ignored in a culpable way. A patient advocate is qualified and able to investigate complaints and to take remedial action. Patient advocates can be of various kinds. The federally funded Office on Aging in most communities can provide elderly individuals with information about benefits they are entitled to, and can coordinate activities of other helping agencies. Adult Protective Services can investigate cases of abuse and neglect in any setting. Most hospitals have a patient care representative who can be contacted to assist patients and their families with complaints about hospital care. In some states, such as New York, there is a health care ombudsperson who can investigate complaints against physicians and hospitals.

Patient advocacy is needed in situations in which there has been a complete omission of attention to the psychosocial aspects of stroke care. Such omission is more likely to occur in a general-hospital setting than in a rehabilitation one, and is more commonly due to failure of communication than to lack of motivation to help.

The wife of a patient recently told me this story:

> Stanley [her husband] went into the hospital after the third stroke. That was the worst one. He never talked or walked after that. None of the doctors ever spoke to me. Not one of them ever returned my telephone calls. The only information I got was from the nurses. They said there was nothing they could do and he would never get any better. Then the hospital said I had to get him out because Medicare wouldn't pay anymore. They said I had to put him in a nursing home 30 miles away. I can't drive on account of my eyes. My daughter has to take off work to drive me. I used to see him every day in the hospital. He's angry now because I don't come every day. He still knows who I am. He holds my hand and doesn't want me to go.

Summary

The mental effects of stroke cause more stress for family caregivers than the physical effects. Family caregivers suffer sleep problems, social isolation, and financial burdens and report experiencing anxiety and depression. In counseling stressed caregivers, practical advice should be offered but may not be accepted. The problems families encounter with health and social agencies may be better handled by advocacy services than by mental health services.

References

Anderson R: The Aftermath of Stroke. Cambridge, UK, Cambridge University Press, 1992

Carnwath TCM, Johnson DAW: Psychiatric morbidity among spouses of patients with stroke. BMJ 294:409–411, 1987

Daly MP, Fredman L: Caregiver stress (letter). J Am Geriatr Soc 41:466–467, 1993

Eagles JM, Craig A, Rawlinson F, et al: The psychological well-being of supporters of the demented elderly. Br J Psychiatry 150:293–298, 1987

Evans RL, Bishop DS, Matlock A-L, et al: Family interactions and treatment adherence after stroke. Arch Phys Med Rehabil 68:513–517, 1987a

Evans RL, Bishop DS, Matlock A-L, et al: Pre-stroke family interactions as a predictor of stroke outcome. Arch Phys Med Rehabil 68:508–512, 1987b

Evans RL, Matlock A-L, Bishop DS, et al: Family intervention after stroke: does counseling or education help? Stroke 19:1243–1249, 1988

Greveson GC, Gray CS, French JM, et al: Long-term outcome for patients and carers following hospital admission for stroke. Age Ageing 20:337–344, 1991

Isaacs B: Five years' experience of a stroke unit. Health Bulletin (Edinburgh) 35:94–98, 1977

Rush EW: Interdisciplinary home care. Home Healthcare Nurse 10:10–11, 1992

Silliman RA, Fletcher RH, Earp JL, et al: Families of elderly stroke patients: effects of home care. J Am Geriatr Soc 34:643–648, 1986

Teroaka J, Burgard R: Family support and stroke rehabilitation. West J Med 157:665–666, 1992

Tóibín C: The Heather Blazing. London, Pan Books, 1992

Wade DT, Legh-Smith J, Langton-Hewer R: Effects of looking after and living with survivors of a stroke. BMJ 293:418–420, 1986

Wright HT: The Matthew Tree. New York, Random House, 1975

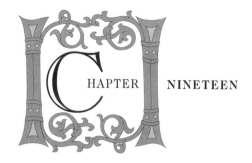

CHAPTER NINETEEN

The Stroke Treatment Team

The acute stroke patient is the focus of dramatic interventions. Such a patient, in an acute-care setting, is supposed either to reward doctors and nurses by getting better, or, if he or she cannot deliver that reward, to die. Stroke patients often do neither, but linger on as a reproach to the medical care system. There have been changes in the medical care system that have recently increased the attention given to patients such as partially recovered stroke victims. These changes have arisen because of the aging of the population, because of new health care reimbursement methods, and because of the development of geriatric and rehabilitation medical specialties. Notwithstanding these changes, the hospital, as a social unit, has not historically been geared toward the chronic patient.

Goodstein (1983) provided an insightful account of what happens when a stroke patient enters a hospital. He theorized that in the general hospital, the staff caregivers and the stroke patient often come to function like a family, and that anger toward the patient who does not get better is an example of the mechanism of projection. Staff members find it difficult to acknowledge chronicity and, as a result, unconsciously assume that the reason the patient does not get better is that they, the staff, are bad and incompetent. They then project this idea of badness onto the patient, and look for evidence that the patient does not want to get well or is uncooperative. Projection may also cause false optimism. The staff wish to succeed, and project this wish onto the patient, encouraging a shared belief that if everyone is good, a magical cure will take place.

These feelings of love and hate that can arise between the patient and the caregivers are sometimes explained as *transference* and *counter-transference*. The term *transference* was originally used by Freud in 1910 to describe a process whereby the patient "directs towards the physician a degree of affectionate feeling (mingled, often enough, with hostility) which is based on no real relation between them and which—as is shown by every detail of its emergence—can only be traced back to old wishful phantasies of the patient which have become unconscious" (Freud 1910/1957, p. 51). The reciprocal feelings of love and hate engendered in the therapist by the patient's transference were called *countertransference*.

Acute-care settings often develop their own culture. Camaraderie and ésprit de corps are present, but are designed to maintain order in the face of crisis rather than provide emotional warmth and support. The group is cohesive, with defined roles, and is hierarchical rather than democratic. When the established authority figures are older male doctors with technical expertise, and newcomers are young female nurses, then acceptance of the hierarchy is so established that little overt conflict arises.

The absence of overt disputes in these traditional male-dominated settings does not mean that there are no tensions. Professionals who help care for stroke patients often suffer emotional strain. Those trained to cure may be frustrated when they feel that all they can do is comfort. Much of the day-to-day care of the institutionalized stroke patient falls upon nurse's aides. Often these personnel come from ethnic groups other than those of the patients, and there may be language barriers and cultural differences that add to the tensions they work under (Tellis-Nayak and Tellis-Nayak 1975).

The traditional family-like hierarchies in acute-care settings have recently been changing, and there has been a trend toward replacing the hierarchy with a team. Introducing a team approach into acute-care settings can make it easier both to avoid confrontations and hostility and to improve efficiency. An advantage of such an approach is that in team meetings, new and junior members are encouraged to speak out. When a new member of a treatment team arrives, he or she may serve a useful role by questioning established methods that are perhaps not well justified but have become customary.

Thurgood (1990) described how good communication and the observations of a junior member of the team led to the elucidation of the cause of an outburst of crying by an aphasic patient. She pointed out, "In many situations junior staff members are reluctant to speak out for fear of 'looking stupid.' The advantage of being in a team is that everyone is viewed as valuable and equal, which gives individuals the confidence to comment and know that the team will welcome their input" (p. 39).

The Interdisciplinary Approach

The use of an interdisciplinary team approach is widespread in rehabilitation, partly because rehabilitation almost always involves the services of more than one discipline (Jaffe 1989). Another impetus to interdisciplinary approaches in diagnosis-related group (DRG)–exempt settings has been the need to document the treatment being given to satisfy third-party insurance payers. Whereas, in the acute-care unit, a fixed payment is provided for the diagnosis of stroke, in the DRG-exempt unit, payment is provided for each day that active treatment is documented. Team meetings are needed to prepare this documentation because the role of each team member must be specified. Outside the institution, the team approach becomes harder to adhere to because the membership of the team widens and the leadership becomes more diffused.

In Britain, the Consensus Statement of the King's Fund Forum recommends that, after discharge from the hospital, or if the stroke patient is not admitted to a hospital,

> [t]he onus is on the general practitioner to coordinate rehabilitation and continuing care services. If the general practitioner does not undertake this personally he or she should nominate a key worker to undertake these responsibilities. . . . The general practitioner or key worker should arrange to see the patient regularly. At the very least this will help to overcome the feelings of isolation and abandonment expressed by so many patients and carers. It should also enable the general practitioner to discover any further medical or social problems. . . . Participants in the rehabilitation process include nurses, physiotherapists, occupational therapists, dietitians, chiropodists, psychologists and doctors. They should work as a team. For the team to work effectively there must be trust and respect for each other's skill. A key worker should be identified for every patient at every stage to coordinate an individual plan and provide education and positive support. (Consensus Conference Panel 1988, pp. 127–128)

Critical Path methodology has been adapted from industrial management for use in stroke rehabilitation (Luttman 1993; Romito 1990). In this approach, the treatment team compiles a timetable with weekly expectations, listing every possible intervention and outcome. Team members then meet weekly to discuss progress and short-term goals.

Preston (1990), in California, described in detail the management of a stroke patient at home by means of a team employed by a home health care agency. The team consisted of nurses, home health aides, physical therapists, occupational therapists, speech pathologists, social workers, and respiratory therapists. The physician, pharmacist, psychologist, patient, and patient's family are also considered members of the team in this model. A case manager is appointed, usually a nurse (the ultimate goal is that the patient becomes his or her own case manager). The process includes assessment, goal setting, and planning followed by implementation and then by evaluation and modification of goals and plans. Preston emphasized that there should be continuous, open communication, preferably carried out as a group process, with written documentation and with each team member aware of the areas being addressed by the other team members.

Although probably cost-effective in the long run, Preston's approach could only be financed in the United States in a system of managed care.

The Mental Health Professional

At what point, if at all, should a mental health professional be involved in stroke care? The answer might depend on what is meant by a mental health professional. Speech therapists and social workers could be included in this category. Neurologists have postdoctoral training in psychiatry, as have physicians recently trained in geriatrics and family practice. It must be admitted that there are psychiatrists and psychologists who are not interested in working with neurologically impaired individuals, although, on the other hand, the burgeoning specialties of neuropsychiatry and neuropsychology attest to the fact that there are many professionals who *are* interested in such work. Specialized neuropsychologists see their function as identifying disabilities, performing neuropsychological testing, and formulating treatment plans, often based on learning theory. In some settings, these specialists may play a leading role even without providing psychotherapy.

In some cases, rehabilitation hospitals have affiliations with psychiatrists or psychologists. These professionals may conduct a liaison service that provides support in activities such as training staff and attending meetings. Sometimes such practitioners see individual patients only in formal consultations requested by a physician.

The work of a psychiatrist in a rehabilitation hospital in England was described by Holland and Whalley (1981). They found that although more patients were admitted with stroke than with head injury, more head-injury patients were referred to the psychiatrist. The head-injury patients were younger than the stroke patients and had a higher incidence of behavioral problems—in particular, aggressive conduct, confusion, and personality change. Holland and Whalley suggested that the predominantly young staff may have identified more strongly with the younger patients, and that this may have influenced the different rate at which head-injury and stroke patients were referred for psychiatric consultation. Patients with chronic neurological disease other than stroke or head injury received the most frequent psychiatric referrals of all, and family distress and the need for family counseling were greater in this group than in the head-injury or stroke groups.

Holland and Whalley suggested three main tasks for the psychiatrist: first, excluding the possibility that the patient is suffering from a specific treatable mental illness; second, offering counseling to the patient trying to adjust to the illness (they suggest this function as one for the psychiatrist on the assumption that he or she "has more time" than the primary physician); and third, offering specific treatments such as behavior modification programs, individual psychotherapy, and family therapy (which might in some settings be the province of mental health professionals other than psychiatrists), drug treatment, and transfer for psychiatric inpatient treatment.

When a patient recovers from stroke without a speech disorder or dementia, there is not always a need for a psychiatrist or psychologist to be continuously involved in direct care; however, every stroke patient deserves a detailed assessment of cognitive capacity and mood at some point.

As the patient begins to recover from a comatose state, assessment with a simple scale such as the Glasgow Coma Scale (Teasdale and Jennett 1974) can be administered by any health care professional. When consciousness is fully regained, the presence and degree of cognitive impairment should be evaluated in more detail with standardized scales. A mental health professional should be involved both in choosing the scales to be used and in training others in their administration, although he or she need not be the one who conducts the actual tests. Many nurses and nonpsychiatric physicians record mental status data in their regular progress notes; however, unless they have had special training, such information is likely to be vague. The narrative account is best used for describing specific behaviors and for quoting actual words the patient used.

For any patient put in a physical restraint, careful and complete documentation of his or her mental state, preferably by a mental health professional, is mandatory. Any stroke patient given any psychotropic medication should be seen by a psychiatrist or by a physician with formal psychiatric training.

Any reasonable program of care for the stroke patient should include a certain minimum of psychosocial treatment that does not demand a mental health professional. Treatment providers should know what is happening regarding patients' jobs and families, where patients are going to be living after leaving the hospital, and who will be looking after them. The medical team must reach a consensus about the extent of the disabilities and their prognosis, and decide whether and how to convey this information to the patient and his or her family. An assessment must be made of the degree of dementia and aphasia present, and of whether the available resources are sufficient to provide care for the patient's disability.

Summary

Professionals who help care for stroke patients often experience emotional strain. The psychological mechanisms of projection and transference may affect caregivers' relationships with the patient. Team approaches can reduce hostility, improve efficiency, and facilitate the formation and documentation of treatment plans. Mental health professionals may be involved in diagnosing and treating specific mental illness, counseling patients attempting to adjust to an illness, developing behavior modification programs, conducting individual psychotherapy and family therapy, administering psychotropic drug treatment, and transferring patients for psychiatric inpatient treatment. When a stroke patient regains full consciousness, a detailed assessment of the presence and degree of any cognitive impairment should be performed, usually by employing standardized scales. Although a mental health professional should be involved both in choosing which scales are used and in training staff in their administration, he or she need not conduct the actual testing. If a patient is put in a physical restraint or given a psychotropic medication, careful and complete documentation of his or her mental state, preferably by a mental health professional, is necessary.

References

Consensus Conference Panel: Treatment of stroke: consensus statement. BMJ 297:126–128, 1988

Freud S: Five lectures on psycho-analysis (1910 [1909]), in The Standard Edition of the Complete Psychological Works of Sigmund Freud, Vol 11. Translated and edited by Strachey J. London, Hogarth Press, 1957, pp 3–56

Goodstein RK: Overview: cerebrovascular accident and the hospitalized elderly—a multidimensional clinical problem. Am J Psychiatry 140:141–148, 1983

Holland LK, Whalley MJ: The work of the psychiatrist in a rehabilitation hospital. Br J Psychiatry 138:222–229, 1981

Jaffe KB: Home health care and rehabilitation nursing. Nurs Clin North Am 24:171–178, 1989

Luttman RJ: The critical path method alone does nothing to improve performance (letter). QRB Qual Rev Bull 19:142–143, 1993

Preston KM: A team approach to rehabilitation. Home Healthcare Nurse 8:17–23, 1990

Romito D: A critical path for CVA patients. Rehabilitation Nursing 15:153–156, 1990

Teasdale G, Jennett B: Assessment of coma and impaired consciousness. Lancet 2:81–84, 1974

Tellis-Nayack V, Tellis-Nayack M: Quality of care and the burden of two cultures. Gerontologist 29:307–313, 1975

Thurgood A: Seven steps to rehabilitation. Nursing Times 86:38–41, 1990

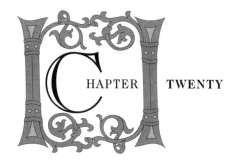

CHAPTER TWENTY

The Spectrum of Care

ew illnesses present greater problems of placement in the spectrum of care than stroke. Stroke patients may be misplaced in acute-care medical facilities, nursing homes, rehabilitation units, psychiatric facilities, day hospitals, or even in their own homes. This tendency for misplacement arises from the variety of disabilities that stroke may cause, but most especially from the presence of dementia and behavioral disturbance. (A summary of basic information about treatment facilities, directed toward family caregivers, is provided in Appendix B.)

In the acute stage, the decision about where to treat a stroke patient is made by one or two people in settings such as an emergency room or a doctor's office. Although the initial decision makers perform an informal assessment of the patient's mental state, that assessment does not go on record as influencing the decision. However, as the patient progresses through the health care system, more professionals get involved, more paperwork is done, and the assessment of the patient's mental state must be more formal, if only to comply with the regulations of government agencies and insurance companies.

Acute-Care Hospitals

Official recommendations in the United States state that all stroke patients should be hospitalized, and that this is a purely medical decision (Consensus Statement 1993). One reason for not hospitalizing is that even with a first stroke there can be doubt as to whether medical intervention will be curative (Alberts et al. 1992). However, the life of any deeply comatose patient may be saved by measures available in intensive care units, such as protection of the airway and control of life-threatening arrhythmias by cardiac monitoring. If coma persists, intravenous fluids may be necessary to prevent death from dehydration. These measures can be provided only in a hospital, and hospitalization may thus save the patient's life. Moreover, hospitals have available a vast array of sophisticated and expensive technology that can make the diagnosis of stroke more precise. The impact of the results from the multicenter National Institute of Neurological Disorders and Stroke (NINDS) trials of thrombolytic therapy has yet to be felt (National Stroke Association 1996).

Nevertheless, 40% of stroke patients in the United States are not hospitalized (Alberts et al. 1992), and the factors leading to institutionalization are often not strictly medical. Instead, a mix of medical, psychiatric, social, and economic factors, which cannot be easily separated, come into play. Often, the fact that a patient has experienced a previous stroke and is already crippled or extremely old or has dementia enters into the decision about where to treat. A major reason for hospitalization is the need for additional nursing care that cannot be provided at home, and when a second stroke occurs in a nursing home, the patient is commonly not transferred to a hospital. Surveys have failed to isolate any strictly technical or medical consideration that drives the decision to hospitalize.

Brocklehurst et al. (1978), in the Manchester area in England, compared stroke patients who were hospitalized (76% of their sample) with those who were not (24%). The most common reason for hospitalization involved the need for nursing care and the existence of social problems in the home. Among the hospitalized patients, 17% were able to walk unaided; among those not hospitalized, 35% were unable to walk. Those with left hemiplegia were mostly admitted to geriatric units rather than medical ones. (Geriatric units in England provide a level of care closer to that of the American nursing facility than of the acute-care general hospital.)

Stroke Units

Specialized acute-care stroke units are found in a few of the larger teaching centers, but most stroke units are rehabilitation units. Just over half of hospital-treated stroke patients in the United States return to their own homes, and most of the rest go to nursing homes. The remaining portion enter specialized rehabilitation units. Most rehabilitation units in the United States are attached to general hospitals, and stroke units form part of these rehabilitation units. There are also about 75 freestanding rehabilitation hospitals accredited by the Commission on Accreditation of Rehabilitation Facilities. (A list of these hospitals can be obtained from the American Rehabilitation Association [address provided in Appendix B].) Sometimes head injury and other neurological rehabilitation is grouped with stroke. The patient progresses from the acute-care unit to less intensive hospital care and then to the stroke unit. In Britain, stroke units are often attached to geriatric services.

The proportion of patients entering stroke units has risen considerably since the enactment, in 1983, of the Medicare Prospective Payment System (PPS) (Dobkin 1991) as part of the Tax Equity and Fiscal Responsibility Act (TEFRA). This legislation introduced the diagnosis-related group (DRG) method of reimbursement for hospitals. The usual DRG payment to an acute-care general hospital for a case of stroke is equivalent to the cost of a 7.5-day stay.

Stroke units are usually classified as rehabilitation units, which (like psychiatric units) are DRG exempt, but their reimbursement from Medicare is limited because it depends on continued demonstration that rehabilitation activities are actively being performed. In fact, most patients in stroke units spend most of their time doing nothing (Lincoln et al. 1989), although this is also true of patients in rehabilitation units in general (Miller and Keith 1973).

Doubt has been cast on the effectiveness of stroke units. That effectiveness is certainly questionable if we insist on objective physical measurements and discount less concrete effects on morale and sense of well-being. Harris (1990) reviewed five studies of outcome in various countries. Two of the studies had no control group, one had an inadequately matched control group, and one had too small a sample size. Harris noted several difficulties in conducting adequate trials of effectiveness: the intuitive belief in the effectiveness of rehabilitation is so strong that denying this service to a control group is felt to be unethical; variability due to factors intrinsic to the stroke may overwhelm the effects of therapy; and different outcome evaluation criteria are possible, including mortality, length of stay, discharge to home, and activities of daily living (ADL) capacity.

It is difficult to be certain, even in a controlled trial, that groups are evenly matched. Stroke units are more likely to admit young patients without dementia who have had a first stroke. Nevertheless, some controlled trials do indicate some benefits.

Stevens et al. (1984) conducted a carefully controlled trial in which physicians caring for acute stroke patients were asked to refer patients they considered fit for and in need of rehabilitation to an inpatient stroke unit. Half of those referred were then selected at random for the unit, and the remainder served as a control group. Patients in the stroke unit were found to receive significantly more occupational therapy and speech therapy than the control subjects. The only statistically significant difference in outcome was in independent dressing skills, which were better in the stroke unit group at 1-year follow-up. There were a number of nonsignificant trends favoring the stroke unit–treated group, but since there were more than 100 subjects in each group, it seems unlikely that failure to show significance was due to insufficient numbers for power requirements. Only physical and ADL improvement was measured; no assessment was performed of mood, morale, psychiatric symptoms, or overall patient and family satisfaction.

Garraway et al. (1980a, 1980b) found that the improvement attained in stroke units tended to be lost after discharge home. One reason for this loss was that families found it easier to do things for the patients than to allow the patients to do for themselves the things they had learned in rehabilitation. Forster and Young (1989) also raised this point, and emphasized the need for adequate communication so that the rehabilitation staff are aware of practical handicapping problems present in the home.

Cost-effectiveness is one measure of the efficacy of stroke units. Blackbeard and Seeman (1990), in New Zealand, examined the cost-effectiveness of a stroke unit, the expenses of which exceeded those of a long-term care hospital only by the additional cost of increased input by physicians, occupational therapists, and physical therapists. The patients admitted would otherwise have gone to a long-term care hospital indefinitely. Patients stayed an average of 4 months in the unit, and most were discharged home or to a less-expensive facility that provided less-intensive care.

Friedman (1990), also in New Zealand, found that the expertise of a stroke treatment team reduced hospital stays, and that this effect was not attributable to improved functional results. The team was skilled in identifying those patients who would not benefit from further hospitalization and transferring them to long-term care facilities. The context of Friedman's study was a stroke unit within a general hospital.

Such objective studies mostly seek to eliminate the placebo—or Hawthorne—effect, in which the sense that something is being done for them makes people feel better. This striving for objectivity may lead to ignoring an important benefit of the units. Even if we call this benefit a placebo effect and say it is only in the mind, that does not mean it does not exist at all.

Nursing Homes

One million eight hundred thousand Americans are in nursing homes (now officially called *nursing facilities),* a common destination for the stroke patient, especially the elderly white female.

OBRA '87 regulations.   The Omnibus Budget Reconciliation Act of 1987 (OBRA '87) was originally intended to stop mentally ill patients from being put in nursing homes. Nevertheless, stroke patients with severe behavioral problems are still being placed in nursing homes. One reason for this is that OBRA '87 made an exemption for dementia, and stroke patients with mental disorders may be diagnosed as having multi-infarct dementia. It may also be decided that the stroke is the primary diagnosis and is a nonpsychiatric medical condition that overrides the psychiatric diagnosis.

OBRA '87 additionally introduced regulations concerning the use of treatments such as psychotropic drugs in nursing homes. The intent of these regulations was to prevent the use of drugs as chemical straitjackets. If psychotropic drugs are used in such settings, there must be documentation of the specific psychiatric condition being treated. Likewise, in order for restraints to be used, it must be documented that alternative measures have been considered.

Nursing homes for younger patients.   Most nursing-home patients are elderly and have dementia, and will never be discharged. Proximity to this population has a demoralizing effect on younger stroke patients without dementia who are placed in nursing homes. Occasionally, a nursing home can be found that specializes in younger patients. Some private organizations provide accredited nursing facilities, reimbursed at the nursing-home rate by Medicaid, for younger patients with head injuries; younger stroke patients may prefer these.

Board-and-care facilities.   A number of young stroke patients gravitate to adult homes, rest homes, or single-room-occupancy hotels (SROs), which take in patients who can provide basic self-care and do not need nursing services. The names used by these institutions are not standardized, and the same name can mean a different level of care in a different state (Birkett 1991, p. 8). Board-and-care facilities do not provide care by registered nurses, although some may offer services such as supervision of medications; most, however, are no more than rooming houses. Because residents are free to come and go, management personnel have little ability to restrict the use of cocaine and cigarettes. The stroke patients who enter these facilities are often those who neither cooperate with medical regimens nor tolerate restrictions.

Psychiatric Hospitals and Units

Many patients with cerebral infarcts are in psychiatric inpatient care of various kinds in the United States. Sometimes patients who present with psychiatric symptoms are admitted to psychiatric units and found after admission to have cerebral infarction. Although cases of this type may be considered misplacements and thought to indicate a failure in diagnosis, they can occur even with conscientious care and full examination.

State hospitals.   In recent years, the place of large state mental hospitals in psychiatric care has waned, but these institutions still contain a considerable residuum of elderly patients.

In 210 state-hospital autopsies done in a recent 10-year period, 91 revealed brain infarcts (Birkett et al. 1992). These were more common among patients originally admitted with a diagnosis of functional psychosis than among those admitted for dementia.

General-hospital psychiatric units.   The place of general-hospital psychiatric units in stroke care is still in flux. Municipal hospitals traditionally admitted indigent and severely disturbed patients on a short-term basis, with the understanding that these individuals would be transferred to a state hospital. Nongovernment general hospitals (with some distinguished and honorable exceptions) were originally reluctant to accept mentally ill patients. The introduction of psychiatric units in voluntary general hospitals was often begun with the understanding that such units would not admit violent or chronically ill patients.

Social and legislative changes have now established the general-hospital psychiatric unit as the primary setting in which mentally ill patients are hospitalized, but there is still a reluctance to treat those with structural brain damage, despite the fact that the general hospital has the best combination of resources for neurological investigation and medical management—resources that have increased tremendously in scope and sophistication. This reluctance may still be based on therapeutic nihilism, as well as on other factors such as nonmedical therapeutic orientation, fear of chronicity and placement problems, and lack of experience in formulating treatment plans for cognitively impaired patients.

Medical-psychiatric inpatient units.   One response to the reluctance of psychiatric units to treat medical conditions has been the development of the "med-psych" unit in some hospitals. Such units specialize in treatment of overlapping medical and psychiatric conditions, and may be organized as primarily medical or primarily psychiatric. Insurance reimbursement usually favors the primarily psychiatric model. Units so far established have been very successful, both economically and in meeting community needs, and may well increase in number in the future. Although they appear to be a logical place to treat stroke patients with mental disorders, census figures at present do not indicate that these units admit many such patients (Fogel and Stoudemire 1986; Goodman 1986; Stoudemire and Fogel 1986).

Care plans.   The care plan for the stroke patient in the DRG-exempt psychiatric or medical-psychiatric unit needs to cover a wide range of problems and involve many disciplines. Special attention must be given to areas of communication and ADL, and specific impairments must be identified and addressed. Because of the many disciplines involved, it is not always practical to insist that every team member be present at every meeting. The psychiatrically oriented team members may have to list the problems that seem to involve communication or mobility, and then seek consultations with speech pathology, physical therapy, occupational therapy, and neurology staff and incorporate these consultations into the care plan. Efforts to maintain a multidisciplinary team approach should nevertheless be maintained. The nonpsychiatric therapists should be encouraged to consider psychological barriers to rehabilitation and to discuss them with the team.

Day Care

Because adult day care is especially useful in enabling family members to get out of the house to go to work or to get a break from the burden of caregiving, it can allow families to keep at home a stroke patient who might otherwise have to be institutionalized. On the other hand, a day-care facility that provides little more than "baby-sitting" may be demoralizing for stroke patients who want active rehabilitation.

Transportation.   Transportation can be a major obstacle to accessing day care, although the degree of difficulty caused by this factor varies from country to country. In North America, the availability of private automobiles is high for those who can drive or get someone to drive them. It can take just as much time and effort for caregivers to organize transportation or get a patient ready for public transportation as to keep the patient home. Multipassenger transport systems, using vans or minibuses, pick up several passengers from different locations in one trip. If the trip becomes too long, patients can get motion sickness (Stokoe and Zucollo 1985).

Day hospitals.   Day hospitals are more common in the United Kingdom than in the United States (Forster and Young 1989) and are usually run by geriatricians, although some younger stroke patients may also attend such facilities. Although these British day hospitals are not designated as stroke treatment centers, stroke is the most common reason for referral and accounts for nearly one-half of those attending. Day hospitals in Britain differ from day centers in that they provide active medical treatment and are more rehabilitation oriented (although not as actively engaged in rehabilitation of young people as the American ones). These hospitals provide what American authors call "transitional rehabilitation" (Tucker et al. 1984).

Hildick-Smith (1984) found that although British day hospitals were as expensive as inpatient care, they were preferred by patients and were easier to recruit staff for. As with many other stroke treatment measures, there is a dichotomy in the perception of benefits. Forster and Young (1989) noted that whereas "the patients enjoy attending and the relatives find it beneficial . . . , there is little objective information available to quantify the benefits of day hospital attendance" (p. 182). Tucker et al. (1984) conducted a randomized controlled trial in New Zealand of British-type day care and found no advantage in ADL capacity and no financial economies. They randomly allocated patients to treatment in a newly opened day hospital, using as a control group patients who continued whatever type of care they were previously getting, whether at home or in the hospital. There was a sustained benefit on mood, indicating that the day hospitals were good for morale, but there was no measurable effect on clinical depression.

Home Care

When sick, most people (although by no means all) would rather be at home than in the best of institutions, and caring for the stroke patient at home rather than in an institution has many advocates. It has not been conclusively shown that home care is less expensive, especially if the emotional drain on the caregivers, who are usually wives, is taken into consideration.

The provision of home care is often haphazard. Even with the uniform nationwide government-financed health care system provided in England by the National Health Service, Greveson et al. (1991) found a marked discrepancy between the need for community services for stroke patients and the availability of such services: "There was no relationship between level of dependency, presence of an informal carer or age of carer and level of support from voluntary or statutory services" (p. 341). For example, one independent man living with a fit brother received Meals on Wheels, while other severely disabled and isolated patients received no help at all.

Helping patients to arrange for home care can require much skill and patience. Paradoxically, finding home care becomes easier once the patient has been hospitalized, because the hospital has professional discharge planners and home care coordinators. The ambulant patient with behavioral problems is often the most difficult to provide for.

Surveys of elderly patients reveal that those who are kept at home are often as sick as those who are institutionalized (Gurland et al. 1983) and that what enables them to stay at home is a multiplicity of support systems. Apart from assistance from the family and the recognized medical and nursing services, independent survival in the community may be facilitated by an informal network of care by which people help each other. Supplementing this informal network with official interventions could even be damaging (Zarit and Zarit 1982)—it is a fragile ecology, and easily wrecked. The network can include the local grocery store that makes deliveries, the next-door neighbor who notices if the mail is not picked up, the convenient taxi service, the friend who comes by to check up, the lodger in the spare room, the weekly cleaning lady, the poker partners, the drinking buddies, the church ladies, and a host of others, each of whom may play only one small part in keeping a disabled person going.

> A woman who is 70, in poor health, and living on Social Security goes every weekday morning to sit with a bedridden neighbor who has had a stroke and is incontinent. She cares for her friend until the woman's daughter comes home from work, and does not get one penny of monetary payment. When the daughter gets home "from work," she takes over. She does not get help from any government agency.

Summary

Although it is medically recommended that all stroke patients be hospitalized, this is not always done. Psychosocial factors probably predominate in the decision. Most hospital-treated stroke patients go back to their own homes, and most of the rest go to nursing homes. OBRA '87 was intended to stop mentally ill patients from being put in nursing homes but made an exemption for dementia. It also introduced regulations concerning the use of psychotropic drugs and restraints in nursing homes. Day hospitals are distinguished from day centers by their provision of active medical treatment and their rehabilitation orientation.

References

Alberts MJ, Perry A, Dawson DV, et al: Effects of public and professional education on reducing the delay in presentation and referral of stroke. Stroke 23:352–356, 1992

Birkett DP: Psychiatry in the Nursing Home. New York, Haworth, 1991

Birkett DP, Desouky A, Han H, et al: Lewy bodies in psychiatric patients. International Journal of Geriatric Psychiatry 7:235–240, 1992

Blackbeard RR, Seeman HMI: Rehabilitation cost effectiveness of stroke (letter). N Z Med J 103:109, 1990

Brocklehurst JC, Andrews K, Morris P, et al: Why admit stroke patients to hospital. Age Ageing 7:100–108, 1978

Consensus Statement: Stroke: the first six hours. Stroke Clinical Updates 4:1–12, 1993

Dobkin DH: The rehabilitation of elderly stroke patients. Clin Geriatr Med 7:507–522, 1991

Fogel BS, Stoudemire A: Organization and development of combined medical-psychiatric units, II. Psychosomatics 27:417–420, 425–428, 1986

Forster A, Young J: Day hospital and stroke patients. International Disability Studies 11:181–183, 1989

Friedman PJ: Stroke rehabilitation in the elderly: a new patient management system. N Z Med J 103:234–236, 1990

Garraway MW, Akhtar AJ, Prescott R, et al: Management of acute stroke in the elderly: preliminary results of a controlled trial. BMJ 280:1040–1043, 1980a

Garraway MW, Akhtar AJ, Hockey L, et al: Management of acute stroke in the elderly: follow-up of a controlled trial. BMJ 281:827–829, 1980b

Goodman B: Combined psychiatric-medical inpatient units: the Mount Sinai model. Psychosomatics 26:179–182, 185–186, 189, 1986

Greveson GC, Gray CS, French JM, et al: Long-term outcome for patients and carers following hospital admission for stroke. Age Ageing 20:337–344, 1991

Gurland B, Copeland J, Kuriansky J, et al: The Mind and Mood of Aging. New York, Haworth Press, 1983

Harris JM: Stroke rehabilitation: has it proven worthwhile? Journal of the Florida Medical Association 77:683–686, 1990

Hildick-Smith M: Geriatric day hospitals: changing emphasis in costs. Age Ageing 13:95–100, 1984

Lincoln NB, Gamlen R, Thomason H: Behavioral mapping of patients on a stroke unit. International Disability Studies 11:149–154, 1989

Miller RH, Keith RA: Behavioral mapping in a rehabilitation hospital. Rehabilitation Psychology 20:148–155, 1973

National Stroke Association: First-ever emergency stroke treatment proven effective. Be Stroke Smart 13:1, 1996

Omnibus Budget Reconciliation Act of 1987 (OBRA), Public Law 100-203

Stevens RS, Ambler NR, Warren MD: A randomized controlled trial of a stroke rehabilitation ward. Age Ageing 13:65–95, 1984

Stokoe D, Zucollo G: Travel sickness in patients attending a geriatric day hospital. Age Ageing 14:308–311, 1985

Stoudemire A, Fogel BS: Organization and development of combined medical-psychiatric units, I. Psychosomatics 27:341–345, 1986

Tucker MA, Davison JG, Ogle SJ: Day hospital rehabilitation effectiveness and cost in the elderly. BMJ 289:1209–1212, 1984

Zarit SH, Zarit JM: Families under stress: interventions for caregivers of senile dementia patients. Psychotherapy: Theory, Research and Practice 19:461–471, 1982

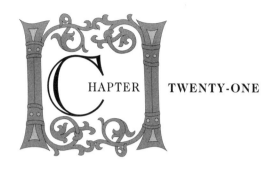

CHAPTER TWENTY-ONE

Legal Issues

Many of the legal issues in stroke overlap with those of geriatric psychiatry, which are discussed in texts such as that of Sadavoy et al. (1991). Legal competence and dementia, for example, are two topics of particular geriatric concern. Stroke, however, may strike at any age and can cause special problems of its own, such as communication impairment.

Legal Competence

Testamentary Capacity

The validity of wills is a topic to which lawyers have given much attention. Spar and Garb (1992) have provided an overview of the law of testamentary capacity in the United States, and the general principles that apply in most jurisdictions.

Lawyers do not expect physicians and nurses to be legal experts, but it is always worth bearing in mind the questions that might be asked about a patient's ability to make a will—not only because of the actual contingency that one might be asked questions after the patient's death relevant to testamentary capacity, but also because the ability to answer such questions is an indication of a good examination. A reasonable mental status or neurological examination will include inquiry about the ability to do simple mental arithmetic and about whether the patient knows where he or she lives, and who his or her relatives are. If such inquiries have been made, it should be possible to help the lawyers answer questions such as whether the testator knew the "nature, situation and extent of his/her property" and "the objects of his/her bounty and their relationship to him/her."

The answers to these questions will detect cases of gross dementia, a condition that is relatively easy to explain to a court. The personality and emotional changes associated with cerebrovascular disease are more nebulous. The case of Woodrow Wilson is discussed in detail in Appendix C to illustrate the quandaries that may arise in such circumstances. Those who have suffered a brain infarct but who do not have severe dementia are often susceptible to sudden and unreasonable rages (see Chapter 11) as well as to acts of what is often vaguely described as "poor judgment." The court may want to know that such susceptibility exists but choose to make its own determination as to what is unreasonable and what is poor judgment. Medical witnesses are sometimes asked questions about the circumstances of an examination that are designed to elicit whether undue influence was exerted upon the patient. For example, physicians are sometimes asked about a patient's apparent attitude toward the relatives or friends who brought him or her to the office. It is therefore helpful to keep a record of such escorts.

Physicians in court are sometimes asked to say how long prior to their examination the patient's mind had been weakened. Unless one is being called (and paid) as an expert witness, a good reply to this question is "I don't know." Another possible reply is to give an estimate of the extent of the incapacity that was caused by vascular disease and to date it either from the clinically identified stroke or from the age of the infarct found at autopsy or on computed tomography (CT). If an opinion on the age of the cerebral infarct based on CT or autopsy findings is called for, it is reasonable to deny expertise on this topic and to suggest calling in a radiologist or pathologist.

In the case of aphasia, any reasonable assessment of speech and understanding will serve. If a good record has been kept, it will contain notes about, for example, how the patient made his or her wishes known, and whether the patient could read or sign his or her own name. The court can decide whether these methods rendered the testator vulnerable to undue influence. (Readers of Alexandre Dumas's *The Count of Monte Cristo*

[1844] will remember the episode of Noirtier's will, in which the will of a paralyzed aphasic person was validated, presumably under the Code Napoleon, by being read in the presence of seven witnesses approved by the testator and sealed by a notary in their presence.)

Like many family disputes, the battles over money can involve a large hidden agenda. Sometimes a child has looked after an invalid parent for years, providing care that would have cost hundreds of thousands of dollars, and is then accused by the other siblings of having taken all the parent's money. It may be possible to point out the financial realities to such families, but usually the pocket calculator is not a powerful enough tool to dig out a deep-rooted sibling rivalry. Although it may seem that counseling and mediation are advisable, sometimes matters have gone too far for any intervention, and lawyers often discourage mental health professionals called in as experts from getting involved in this aspect.

Contractual Capacity

Patients may enter into contracts that someone later wants to void on the basis of incompetency. If the patient is alive but now obviously incompetent, the question will arise of how long this state has existed. Many of the same considerations arise in contractual capacity as in testamentary capacity, and the health care provider can expect to be asked the same kinds of questions in court. One difference is that courts generally expect a lesser degree of competency for making a will than for entering into a business contract. The courts assume that someone making a will has had time to think, and they are reluctant to overturn the testator's expressed wishes. Conversely, because they assume that entering into a business contract demands quick thinking and the ability to withstand pressure (qualities that require a higher degree of competency), such contracts are more easily disputed. Contract disputes are usually based more purely on technical legalities and money matters, and do not have the highly charged emotions that characterize will disputes, because will disputes pitch family members against one another. In some jurisdictions, there are provisions (enacted so as to protect the supposedly gullible elderly population from high-pressure sales pitches) whereby contracts entered into under sales pressure can be rescinded if this is done within a short period of time. A local Office on Aging or Adult Protective Services can provide assistance with such problems.

Handwriting often changes because of a stroke, and, if signatures are not notarized, medical opinion may be sought about their integrity. Such an opinion is easier to give if the patient's ability to read and write was checked in the initial examination, thus providing a baseline writing sample.

Legal Guardianship and Power of Attorney

Various legal ways exist for one person to make decisions on behalf of another. Appointment of a legal guardian is one of these ways, but there are cheaper and simpler ones. For example, a short form is available from the local Social Security office to appoint a representative payee for Social Security benefits. Many pension funds and insurance companies have their own forms for such purposes.

If the family situation and financial affairs are not too complicated, giving power of attorney to a relative is easier than getting a legal guardian appointed. The power-of-attorney procedure covers cases of right hemiplegia with aphasia and without dementia. The patient must be willing to grant the power of attorney. A patient might be so severely mentally impaired as to be incompetent to give power of attorney, so sometimes a physician's letter is needed saying that the patient knew he or she was giving power of attorney. If such a letter is required, the physician should seek evidence that the patient is able to recognize family members and knows what is being signed.

These simple procedures can be applied only if there is no dispute. If there is doubt or disagreement, such as an argument within the family over who is to have power of attorney, then the advice of a lawyer will be needed concerning other options. For some transactions, such as those involving real estate or large amounts of money, the power-of-attorney signature may not suffice.

For patients with more money and more complicated financial affairs, a legal guardian may have to be appointed. In addition to being expensive and prolonged, this procedure can have unintended consequences:

> A confused man was found in a bus station carrying $50,000 in cash. He was taken to a mental hospital for his own safety, and lawyers were appointed to decide what to do with the money. By the time the matter was settled, the man's hospital and attorney fees had exceeded $50,000.

There is considerable variation among jurisdictions in the legal procedures for surrogate decision making. The persons appointed to look after funds have various titles, such as conservators or guardians. Some jurisdictions differentiate between guardians of the property and guardians of the person. The latter are empowered to make medical as well as financial decisions.

The subject of guardianship is complex and occupies long sections of legal texts, but health practitioners and social workers need to know something about it. Knowledge can often be acquired by studying the documentation of a patient who has already had a guardian appointed. Local chapters of the Alzheimer's Association often hold instructional meetings and offer publications and lists of interested attorneys. Many areas of legal competence are explained in free brochures obtainable from the American Association of Retired Persons (AARP; see list of addresses in Appendix B). These include "Health Care Powers of Attorney," "Tomorrow's Choices," and "A Matter of Choice."

Informed Consent

The issues in consent to medical treatment are similar to those in guardianship. If the patient is not competent, some kind of arrangement for a surrogate decision maker must be made. The provisions of the Patient Self-Determination Act of 1991 are described in Chapter 23 (see "Intensity of Care"). Compared to decisions about financial guardianship, decisions about health care are usually less formal and more colored by medical contingency. Urgent medical necessity can override legal barriers, but there may be doubt about what constitutes urgent medical necessity. Quite often what matters in practice is not what the law says but what those involved think the law says. If a physician thinks he or she cannot do an emergency tracheotomy without a psychiatric opinion about the patient's capacity to give informed consent, then it may be best to give the psychiatric opinion quickly and argue later.

Research into stroke-related mental disorders, particularly vascular dementia, faces a dilemma in obtaining the informed consent of participants. If fully informed consent by the patient/subject is insisted upon, research into dementia would be at an impasse. Important considerations are obtaining the consent of a surrogate and ascertaining the patient's previously expressed wishes. Individual investigators are typically subject to an institutional review board (IRB) that considers the ethics of the use of human subjects, and most journals and grant-awarding bodies require evidence of approval by an IRB before endorsing a project. Most IRBs are guided by publications such as that of the National Commission for the

Protection of Human Subjects of Biomedical and Behavioral Research (1978), although these do not cover all contingencies (Sachs et al. 1993).

Criminal Intent

The relationship of local brain lesions to the insanity defense has been extensively discussed in the literature (Simon 1992) but is seldom relevant in stroke because, in stroke cases, it is rare for mental health practitioners to be called upon in the traditional role of providing help with a psychiatric defense. In dementia, the issue is usually that of a patient's competency to stand trial at all. If the dementia patient cannot instruct counsel and cannot understand the nature of the trial, then the courts do not proceed. This decision not to proceed criminally is often made by police officers in obvious cases. In the unlikely event of a trial, such a defendant might be found not to know the nature of his or her actions. This is an ancient common-law defense, preceding even the McNaughton Rules, and inquiry into the nuances of criminal responsibility is not conducted.

An individual's stroke-related handicap is often evident to the layperson, and its presence leads law enforcement agencies to seek a medical, rather than a punitive, response to crime. Cases may arise in the future where the evidence of cerebral infarction is disputed, such as those with magnetic resonance imaging (MRI) rarefactions discussed in Chapter 2, but if the infarct is definite, courts are very ready to accept it as explaining aberrant behavior.

A further consideration mitigating punitive judicial zeal is the understandable reluctance of the courts to imprison individuals who are elderly and infirm. Stroke patients are often in this category.

For all of these reasons, the usual requests from the legal to the medical profession are for help with placement and supervision, rather than for provision of a psychiatric defense. Providing such help can be an onerous role, calling for ingenuity in orchestrating multiple links among social, medical, psychiatric, and probation services.

An elderly stroke patient had an obvious hemiparesis and speech impairment, but was fully ambulant and not grossly demented. He patrolled his neighborhood stores shoplifting anything that took his fancy. Whenever arrested, he would be returned to his family by the police or the court, with the admonition that they should look after him and seek proper medical care. The situation was eventually resolved by placing the patient in an adult home in a rural area that was not within walking distance of any stores.

Psychiatric Aspects of Malpractice in Stroke

Patients are unlikely to sue physicians with whom they have a good and continuing relationship, and for this reason the emphasis on high technology—rather than human contact—at the onset of the illness produces a special legal hazard in stroke. The patient can feel a sense of abandonment after the acute episode. When a stroke patient is rushed to the hospital, a hospital-based specialist often takes over treatment, and the family sees the wonders of the latest diagnostic methods—wonders that can raise their expectations of equally wonderful treatment methods. If the patient survives, he or she may be transferred to less–well-funded chronic facilities. Such transfer is more likely for those too severely impaired to come to the specialist's private office as an outpatient. The patient thus loses touch with the physician responsible for the initial hospital treatment, who may then become a target of anger.

This anger can be mitigated if the primary care physician remains obviously in charge throughout treatment. Another way to prevent this sense of abandonment is for the specialist to follow patients who go to nursing homes. In addition to being a good malpractice suit–prevention practice, such a strategy can be a good learning experience.

Raising false expectations about treatment can set the stage for a lawsuit, but at the other extreme, therapeutic nihilism, although it may be scientifically honest, can cause a litigation response:

> A 55-year-old man, previously in good health, was admitted to a hospital with a stroke affecting the brain stem. The physician told his family there was no effective treatment. They telephoned the physician repeatedly and desperately through the night, and were told the same thing. The patient became quadriplegic, and the physician was sued.
>
> Expert evidence supported his contention that there was no specific treatment that would have made any difference, and that reasonable care had been given. The plaintiff's attorneys produced evidence of several treatments that had been rated as possibly effective, although none were of proven benefit. The attorneys brought enthusiastic advocates of these treatments to the witness stand.
>
> The patient was wheeled into court in a quadriplegic condition, which profoundly affected the jurors. A million-dollar verdict was returned against the physician.

One of the most common lawsuits in stroke is for neglected subarachnoid hemorrhage—a patient with a severe headache is misdiagnosed as having tension headache or migraine (see Chapter 8). If such a case comes to court, the diagnostic error is difficult to defend. Nevertheless, what leads to the lawsuit is often not the technical error but rather the negative attitudes the patient encounters when he or she seeks help, perhaps including insinuations that he or she is attempting to obtain addictive drugs or is malingering.

In long-term care situations, litigation and anger are commonly directed against institutions rather than individual practitioners. Some cases involve failure to prevent falls and wandering (Tammalleo 1988). Fear of such litigation, whether justified or unjustified, often leads to use of physical restraints. A strong sentiment against the use of physical restraints is incorporated into Omnibus Budget Reconciliation Act of 1987 (OBRA '87) regulations and may find expression in litigation.

Noncompliance with antihypertension treatment.   A stroke does not become imminent because of a single high blood pressure reading, but in cases when a patient who has a stroke has previously had a high reading, or has seen a physician who did not take his or her blood pressure, there have been lawsuits on the grounds that the stroke could have been prevented (Hinkle 1993). The issue then often turns on the patient's behavior and willingness to comply with treatment for the high blood pressure. Careful assessment of these psychological aspects, as well as the recording of other stroke risk factors, can help prevent such actions from being brought.

> A 33-year-old man with a history of smoking and cocaine use was involved in a fight, and was treated for his injuries by a physician who did not take his blood pressure. Two months later, the patient had a cerebral hemorrhage, and the physician was sued for failing to take action to prevent this. The physician claimed that the patient would have been unlikely to follow advice about stroke prevention.

The Impaired Professional

Failure to return to work after a stroke is usually regarded as an adverse outcome, but return to work can cause its own troubles when that work involves responsibility for others (see Appendix C). The stroke patient's colleagues may face the dilemma of discriminating against a co-worker on the basis of handicap or tolerating professional incompetence:

> An anesthesiologist had a stroke with left hemiplegia. He returned to work and made several errors, including a fatal injection of a high dose of a drug

he had mistaken for another one. The family of the deceased patient sued the hospital and the anesthesiologist's partners for allowing him to work.

Periodic relicensure and recertification requirements by licensing and specialty boards may lift some of the burden of decision from colleagues in such cases. It is reasonable to ask for medical certification of fitness to return to work, but intransigent stroke patients who are themselves physicians can often circumvent a request of this kind through strategies such as arranging for a physician who is a close friend to provide certification. The physician providing certification should find out if he or she has authority from the physician-patient to discuss the case with colleagues. If this full authority is refused, then it should be explained that the usefulness of certification is limited. The physician-patient should not be denied the opportunity to enter psychotherapy under a guarantee of confidentiality, but having done so, must not expect the psychotherapist to certify his or her professional competence. Frank and open communication between those concerned is probably the best safeguard. Efforts should be primarily directed toward breaking the conspiracy of silence. Once this is broken, the issues will often resolve themselves. Objective tests of professional competency can then be arranged and the results discussed with the physician-patient and those who share responsibility for his or her work.

Summary

Questions asked about testamentary capacity relate primarily to whether the testator knows how much property he or she has, and who his or her relatives are. Stroke patients who do not have obvious dementia may have personality changes that affect their testamentary capacity. In the case of aphasic patients, a record should be kept of how the individual makes his or her wishes known, and of the individual's ability to read and write. Handwriting is often altered because of a stroke.

Methods for handling the financial affairs of incompetent patients vary from jurisdiction to jurisdiction. The persons appointed to look after funds may be called conservators or guardians. Giving power of attorney to a relative is cheaper and easier than having a legal guardian appointed.

In criminal matters, the courts do not proceed if a dementia patient cannot understand the nature of the trial. A patient's stroke-related impairment is often evident to the layperson, and the usual requests to the medical profession are for help with placement and supervision rather than for a psychiatric defense.

The concentration of high technology at the onset of the illness produces a special malpractice hazard in stroke because patients often feel abandoned after the acute episode. The danger of lawsuits arises from failure in physician-patient relationships.

Litigation against institutions may involve failure to prevent falls and wandering, but OBRA '87 regulations limit the use of physical restraints.

The colleagues of a professional who is mentally impaired by stroke may face the dilemma of either discriminating against a co-worker on the grounds of handicap or tolerating professional incompetence.

References

Hinkle BJ: The challenge of crescendo hypertension. Medical Malpractice Prevention 8:12–15, 1993

National Commission for the Protection of Human Subjects of Biomedical and Behavioral Research: The Belmont report: ethical principles and guidelines for the protection of human subjects of research (DHEW Publ No OS-78-0012). Washington, DC, Department of Health, Education and Welfare, 1978

Omnibus Budget Reconciliation Act of 1987 (OBRA), Public Law 100-203

Sachs GA, Rhymes J, Cassel CK: Biomedical and behavioral research in nursing homes: guidelines for ethical investigations. J Am Geriatr Soc 41:771–777, 1993

Sadavoy J, Lazarus LW, Jarvik LF (eds): Comprehensive Review of Geriatric Psychiatry. Washington, DC, American Psychiatric Press, 1991

Simon RI: Ethical and legal issues in neuropsychiatry, in American Psychiatric Association Textbook of Neuropsychiatry, 2nd Edition. Edited by Yudofsky SC, Hales ER. Washington, DC, American Psychiatric Press, 1992, pp 773–800

Spar JE, Garb AS: Assessing competency to make a will. Am J Psychiatry 149:169–174, 1992

Tammalleo AD: Patient wanders off: killed by daughter—*Fields v. Senior Citizens Center Inc.* Regan Report on Nursing Law 29:2, 1988

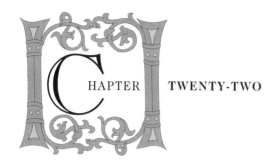

CHAPTER TWENTY-TWO

Economic and Financial Issues

Diseases that kill people rapidly and at an advanced age are not necessarily the most costly to the community; however, stroke also produces prolonged disability, much of which is mental. Half a million people suffer strokes annually, and two-thirds of them survive to face a long and disabling illness. According to some estimates, the cost of stroke in the United States is $25 billion each year (American Heart Association 1991), but this figure is probably too low because the proportion of dementia that is vascular is not certain (see Chapter 16), and dementia represents a major financial burden, both to the taxpayer and to the individual so affected.

The Psychiatric Component of Stroke Care Costs

The need for care after the acute stroke is probably determined more by mental than by physical disability. Surveys done in nursing homes, the largest and most expensive component of government-funded stroke aftercare, indicate that these facilities are, in effect, mental hospitals (G. D. Cohen 1994). Although the cost of the initial acute care is high,

351

it is generally agreed that the cost of even the most sophisticated stroke workup is far less than that of stroke aftercare (Shriver and Prockop 1993). This does not mean that the initial acute care is more cost-effective. In fact, cost-effectiveness may mandate diverting money from medical areas of acute care to psychosocial areas of aftercare (Cochrane et al. 1991).

Returning to work after a stroke other than a single transient ischemic attack (TIA) or a reversible ischemic neurological defect (RIND) is unusual. The obstacles to successful rehabilitation are, as seen in Chapter 10, largely the result of the mental state of the patient. The unemployability of the stroke patient is probably due to mental rather than physical disability. Physical illnesses, such as heart attacks, usually cause more disability in low-paying occupations; well-paid professionals or executives will usually return to work after a heart attack, but are less likely to do so after a stroke.

Financial Impact on the Individual

On an individual level, stroke is a pecuniary disaster. The cost of medical care itself is obviously one of the greatest financial burdens in stroke but does not seem to be the primary one. Surveys in countries, such as Britain, with state-financed medical care systems reveal that financial stress is just as severe there as in the United States (Anderson 1992).

There are a large number of less-obvious expenses in addition to the direct medical costs. Transportation expenses and time spent traveling are a major imposition, especially when the stroke patient was the only car driver in the family and when public transportation cannot be used.

The earning power lost is not only that of the patient. Family members sometimes give up work to look after the patient. This is most commonly done by wives who stay home to look after husbands. Thus, both incomes are lost, and poverty is added to the other problems.

Cocaine-Related Stroke

The economics of cocaine-related stroke merit separate consideration. Much of the damage done by cocaine, to the individual and the community, arises from the cost of the drug itself. Cocaine users who have had strokes are often indigent, with no money, no insurance, and no Medicaid. Patients may be less overtly concerned about this circumstance than their caregivers are, so that part of the rehabilitation process is getting the patients back in touch with economic reality. Although the youth of these patients improves their rehabilitation prospects in some respects, their drug use history limits their employability.

Units that treat many patients with cocaine-related stroke, in areas of high cocaine use, will often have a cadre of staff who have become expert in dealing with the various aspects of this condition, including the financial. These staff members represent a valuable resource for units that see only occasional cases of stroke caused by cocaine use. Such specialists can be called into consultation for individual cases or provide in-service instruction.

Medicare, Medicaid, and Stroke

Some of the basic information on paying for care needed by families is listed in Appendix B, and the principal government programs for financial support are summarized in Table 22–1. The anomalies of Medicaid nursing-home coverage and the "spend-down," whereby the patient has to become impoverished to be covered, are well known. Medicare will not normally pay for nursing homes or home aides. When the patient is severely ill, it may be possible to get coverage in a hospice program (Thal 1993).

Several economic factors enter into the decision to place a stroke patient in a nursing home. In some cases, the Medicaid-covered nursing-home care enables a family member to keep working at a relatively high-paying job, and there is thus a financial incentive to institutionalization. On the other hand, in a low-income family, the patient's Social Security check may be an important item in the family budget, and there is a financial disincentive to institutionalization.

The implications for Medicare hospital coverage of the Tax Equity and Fiscal Responsibility Act (TEFRA) and diagnosis-related groups (DRGs) are discussed in Chapter 20. The acute-care general hospital is subject to the diagnosis-related restriction. Psychiatric and rehabilitation units are DRG exempt as long as they provide active treatment.

Several authors have published reviews of Medicare coverage for geriatric psychiatry in general (e.g., Gottlieb 1991). Historically, Medicare has discriminated against psychiatric treatment, but recent changes have reduced this discrimination and in some cases reversed it. For example, the fee for psychotropic medication management (coded as 90862) is

Table 22–1.   Summary of principal government programs relevant to community services

Program	Service	Eligibility
Old Age Survivors and Disabled Insurance (OASDI; 1935)	Social Security benefits	All persons 65 and older, disabled workers, and dependent survivors when worker dies; reduced amounts for retirees aged 62, widows aged 60, and disabled aged 50
Supplemental Security Income Program (1972)	Supplemental payments to bring persons to poverty threshold; states have option to pay for domiciliary care homes and personal home care	Indigent persons 65 and older, disabled, and blind
Title XVIII of the Social Security Act (1965)	Medicare, which includes hospital costs, physicians' fees, skilled nursing facility (limited), home health care, and hospice care	Persons 65 and older and those under 65 who receive Social Security disability
Title XIX of the Social Security Act (1965)	Medicaid, which includes medical services, skilled nursing care (unlimited), and home health care; optional by state: adult day care, drugs, and intermediate care facility	Indigent aged, disabled, blind
Social Services Block Grant (1981) (formerly Title XX of the Social Security Act [1975])	Varying levels by state: chore services, congregate meals, home-delivered meals, homemaker, seniors centers, protective services	Indigent persons (all ages) up to 115% of state median income
Older Americans Act (OAA; 1965)— Title III	Services vary by state: congregate meals, home-delivered meals, home health care, chore services, seniors centers, friendly visiting	All persons 60 and older; low-income persons are special targets

(continued)

Table 22–1. Summary of principal government programs relevant to community services *(continued)*

Program	Service	Eligibility
Older Americans Act (OAA; 1965)— Title V	Community employment (e.g., senior aides, Green Thumb)	Indigent persons 55 and older
ACTION (1971)	Federal agency established to coordinate volunteer programs; programs for aged include Foster Grandparents, RSVP, and Senior Companions	Some programs open only to indigent
Section 202 Housing (1959)	Low-interest loans for construction of low-rent housing	Nonprofit sponsors
Section 8 (1974)	Rent subsidies to cover difference between fair market rent and 30% of participants' income	Low-income elderly
Food Stamp Program (1964)	Department of Agriculture program for purchasing foods at lower prices	Low-income persons

Source. Adapted from Huttman 1985; Maddox 1987; Skolnick and Warrick 1985. Reprinted from Cohen C: "Integrated Community Services," in *Comprehensive Review of Geriatric Psychiatry.* Edited by Sadavoy J, Lazarus LW, Jarvik LF. Washington, DC, American Psychiatric Press, 1991, pp. 617–618. Copyright 1991, American Psychiatric Press, Inc. Used with permission.

now higher than that for a regular nursing-home visit. Much depends on local interpretation by the insurance companies (carriers) administering Medicare.

> A patient with a long history of paranoid delusions and hallucinations was put in a nursing home following a stroke. She was capable of walking and of some self-care, but her family was unable to manage her at home because of her mental condition, for which she took an antipsychotic medication. The patient's physician billed Medicare for code 90862, listing the primary diagnosis as stroke. The Medicare carrier rejected this claim and would pay only for a nursing-home visit. However, when the claim was resubmitted with a primary psychiatric diagnosis, the carrier agreed to pay for the psychotropic medication management.

Some of the recent Medicare changes also allow for payments to psychologists and social workers. Payment for psychotherapy remains limited, and it is difficult to obtain reimbursement for meetings with families and caregivers.

It is a common finding that stroke patients and their families do not receive the public benefits to which they are entitled. Expertise by the treatment team in this area can often be more useful than technical medical expertise. Help can be obtained from groups such as the National Stroke Association, both through direct information to the patient and through instruction to the treatment team. All members of the stroke treatment team should have some knowledge of the intricacies of Medicaid, Medicare, and the various transfer payment programs, such as Social Security Supplementary Security Income (SSI) and Social Security Disability Income (SSDI). At least one member of the treatment team should be an expert on these programs and should be prepared either to act as a patient advocate or to recommend someone else to fulfill that function.

Stroke Prevention

The behavioral aspects of stroke risk factors (discussed in Chapter 3) have economic implications. There are two approaches to reducing the incidence of a disease in the community; the "mass" and the "high-risk." The mass approach uses lifestyle modification to achieve modest reductions in the level of the risk factor in every individual in the population. The high-risk approach, on the other hand, first selects those individuals at greatest risk and then targets them for active intervention. An example of a high-risk approach would be surgical treatment of carotid artery disease to prevent stroke. An analysis of the currently available data suggested that reduction of the two factors of hypertension and cigarette smoking by a mass approach is the most cost-effective strategy for stroke prevention (Gorelick 1994).

Summary

Stroke costs $25 billion each year in the United States.[1] Half a million people have strokes annually, and two-thirds of them survive. The precise incidence of vascular dementia is not known. Most disability after a

---

[1]This figure adds together all the costs of care, by whomsoever paid, and the losses in earnings.

stroke is mental rather than physical. The cost of the initial acute care is less than that of stroke aftercare, much of which is needed because of mental infirmity. There are many expenses besides the direct costs of medical care. Family members sometimes must give up working to look after the stroke patient.

Cocaine users with strokes are often indigent and resist involvement in government programs. Medicare will not usually pay for nursing homes or home aides. Medicare has discriminated against psychiatric treatment, but recent changes have reduced this. Much depends on local interpretation by the carriers.

Knowledge of entitlements to Medicaid, Medicare, Social Security, and other benefits can be more useful to the patient than technical medical or psychiatric expertise. Information can be obtained from groups such as the National Stroke Association. Reduction of hypertension and cigarette smoking by a mass approach is the most cost-effective strategy for preventing stroke.

References

American Heart Association: Heart and Stroke Facts. Dallas, TX, American Heart Association, 1991

Anderson R: The Aftermath of Stroke. Cambridge, UK, Cambridge University Press, 1992

Cochrane M, Ham C, Heginbotham C, et al: Rationing: at the cutting edge. BMJ 303:1039–1042, 1991

Cohen C: Integrated community services, in Comprehensive Review of Geriatric Psychiatry. Edited by Sadavoy J, Lazarus LW, Jarvik LF. Washington, DC, American Psychiatric Press, 1991, pp 613–634

Cohen GD: The health care reform debate about primary care providers. American Journal of Geriatric Psychiatry 2:93–94, 1994

Gorelick PB: Stroke prevention: an opportunity for efficient utilization of health care resources during the coming decade. Stroke 25:220–224, 1994

Gottlieb GL: Financial issues, in Comprehensive Review of Geriatric Psychiatry. Edited by Sadavoy J, Lazarus LW, Jarvik LF. Washington, DC, American Psychiatric Press, 1991, pp 667–686

Huttman ED: Social Services for the Elderly. New York, Free Press, 1985

Maddox GL: Mutual support groups, in The Encyclopedia of Aging. Edited by Maddox GL. New York, Springer, 1987, p 465

Shriver ME, Prockop LD: The economic approach to the stroke work-up. Curr Opin Neurol Neurosurg 6:74–77, 1993

Skolnick B, Warrick P: The Right Place at the Right Time: A Guide to Long-Term Care Choices. Washington, DC, American Association of Retired Persons, 1985

Thal AE: Health care for end-stage dementia (letter). J Am Geriatr Soc 41:888, 1993

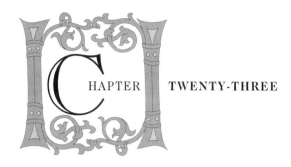

CHAPTER TWENTY-THREE

Ethical Issues

Although many of the ethical issues in stroke are not unique to stroke, some aspects are specific to the illness. Stroke is a disease that bestows an easy death but a hard life. Those who die of stroke may well "cease upon the midnight with no pain." Those who survive it face a life of lessened quality. Judgment of the quality of life in stroke is hindered by communication disorders as well as by dementia and other mental changes. Such judgment is largely intuitive, and depends much on good rapport and prolonged contact with a patient, but there are also several scales that can be used. One of these—the Frenchay Activities Index (Holbrook and Skilbeck 1983)—was especially designed to measure quality of life in stroke patients (de Haan et al. 1993).

The Right to Die

For some years, it would have been unusual to consider suicide as an ethical issue, although it was at one time regarded as a sin, and, until the pioneering studies of Durkheim (1897/1966), was seen as a logical but culpable response to intolerable adverse circumstances. Durkheim studied the epidemiology of suicide, and his explanations were sociological. Psychiatry has tried to regain the ground from sociology by pointing out the role of mental disorders such as depression, alcoholism, and schizophrenia in suicide. Recent general reviews include those of Jacobs (1992) and of Bongar (1992).

Attention to suicide as a logical act has increased, with advocacy of suicide as a legitimate response to incurable physical illness (Humphry 1991), and the area disputed between psychiatry and sociology is now again being reclaimed by ethics. Among the objections to views such as those of Humphry has been the possibility that treatable psychiatric illness may cause an individual to wrongly perceive his or her situation as hopeless.

This issue has come to the fore in discussions of the suicide of Bruno Bettelheim. He was 86 years old, had had a stroke, and was in a nursing home. Finkel (1991) has suggested that Bettelheim committed suicide because of depression that might have been a biological consequence of the stroke and that should have been treated to prevent the suicide. Others have seen Bettelheim's suicide as a rational act, implying that it is so terrible to be old and have suffered a stroke that one might as well die.

In favor of Finkel's view is the fact that the most severely afflicted stroke patients are not the ones likely to commit suicide. Suicide is rare among those with dementia. The severely paralyzed also do not kill themselves, although it is true that this might be because of lack of capacity to do so. Suicide in stroke is thus more likely among individuals with milder illness.

Against Finkel's view is the fact that suicide has not been shown to be more common in stroke survivors than in the general population. Even if an excess of suicide were demonstrated, it might not be proof of an excess of biological depression. Stroke is associated with other known suicide risk factors, such as the presence of chronic medical illness, old age, and social isolation. In clinical practice, the practitioner must bear this in mind. If other risk factors such as male sex, previous suicide attempts, alcoholism, and access to means of suicide are also present, the possibility of suicide requires careful consideration.

Forcible Treatment

Traditionally, patients in acute-care medical settings who pulled out intravenous tubes or took off monitor electrodes were dealt with coercively. Sedation was used without psychiatric consultation. Staff would assume that the patient's resistance was temporary and due to a transient confusional state, and that the medical interventions were life-saving and necessary. These assumptions have increasingly been questioned, partly because of the rising number of patients, even in nominally acute-care settings, who are elderly and have multiple physical and mental afflictions. Many stroke patients fall into this category.

Enteral feeding.   Enteral feeding is often seen as a paradigm of intrusive and extraordinary attempts to keep patients alive. Controversy has centered on whether this intervention improves the patient's comfort and whether it is really effective in prolonging life (Rousseau 1993). Sometimes patients try to pull out their tubes, and psychiatric opinion may be sought concerning a patient's reasons for doing so.

A point of particular relevance to stroke is that enteral feeding may be a temporary part of active treatment. There is often swallowing difficulty in stroke. A nasogastric tube may be inserted temporarily and, if swallowing does not rapidly return, may be replaced by a percutaneous gastrostomy (PEG). These measures are meant to improve the patient's comfort and to expedite recovery.

Forcible medication.   Forcible medication decisions often concern psychiatric medications, and can involve stroke-related issues:

> A manic patient refused to take lithium and developed grandiose delusions. Because he continued to take his blood pressure medication, was cheerful, and was not violent, it was elected not to seek forcible medication. Subsequently, however, under the influence of his delusions, the patient began refusing to take his blood pressure medication. When his blood pressure rose to 180/110, with left-ventricle hypertrophy, an application was then made to the court, under New York State law, for forcible administration of antipsychotic medication. The patient was given a single injection of a depot neuroleptic (the dose being calculated from his previous known tolerance) and thereafter agreed to take his blood pressure medication.

Physical restraints.   The stroke patient is, paradoxically, more likely to be physically restrained in a nonpsychiatric medical setting than in a psychiatric one. This is because psychiatric facilities normally have stringent regulations set up concerning the use of such restraints. Nursing homes are also now subject to considerable regulation regarding the use of physical restraints under the Omnibus Budget Reconciliation Act (OBRA '87). Restraints are sometimes used casually on acute medical floors of general

hospitals. Use of physical restraints in these settings should be accompanied by full documentation of the patient's mental state.

Diet and smoking restriction.   One of the most important concerns in
treating stroke is preventing another stroke. Stroke-prevention measures
are often restrictions. If the patient is hopelessly crippled and has dementia, is it justifiable to take away his or her few remaining pleasures? Should
an 80-year-old in a nursing home be made to adhere to a low-cholesterol
diet and refrain from smoking? Consider the following:

> An 82-year-old patient in a nursing home does not know where she is or what
> the date is, but still likes to read and seems cheerful. She has had a transient
> ischemic attack (TIA), is in atrial fibrillation, and is obese to an extent that
> limits her walking. Despite having high blood sugar and high blood choles-
> terol, she does not adhere to a prescribed diet. She is at high risk for a stroke
> because of her atrial fibrillation. The risk could be reduced by anticoagulant
> medication, but anticoagulation also has risks and inconveniences.

One opinion is that if diet and smoking are not restricted, then other
medical intervention, such as medications that might have side effects,
may also be withheld. This is a logical position, but not everyone agrees
with it. Alert and ambulant office patients can choose to disagree and to
exercise their own choices. With dementia patients or institutionalized
patients, health professionals must try to arrive at a consensus. The caregivers should be given full information about both the benefits of the
restriction and the adverse effects of the medication. Providing such information involves time spent educating the caregivers—by training if
they are paid, and by counseling if they are family members.

Intensity of Care

At the time of occurrence of the stroke, decisions must be made about
the intensity of care to be offered. The Patient Self-Determination Act of
1991 was meant to facilitate the creation of advance directives. This act
requires that all persons admitted to a hospital or nursing home be told
of their right to refuse treatment, and be given the opportunity to appoint someone to make such a decision for them if they become incapable. (The act's provisions are further described in free brochures obtainable from the American Association of Retired Persons [AARP; address
available in Appendix B]. These include "Health Care Powers of Attor-

ney," "Tomorrow's Choices," and "A Matter of Choice.") States can still draft their own documents, such as living wills, durable powers of attorney, and "do-not-resuscitate" (DNR) orders, but the enactment of the federal legislation has caused most states to simplify their laws and to allow for informal documentation of a patient's previously expressed wishes.

An impediment to the use of the simple advance directives provided for in the Patient Self-Determination Act is that stroke patients are usually mentally impaired or unconscious when brought into the hospital. Stroke patients for whom DNR orders are most likely to be written are those with mental impairment (King et al. 1993). In the absence of an advance directive, the patient's previously expressed wishes must be ascertained and a surrogate decision maker appointed—a process that can vary from state to state. In some jurisdictions, such as New York, a psychiatrist must be called in to determine whether a patient is competent to appoint a surrogate decision maker. No standardized method exists for making such a determination (Gerety et al. 1993).

In *In re guardianship of Browning* (1990), the question was raised of whether a patient who had become mentally incompetent by reason of a stroke should now be regarded as having an incurable terminal condition. The Florida court, deciding that she could, allowed termination of nasogastric feeding in accordance with the patient's previously expressed wishes.

Decisions about intensity of care in stroke remain fraught with the ambiguity of determining when the value of a particular individual's quality of life is a decision-making factor. "Common sense" is sometimes advocated in these situations, but common sense is often a synonym for conforming to commonly held opinion. A team approach can be a way to find out what the commonly held opinion is. What looks like avoidance of extraordinary measures to one team member may look like euthanasia to another. Informal polling to find out what "common sense" dictates can be easier when a family is involved, but becomes more complicated if family members disagree with each other. The "daughter from California" syndrome (Molloy et al. 1991) occurs when, after the available family members have agreed on a course of action or inaction for a patient, another relative turns up who has a different opinion. In theory, a legal order of priority exists, with the spouse's wishes taking precedence over others'. In practice, however, the family member who demands the most active treatment wins, because health professionals find it safer to risk being criticized for giving too much care rather than too little.

A physician was summoned to a nursing home to examine a resident who had become comatose. The patient, an 82-year-old woman, had spent much of her life in mental hospitals with chronic schizophrenia. She had been in the nursing home for several years and had remained aphasic with a right hemiplegia. There was no family whatsoever. The patient had not eaten breakfast that morning, although she took some fluids. Now she was not responding.

On examination, the patient had a dense right hemiplegia with contractures. Although she did not respond to speech, her eyes were open and she repositioned her left limbs when they were moved. Oxygen was being given by nasal cannula. Some of the staff at the nursing home felt she should be moved to the hospital, but others disagreed. On discussion, it emerged that those who had wanted her hospitalized were concerned that she would become dehydrated and suffer from thirst. The physician suggested monitoring for dehydration by measuring serum electrolytes and osmolality, and giving fluids by a nasogastric tube. All were satisfied with this course of action, and it was decided to keep her in the nursing home. Her coma deepened progressively, and a few hours later she died.

Summary

Causes of suicide may be sociological or psychiatric. There has been a recent movement to regard suicide in the face of severe illness as justifiable. Suicide in stroke is more likely among those with mild illness and with good potential for recovery. Use of physical restraints must be accompanied by full documentation of the patient's mental state. Stroke-prevention measures often restrict pleasure in life, and their use in patients with severe handicaps or dementia may be questioned. The Patient Self-Determination Act of 1991 requires that everyone admitted to a hospital or nursing home be told of their right to refuse treatment and be given the opportunity to appoint someone to make such a decision for them in the event that they become incapable. A spouse usually has legal precedence in decision making, but other family members' opinions may need to be considered. A team approach can be used to arrive at a commonsense decision about the intensity of care to be provided.

References

Bongar B (ed): Suicide: Guidelines for Assessment, Management, and Treatment. New York, Oxford University Press, 1992 de Haan R, Aaronson N, Limburg M, et al: Measuring quality of life in stroke. Stroke 24:320–327, 1993

Durkheim E: Le Suicide: étude de sociologie. Paris, Alcan, 1897. Translated as: Suicide: A Study in Sociology. New York, Free Press, 1966

Finkel S: Old people and suicide. Psychiatric News 26(22):3, November 15, 1991

Gerety MB, Chiodo LK, Kanten DN, et al: Medical treatment preferences of nursing home residents: relationship to function and concordance with surrogate decision-makers. J Am Geriatr Soc 41:953–960, 1993

Holbrook M, Skilbeck CE: An activities index for use with stroke patients. Age Ageing 12:166–170, 1983

Humphry D: Final Exit. Secaucus, NJ, Hemlock Society, 1991

In re guardianship of Browning, 568 So 2d 4,8,17 (Fla 1990)

Jacobs D (ed): Suicide and Clinical Practice. Washington, DC, American Psychiatric Press, 1992

King JJ, Doukas DJ, Gorenflo DW: Do not resuscitate orders for cerebrovascular accident patients (letter). Stroke 23:1032–1033, 1993

Molloy DW, Clarnette RM, Braun EA, et al: Decision making in the incompetent elderly: "the daughter from California syndrome." J Am Geriatr Soc 39:396–399, 1991

Omnibus Budget Reconciliation Act of 1987 (OBRA), Public Law 100-203

Rousseau P: Enteral feeding in the aged (letter). J Am Geriatr Soc 41:1370, 1993

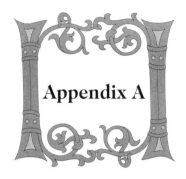

Appendix A

Basic Anatomy of Stroke

The brain is divided into an upper part, the cerebrum, and a lower part, the brain stem, which includes the medulla, pons, midbrain, and cerebellum. In the cerebrum, the gray matter, containing the nerve cell bodies, forms an outer layer called the *cortex*. The white matter, consisting of long nerve cell processes (nerve fibers, axons), is inside. The cerebrum is divided into two halves, the cerebral hemispheres. These are connected by a thick band of white matter called the *corpus callosum* (Figure A–1). Fluid-filled spaces within the brain are called *ventricles,* the largest being the lateral ventricles (Figure A–2). There are also some masses of gray matter deep within the cerebrum. The largest of these are the thalamus, the hypothalamus, and the basal ganglia.

The internal capsule (Figures A–3 and A–4) is the main tract of white matter connecting the cerebrum to the lower parts of the nervous system. It consists of nerve fibers running vertically between the lenticular nucleus laterally (i.e., on the outside) and the thalamus and head of the caudate nucleus medially (i.e., on the inside). The front part (anterior limb) of the internal capsule carries motor impulses downward. The back part (posterior limb) carries sensations upward. The middle part is called the *genu.*

The uppermost part of the brain stem is the midbrain. Below this are

367

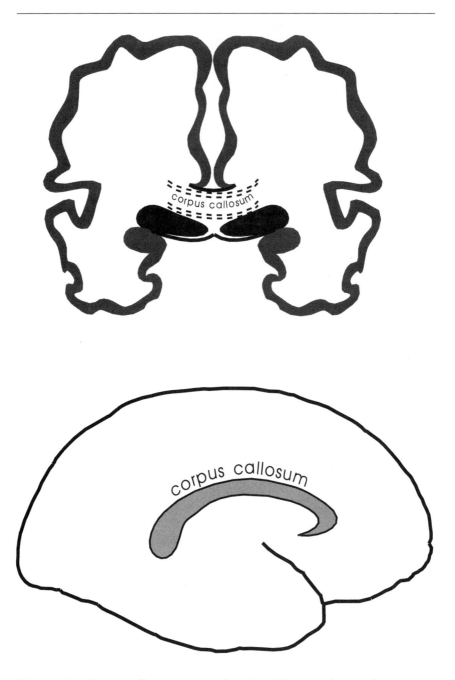

Figure A–1.   Corpus callosum in coronal section *(above)* and sagittal section *(below)*.

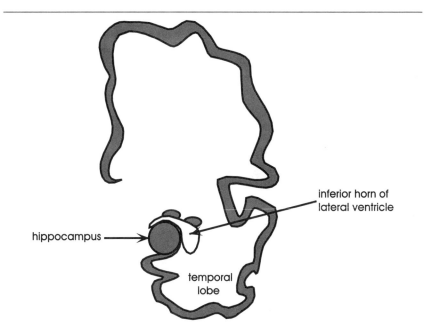

Figure A–2.   Hippocampus in relation to the temporal lobe in coronal section.

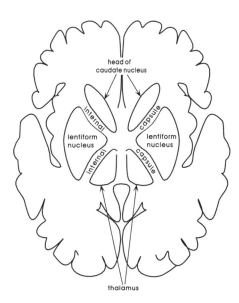

Figure A–3.   Transverse section, showing the internal capsule, the lentiform nucleus, and the head of the caudate nucleus.

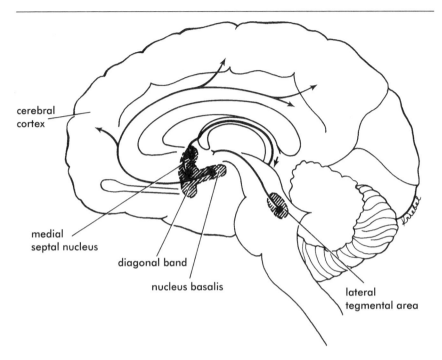

Figure A–4.   Cholinergic projection systems in the brain.
Source.   Adapted from Hyman SE, Nestler EJ: *The Molecular Foundations of Psychiatry.* Washington, DC, American Psychiatric Press, 1993, p. 88. Copyright 1993, American Psychiatric Press, Inc. Used with permission.

the pons and then the medulla, which merges with the spinal cord. The cerebellum is behind the midbrain and pons.

Four large arteries enter the skull to supply the brain. These are the internal carotid arteries in front and the vertebral arteries farther back. The two vertebral arteries unite in front of the brain stem to form the basilar artery, and then divide again to form the posterior cerebral arteries. Connections between branches of these arteries form the circle of Willis.

Cortex

The surface of the cortex shows bulges called *gyri*, separated by grooves called *sulci*. Some of the sulci divide the cortex into lobes: the frontal lobe, the parietal lobe, and the occipital lobe (Figure A–5). The central sulcus (Figure A–6) on the outer surface runs vertically and separates

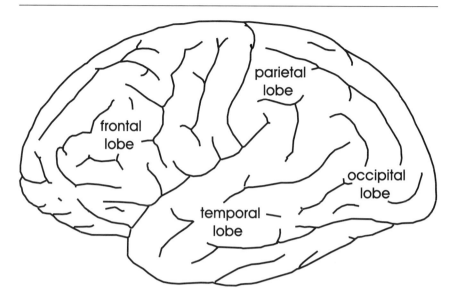

Figure A–5.   Lateral view of the surface of the cerebral cortex, showing division into lobes.

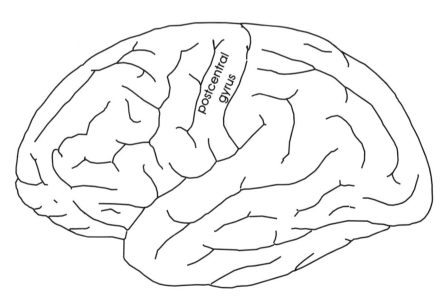

Figure A–6.   Lateral view of the surface of the cerebral cortex, showing the postcentral gyrus, bounded in front by the central sulcus and forming part of the parietal lobe.

the parietal lobe from the frontal lobe. The lateral sulcus, or Sylvian fissure (Figure A–7), runs horizontally and separates the temporal lobe from the frontal lobe.

Frontal lobe.   The frontal lobe is the part of the cerebrum in front of the central sulcus (Figure A–6). The motor areas of the cerebral cortex occupy a part of the frontal lobe immediately in front of the central sulcus. Damage to the precentral gyrus, or in the tracts leading down from it to the spinal cord, produces upper motor neuron paralysis of the opposite side of the body (hemiplegia). The lower back part of the left frontal lobe is Broca's area (Figure A–7) and is concerned with producing speech. Damage to the parts of the frontal lobe in front of the main motor areas, the prefrontal areas, can occur without any obvious paralysis or loss of physical function.

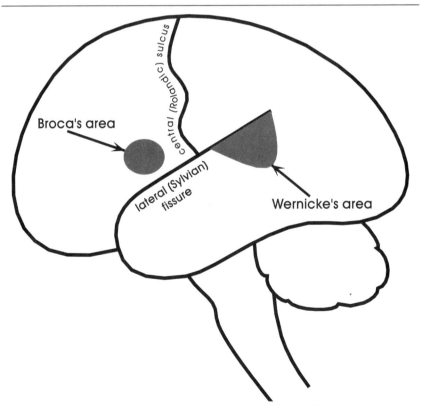

Figure A–7.   Broca's area and Wernicke's area in left hemisphere.

Parietal lobe.   The parietal lobe lies above the Sylvian fissure, behind the central sulcus, and in front of the occipital lobe (Figure A–5). The postcentral gyrus, immediately behind the central sulcus (Figure A–6), receives sensations of touch. The rest of the parietal cortex is also concerned with receiving sensation. The angular gyrus (Figure A–8) is an area on the lateral surface of the parietal lobe, near the junction with the occipital and temporal lobes. The supramarginal gyrus (Figure A–8) is in front of the angular gyrus.

Temporal lobe.   The temporal lobe is below the parietal and frontal lobes and in front of the occipital lobe. Wernicke's area is in the upper back part of the left temporal lobe, impinging on the parietal lobe below and behind Broca's area (Figure A–7).

Hippocampus.   The hippocampus is a set of intermingled layers of nerve cells and fibers within the temporal lobe (Figures A–2 and A–9).

Brodmann's areas.   In addition to topographically, the lobes can also be divided according to the cell architecture seen under the microscope. The divisions made on the basis of microscopy are called *Brodmann's areas* and are numbered arbitrarily from 1 to 43.

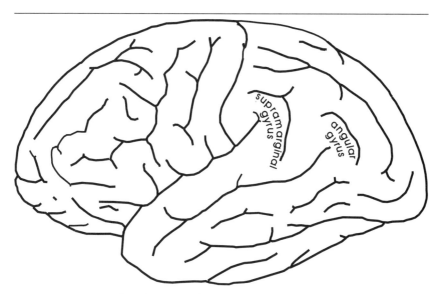

Figure A–8.   Lateral surface view of cerebral cortex indicating location of angular and supramarginal gyri.

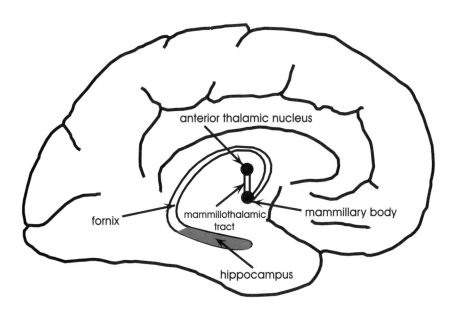

Figure A–9.   Hippocampus in relation to the structures of the limbic system.

The Basal Ganglia (Basal Nuclei)

The basal ganglia include the caudate nucleus and lenticular nucleus. (Several other structures, such as the amygdala, the subthalamic nucleus, and the substantia nigra, are sometimes also included). These lie in close relationship to the thalamus and to the internal capsule (Figures A–3, A–10, and A–11). The globus pallidus is the inner (medial) part of the lentiform nucleus. The corpus striatum (Figure A–11) comprises the caudate nucleus together with the globus pallidus. The amygdala (amygdaloid body) is an almond-shaped (amygdaloid) mass of nerve cells near the end of the tail of the caudate nucleus within the temporal lobe of the brain (Figure A–12). The subthalamic nucleus (body of Luys, corpus luysii) lies above the midbrain and below the thalamus.

Thalamus

The thalamus (Figure A–13) is an area of gray matter deep in the brain, behind the head of the caudate nucleus, that receives sensation from all parts of the body. Smell is the only sensation that bypasses the thalamus. It is divided internally by sheets (laminae) of white matter. These form a Y in transverse section with the tail of the Y pointing backward. Separate nuclei are designated according to their relationship to these laminae (Figure A–14). The lateral and medial geniculate bodies form the back of the thalamus.

Tracts of nerve fibers bringing touch and pain sensations (the medial lemniscus and spinothalamic tracts) end here (in the ventral posterior lateral nuclei) and so do those bringing vision and hearing (in the lateral and medial geniculate bodies). The mammillothalamic tract connects the anterior nucleus of the thalamus with the mammillary body of the hypothalamus, and constitutes part of the limbic system. The thalamus also receives tracts coming from the cerebellum and corpus striatum and has widespread cortical connections. Nerve cells in the dorsal medial (mediodorsal) thalamic nuclei (Figure A–14) degenerate after infarction of the frontal lobe, indicating a functional connection between these areas.

Hypothalamus

The hypothalamus is a mass of gray matter below the thalamus, above and in front of the midbrain (Figure A–15). The mammillary body (Fig-

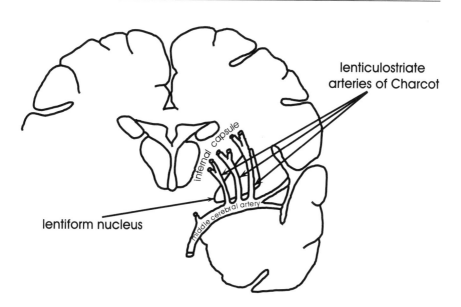

Figure A–10.   Middle cerebral artery with lenticulostriate arteries of Charcot.

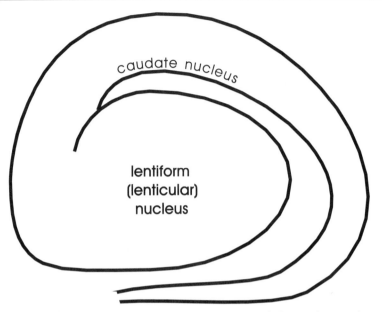

Figure A–11.   Lateral view of the lentiform nucleus and the caudate nucleus.

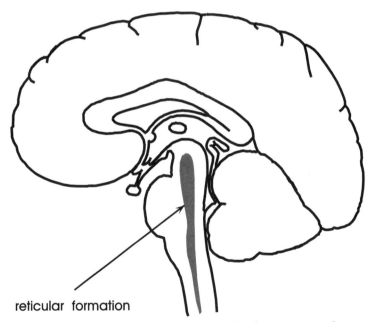

Figure A–12.   Approximate location of the reticular formation in relation to the sagittally cut brain.

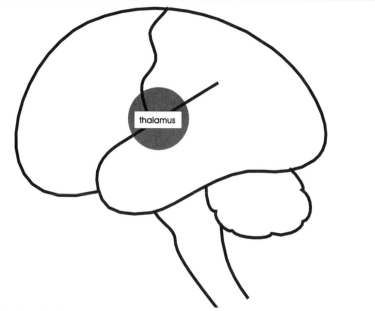

Figure A–13.   Thalamus in relation to the whole brain.

ure A–16) is a group of nerve cells in its lower part. The mammillotha-lamic tract connects the mammillary body with the thalamus. The me-dial forebrain bundle (Figure A–17) connects the hypothalamus with several other parts of the brain. The dorsal longitudinal bundle runs from the hypothalamus down through the brain stem and probably con-veys hypothalamic control to the autonomic nervous system.

The hypothalamus mediates between the brain and two systems not under conscious control—the autonomic nervous system and the endo-crine glands.

Midbrain

The midbrain contains vertically running tracts of nerve fibers connect-ing the cerebrum with the spinal cord. Its front part is formed by the basis pedunculi, behind which is the group of nerve cells called the *sub-stantia nigra* (Figure A–18). The inferior colliculus on the back (Fig-ure A–7) receives hearing sensation. The midbrain also contains the origin of the third or oculomotor cranial nerve (Figure A–19), which controls movements of the eye and contraction of the pupil.

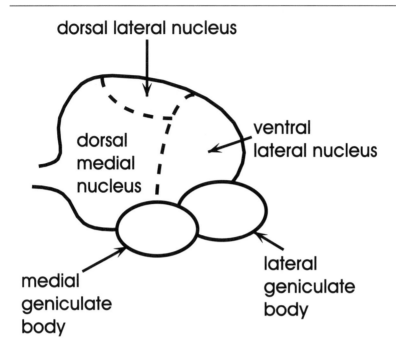

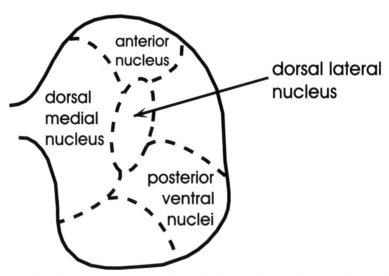

Figure A–14.   Thalamus seen from behind *(top)*, showing the lateral and medial geniculate bodies, and from above *(bottom)*, showing the location of some of the nuclei.

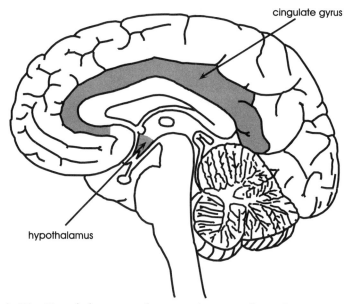

Figure A–15. Hypothalamus in relation to the sagittally cut brain.

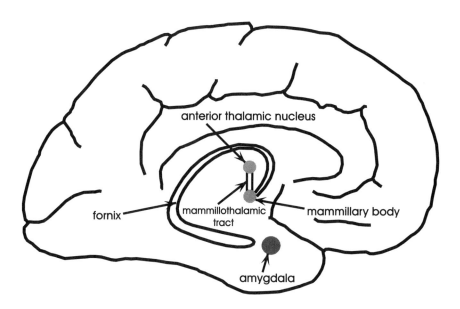

Figure A–16. Amygdala in relation to the structures of the limbic system.

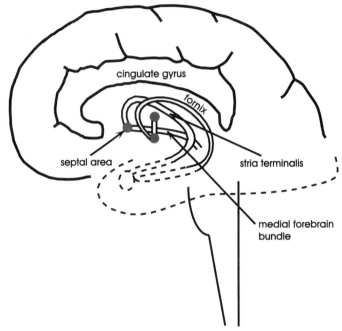

Figure A–17. Limbic system connections.

Pons and Medulla

The pons is the part of the brain stem above the medulla, below the midbrain, and in front of the cerebellum. The medulla merges into the spinal cord, and contains vital centers controlling breathing and heart rate.

Cerebellum

The cerebellum lies behind the pons and below the cerebrum. Its structure resembles the cerebrum in having outer gray matter and inner white matter. It is concerned with control of balance and coordination of fine movement.

Motor Pathways

The primary motor cortex lies anteriorly to the central sulcus. Fibers from nerve cells in this area go down in the anterior limb of the internal capsule to the brain stem, where a crossing over takes place. They then travel down in the spinal cord to reach their effector organs.

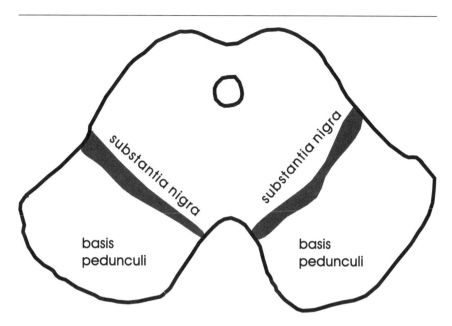

Figure A–18. Transverse section of the midbrain, showing the substantia nigra.

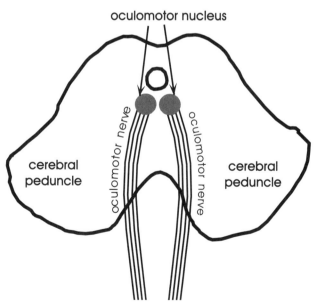

Figure A–19. Transverse section of the midbrain, showing the relationship between the third (oculomotor) nerve and the cerebral peduncle.

The basal ganglia, the substantia nigra, the subthalamic nucleus, and the cerebellum are also concerned with movement.

Extrapyramidal system.   The term *extrapyramidal system* was introduced by Samuel A. Kinnier Wilson for a set of nervous mechanisms for control of movement supposed to be deranged in conditions such as Parkinson's disease and Huntington's chorea. It includes the corpus striatum, which receives input from the cortex, the substantia nigra, and the subthalamic nucleus (corpus luysii); and gives output to the anterior ventrolateral nucleus of the thalamus, from which output goes to the motor cortex.

Sensory Pathways

Bodily sensations travel up in nerve fibers from the spinal cord, crossing at various levels, to reach the medial lemniscus, which goes to the thalamus. Sensations arriving in the thalamus are not yet conscious, and, in order for them to rise to consciousness, the thalamus must pass them up to the parietal lobes. Bundles of nerve fibers go up, in the internal capsule, from the thalamus to the parietal lobe cortex. Touch sensation, or at least light touch sensation, goes to the postcentral gyrus. Proprioception is probably sensed farther back in the parietal lobe.

Vision.   Visual sensations from the eye and optic nerves go to the optic chiasma (Figure A–20), where they partially cross over. This crossing causes objects in the right half of the field of vision to be seen by the right side of the brain, and vice versa. From the optic chiasma, the optic tracts go to the lateral geniculate bodies. The geniculocalcarine tract (optic radiation) carries visual sensation from the lateral geniculate bodies (Figure A–20) to the occipital cortex. There are two main pathways forward from the occipital cortex. The upper (superior longitudinal fasciculus) carries the visual input to the parietal lobes (Brodmann's area 7). The lower (the inferior longitudinal fasciculus) carries visual input to the temporal lobes (Brodmann's area 37). There is also a third pathway on the left, in between the other two, carrying visual information to the angular gyrus (Brodmann's area 39).

Hearing.   Hearing travels upward in the lateral lemniscus from the cochlear nuclei. The two lateral lemnisci are connected across the middle of the pons by the nerve fibers of the trapezoid body *(corpus trapezoideum)* so that sound heard in one ear is bilaterally represented from here up. The hearing sensations then go up to the medial geniculate bodies of the thala-

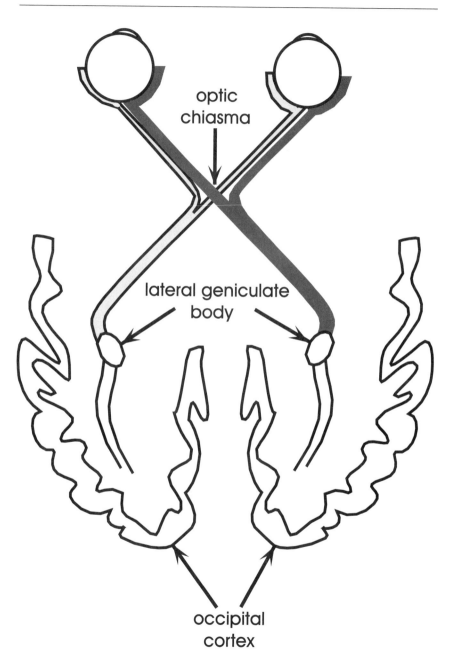

Figure A–20.   Transverse section, showing pathway of vision from the retina to the occipital cortex.

mus (Figure A–7) and from there to Heschl's area of the temporal cortex (Figure A–12).

Reticular formation.   The reticular formation (Figure A–12) is a network of white and gray matter extending from the medulla into the thalamus. It is probably concerned with maintenance of consciousness.

Neurotransmitter Production Sites

The sites of production of some neurotransmitters, such as glycine, glutamic acid, and gamma-aminobutyric acid, are widespread. Dopamine is largely produced in the substantia nigra (Figures A–18 and A–21); cat-

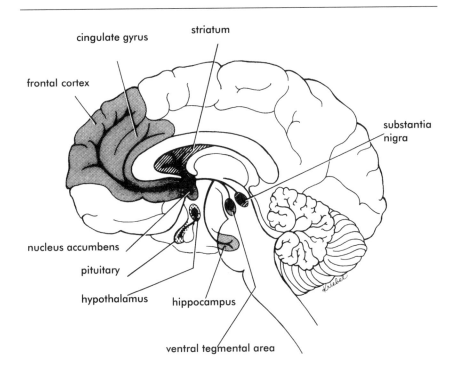

Figure A–21.   Dopaminergic projection systems in the brain.
Source.   Adapted from Hyman SE, Nestler EJ: *The Molecular Foundations of Psychiatry.* Washington, DC, American Psychiatric Press, 1993, p. 77. Copyright 1993, American Psychiatric Press, Inc. Used with permission.

echolamines (other than dopamine) are produced in the locus coeruleus, at the upper end of the pons (Figure A–22); acetylcholine is produced in the nucleus of Meynert (Figure A–4); and serotonin is produced in gray matter (raphe nuclei) in the pons and medulla (Figure A–23). Usually the receptor sites are more diffusely distributed, but some of these can also be mapped, as can the pathways the neurotransmitters follow to them.

Limbic System

The term *limbic system* is applied to a set of connections deep within the cerebrum. Tracts of white matter run from the mammillary bodies forward and then upward, backward, down again, and forward again to the amygdala. This interconnected system is thus approximately C-shaped,

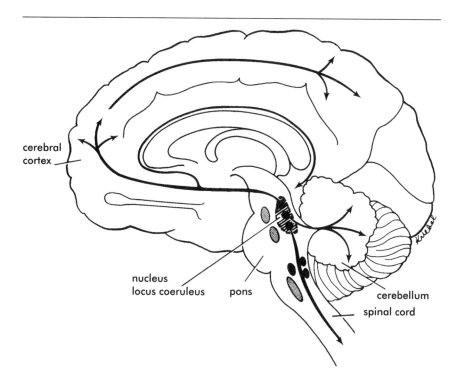

Figure A–22.   Noradrenergic projection systems in the brain.
Source.   Adapted from Hyman SE, Nestler EJ: *The Molecular Foundations of Psychiatry.* Washington, DC, American Psychiatric Press, 1993, p. 78. Copyright 1993, American Psychiatric Press, Inc. Used with permission.

with branches and bifurcations. Limbic system components are the *fornix*, the *stria terminalis*, the *mammillothalamic tract*, the *cingulum*, and the *medial forebrain bundle* (Figure A–17).

Autonomic Nervous System

The autonomic nervous system lies mostly outside the brain and spinal cord, and is not under conscious control. It is divided into the parasympathetic and sympathetic systems. The *parasympathetic system* is partly controlled by the vagus nerve, which originates in the medulla. Parasympathetic impulses also exit from the spinal cord lower down and travel in the nervi erigentes to the genitalia. The parasympathetic system is cholinergic, using acetylcholine as a neurotransmitter.

The *sympathetic system* is distinguished from the parasympathetic system by having epinephrine as its neurotransmitter and by a different anatomical arrangement. The sympathetic nerves exit from the spinal

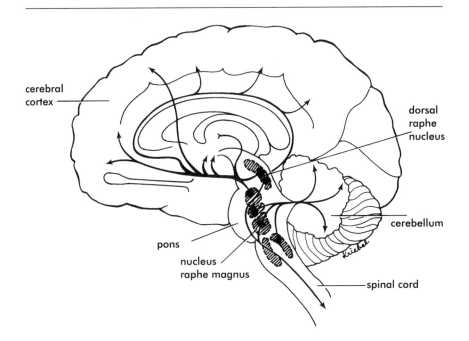

Figure A–23.   Serotonergic projection systems in the brain.
Source.   Adapted from Hyman SE, Nestler EJ: *The Molecular Foundations of Psychiatry.* Washington, DC, American Psychiatric Press, 1993, p. 86. Copyright 1993, American Psychiatric Press, Inc. Used with permission.

cord at several different levels and form plexuses (ganglia) close to the spine.

Carotid Artery

Blood comes into the front of the brain from the carotid arteries. The common carotid artery, which can be felt in the neck, divides into the

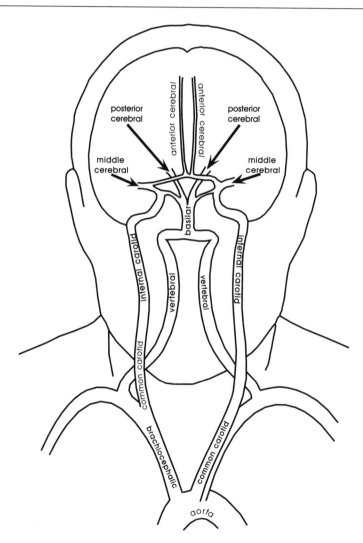

Figure A–24. Arteries supplying the brain, seen from the front.

external carotid artery and internal carotid artery (Figures A–24 and A–25). The internal carotid artery divides inside the skull into the anterior and middle cerebral arteries. The anterior cerebral artery (Figures A–24, A–25, and A–26) supplies the front of the brain. The two anterior cerebral arteries are connected by the anterior communicating artery.

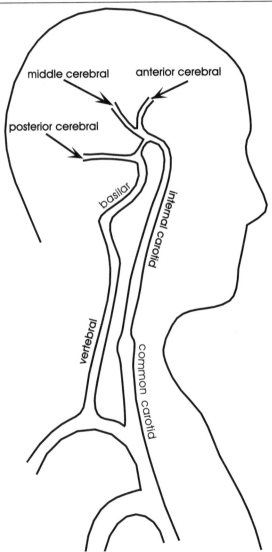

Figure A–25.   Arteries supplying the brain, seen from the right.

The middle cerebral gives off the lenticulostriate arteries of Charcot (Figure A–10) supplying the basal nuclei, thalamus, and internal capsule.

Vertebrobasilar Arteries

The vertebral artery (Figures A–24 and A–26) enters the skull from the neck, gives off the posterior inferior cerebellar artery, then joins with its counterpart of the opposite side to form the basilar artery. The basilar artery divides into the posterior cerebral arteries, which supply the back of the cerebrum. The posterior communicating artery connects the carotid artery with the posterior cerebral artery, and forms part of the circle of Willis (Figure A–26).

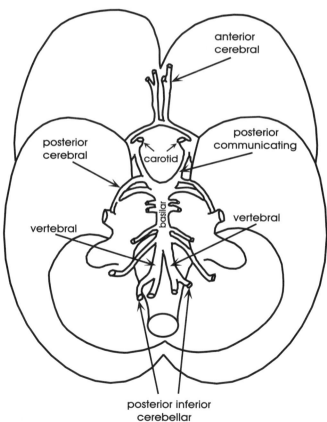

Figure A–26.   Arteries supplying the brain, seen from underneath.

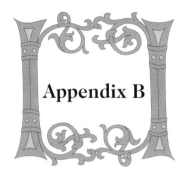

Appendix B

Resources for Family Caregivers

A patient's initial hospital care is usually paid by Medicare, Medicaid, or regular hospital insurance. Information about Medicare coverage can be obtained from a Social Security office. Patients younger than 65 years of age who are disabled may be eligible for Social Security if they have ever made Social Security contributions, and after receiving these benefits for 2 years they may be eligible for Medicare. These are regular Social Security benefits. Supplemental Security Income (SSI) is a type of federal welfare program in which payments are made for people who have not contributed to Social Security (see Table 22–1).

Finding Coverage for Posthospital Care

Payment for care after the hospital can come from several sources. A family that wants to take part in decision making should contact the hospital discharge planning department as soon as possible to discuss where the patient will be going and who will pay for care. The patient may go back home, to a rehabilitation unit, or to a nursing home.

Nursing-home care. The Omnibus Budget Reconciliation Act of 1987 (OBRA '87) was intended to halt the practice of putting mentally ill people in nursing homes, but made an exemption for dementia. Patients with mental symptoms who are going to go to nursing homes will therefore need a dementia assessment while in the hospital.

Medicare will not normally pay for nursing homes or home aides. When a patient is terminally ill, it may be possible to get Medicare coverage in a hospice program. Adult homes and rest homes can accommodate patients who can provide basic self-care and who do not need nursing services. Nursing-home care is covered by Medicaid after the "spend-down."

Home care.   Medicare will sometimes help to pay for patient care at home if hospitalization may be reduced in length or avoided thereby. In practice (although not overtly stated in the Medicare regulations), only patients who have recently been discharged from the hospital can receive such coverage. A doctor must certify the need for home health services and provide a plan of care, and the services must be provided by skilled professionals and be intermittent and part-time, not long term. Some of the Medicare regulations (e.g., the stipulation that the patient must be homebound) tend to exclude mentally disabled patients. Sometimes the physician's certification will disguise a patient's mental disability as a physical one so as to receive home care coverage. For example, blood pressure recording and injections may be ordered because they will be covered, whereas estimates of mental condition will not.

Although partially federally funded, the Medicaid program is administered by the individual states. For this reason, Medicaid payment for home care varies depending on geographical location. In general, Medicaid is more likely to pay for services that reduce the use of nursing-home care. Thus, Medicaid may pay for services such as those of nursing aides or home help on a long-term basis. Some private insurance carriers will cover home care.

Most provision for home care, whether financed by Medicare or Medicaid or by private insurance, is through agencies. An agency may be a government-funded visiting nurse association, an independent (nonprofit or commercial) organization, or an agency run by a hospital. Although designated as "nursing" agencies, such organizations will often provide a range of services, including physical therapists and home aides. When funds are available, if the situation is urgent and there is doubt about the level of care needed, a convenient method is to look in the Yellow Pages under the heading "Nursing" and then contact a commercial agency to send someone on a temporary basis. The agency is paid more than the employee is, but is usually able to provide help on short notice and for a brief time period. The agency can then help to estimate the amount of care the patient needs on a long-term basis.

The ambulant patient with behavioral problems is often the most difficult to obtain home help for. Many of the problems in this population are common to all dementia patients, and are discussed in "Steps to Finding Home Care," a booklet offered by the Alzheimer's Association (address in list at end of this appendix).

Day care.   Information about the availability of day care can be obtained from the National Institute on Adult Daycare (address in list at end of this appendix). Day hospitals are distinguished from day centers by the provision of active medical treatment and by a rehabilitation orientation. Day care for those with primarily mental disabilities should be provided by a local community mental health center. Such centers are listed in the *Mental Health Directory,* published by the U.S. Department of Health and Human Services.

U.S. Organizations and Publishers

Organizations

Several of the publications mentioned below contain further lists of addresses and telephone numbers. *The Stroke Fact Book,* by C. Foley and H. F. Pizer, published by Bantam Books, New York, 1985, and *Stroke: A Handbook for the Family,* by G. Mulley, published by the Council of Health Service Agencies (CHSA), London, 1990, each provide comprehensive listings of community services and entitlements for stroke victims. The University of Virginia Medical Center's stroke hotline (see below for number) provides similar information.

- **Alzheimer's Association** (formerly Alzheimer's Disease and Related Disorders Association), 919 North Michigan Avenue, Suite 1000, Chicago, IL 60611-1676; 1-800-272-3900
  Publishes "Steps to Finding Home Care" ($1.00).
- **Alzheimer's Disease International (ADI)**, 12 South Michigan Avenue, Chicago, IL 60603-4008; (312) 335-5777
- **American Association of Retired Persons (AARP)**, 601 E Street NW, Washington, DC 20049-0002; (202) 434-2277
  Provides free brochures on legal issues: "Health Care Powers of Attorney," "Tomorrow's Choices," and "A Matter of Choice."

- **American Association of Sex Educators, Counselors and Therapists (AASECT)**, 435 North Michigan Avenue, Suite 1717, Chicago, IL 60611-4008; (312) 644-0828
- **American Heart Association**, 7272 Greenville Avenue, Dallas, TX 75231-4596; (214) 373-6300
- **American Rehabilitation Association** (formerly National Association of Rehabilitation Facilities), 1910 Association Drive, Suite 200, Reston, VA 22091-1502; (703) 648-9300
  Provides a list of freestanding rehabilitation hospitals accredited by the Commission on Accreditation of Rehabilitation Facilities.
- **American Speech-Language-Hearing Association (ASHA)**, 10801 Rockville Pike, Rockville, MD 20852-3279; (301) 897-5700
- **National Association for Music Therapy**, 8455 Colesville Road, Suite 930, Silver Spring, MD 20910-3319; (301) 589-3300
  Provides information about the availability and training of music therapists.
- **National Easter Seal Society**, 230 West Monroe Street, Chicago, IL 60606-4703; (312) 726-6200
  Publishes "First Aid for Aphasics" ($1.00).
- **National Institute on Adult Daycare (NIAD)**, c/o National Council on the Aging, 409 3rd Street, S.W., 2nd Floor, Washington, DC 20024-3212; (202) 479-6682
- **National Stroke Association**, 8480 East Orchard Road, Suite 1000, Englewood, CO 80111-5015; (800) 787-6537
  Publications include "Adaptive Resources Guide" (free), "Communication Difficulties" ($3.00), *Disability Workbook for Social Security Applicants* ($14.95), "Family Care-Givers Guide" ($6.00), "Home and Work Adaptations" ($1.00), "Living at Home After a Stroke ($1.25), *Pathways—Moving Beyond Stroke and Aphasia* ($19.50), *The Road Ahead: A Stroke Recovery Guide* ($16.50), "Stroke Questions and Answers" ($1.50), "Suggestions for Communication With an Aphasic Person" ($0.50), "Understanding Speech and Language Problems After Stroke" ($4.00), and "What Every Family Should Know About Stroke" ($0.25).
- **Sexual Information and Education Council of the United States (SIECUS)**, 130 West 42nd Street, Suite 350, New York, NY 10036-7802; (212) 819-9770
- **Sexuality and Disability Training Centers:**
  Boston University Medical Center, 88 East Newton Street, Boston, MA 02118-2393; (617) 638-7358;

University of Michigan Medical Center, Department of Physical Medicine and Rehabilitation, 1500 East Medical Center Drive, Ann Arbor, MI 48109-0042; (313) 936-7067

- **Stroke Clubs International (SCI)**, 805 12th Street, Galveston, TX 77550-5032; (409) 762-1022
- **University of Virginia Medical Center stroke hotline**, (804) 295-9557

Publishers in Health Care Topics

- **Abbey Press**, Hill Drive, St. Meinrad, IN, 47577; (800) 325-2511
- **Health Edco**, P.O. Box 21207, Waco, TX, 76702-1207; (800) 299-3366, ext. 295

U.K. Organizations

- **Action for Dysphasic Adults (ADA)**, Canterbury House, Royal Street, London SE17 1NJ
- **Carers' National Association**, 29 Chilworth Mews, London W2 3RG
- **College of Speech Therapists**, 6 Lechmere Road, London NW2 BU
- **Council of Health Service Agencies (CHSA) Advice Center**, CHSA House, Whitecross Street, London EC1Y 8JJ

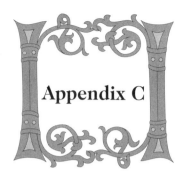

Appendix C

Wilson, Roosevelt, Churchill, Hitler, and Stalin

Cerebrovascular brain disease has had a remarkable place in 20th-century history. All three of the Yalta participants were destined to die of stroke. Two of them would die of this disease while still in office. One was probably experiencing the mental effects of vascular disease at the time of the Yalta meeting. Winston Churchill, Franklin Roosevelt, and Woodrow Wilson were under the scrutiny of astute observers able to make good records of the nuances of intellectual change. Our knowledge of the medical and mental status of Joseph Stalin and Adolf Hitler is more scanty.

Stalin. Stalin withdrew from public appearance after October 1952. Prior to that, there had been no noteworthy change in his behavior. According to the *Pravda* account, he suffered a brain hemorrhage "due to hypertonia and arteriosclerosis" on the night of March 2, 1953, with paralysis of the left side and loss of consciousness. He remained in a coma and died 3 days later.

Hitler. Hitler eventually died by his own hand, and no autopsy was done. The racist doctrines of Nazism have a paranoid tinge but were being expressed in his vigorous youth. During the war years, he was moderately hypertensive, with electrocardiogram (ECG) abnormalities interpreted as showing coronary artery disease. From 1944, his bouts of rage and irrational behavior increased. This was attributed by many observers to the effects on him of the plot against his life, which made him increasingly suspicious of those around him. The most consistent neurological sign noted was shaking. This has sometimes been tentatively attributed to Parkinson's disease, but no somatic tremor is evident on an ECG of June 1943. He was described in April 1945 as barely able to walk, with a stooped back and a shuffling gait, his right leg dragging, his head shaking, and his left hand violently trembling on the limp dangling arm (Irving 1983, p. 272).

Wilson

The story of Woodrow Wilson has been told by several biographers (Nordholt 1991; Smith 1960/1980). There is also a posthumously published study of Wilson by Sigmund Freud, written in collaboration with Wilson's vehement critic William Bullitt, in which Freud interpreted the president's character largely in terms of his relationship to his father. Freud explained the behavioral effects of the stroke as being due to a withdrawal of libido from love-objects in the external world (Freud and Bullitt 1967).

President Wilson became ill at the Paris Peace Conference, in April 1919. It had been noticed that he was talking at unusual length and interrupting himself with laughter, and had developed a tic on one half of his face. Then he ran a fever with diarrhea and was asleep for 3 days. When he awoke, he developed ideas that furniture was being stolen from the house he was staying in and that the servants were all spies. He became bad-tempered and secretive but continued to conduct the affairs of the United States and to compose coherent speeches. Thereafter, he was, in the opinion of many, less skilled as a politician. His unwillingness to compromise was a factor—although this is also matter of opinion—in America's not joining the League of Nations (Smith 1960/1980). From this point on, there was an impression that he looked ill, was harder to get along with, and was not the man he had been. On several occasions, he stopped in the middle of speeches as if unable to find words. On other occasions, he was moved to tears in public. His handwriting deteriorated. In September 1919, at the age of 63, he undertook a strenuous speaking tour, during the course of which he was plagued by increasingly severe headaches; then suddenly he developed weakness of the left side of his body. He remained able to speak and to walk with support, but a week later he became unconscious, and on return to consciousness he had a compete left hemiplegia. From that point on until the end of his second 4 years in office in 1921, his wife, his secretary, and his physician, Dr. Grayson, strictly limited access to him. His physicians used expressions such as "nervous exhaustion" to avoid having to define exactly the extent to which the illness was physical or mental. He was not aphasic, but messages sent to him were answered by his wife with statements beginning, "The President says."

If he had become completely demented, or even completely aphasic, then the dilemmas would have been easier. A particular perplexity was that, at moments when the decision had been made to take over his duties, he was liable to snap out of his haze and vigorously and clearly assert his wishes. When attempts were made to take over the government from him, he thwarted them. At first, cabinet meetings were held by Lansing, the secretary of state, in his absence, but then the president sent a signed and typed letter accusing Lansing of conspiring against him and usurping his authority, and made the secretary resign.

In April 1920, he emerged to take part in a cabinet meeting. He was rambling and forgetful, frequently repeating weak jokes. He became vindictive and bitter, quarreled with old friends, and made many enemies. He was persuaded with difficulty not to run again for office.

Wilson lived until 1924, became able to walk again, and never became grossly demented. He made attempts to practice law again and to write, but his attempts were feeble and embarrassing to others, although not to himself. He attributed these new failures to the poor judgment of others and his own high principles.

Roosevelt

The case of Franklin Delano Roosevelt presents many interesting parallels to that of Wilson. President Roosevelt had been chairbound by poliomyelitis from childhood. In the last year of his life, he suffered from high blood pressure and had a heart attack. He was under such treatment as was then available for congestive heart failure. His doctors apparently concealed the severity of his illness, not only from the public but also from Roosevelt himself. One physician said, "He is irascible and becomes very irritable if he has to concentrate his mind for long. If anything is brought up that wants thinking he will change the subject" (Bishop 1974, p. 295). There were changes in his signature and voice. Nonmedical observers said that the corner of his mouth drooped, and that there were times when he forgot what he had been talking about. It was in this state that he represented his country to decide the fate of the world at Yalta, where Churchill's physician, Lord Moran, noted that the president had "all the symptoms of hardening of the arteries of the brain in an advanced stage" (Bishop 1974, p. 294). Nevertheless, his doctors denied that he had had a stroke prior to the one that caused his sudden collapse and death at the age of 63. No autopsy was performed, but undertakers found that his carotid arteries could not be perfused for embalming.

Churchill

Winston Churchill at Yalta was hale and hearty at the age of 70. In 1949, while out of office, he had a mild stroke that affected his right side and caused him difficulty walking and signing his name. No mental symptoms were noted, and he was subsequently reelected prime minister at the age of 76. A second stroke in June 1953 affected his left side. Following this, he was noted to tire quickly and had spells of depression, but painted, wrote, and remained politically active. It was not until March 1954 that people noticed he was unsure of himself and unable to finish his sentences. He resigned from the office of prime minister a month later, but continued as an ordinary member of parliament. There were several further strokes, but letters handwritten by him at the age of 88 were clear and coherent. When he was 89, his daughter committed suicide, and another daughter who told him of this wrote, "The lethargy of extreme old age dulls many sensibilities and my father took in only slowly what I said to him, but then he withdrew into a great and distant silence" (Gilbert 1991, p. 958).

References

Bishop J: FDR's Last Year. New York, William Morrow, 1974

Freud S, Bullitt WC: Thomas Woodrow Wilson. Boston, MA, Houghton Mifflin, 1967

Gilbert M: Churchill: A Life. New York, Henry Holt, 1991

Irving D: The Secret Diaries of Hitler's Doctor. New York, Macmillan, 1983

Nordholt JWS: Woodrow Wilson: A Life for World Peace. Translated by Rowen HH. Los Angeles, CA, University of California Press, 1991

Smith G: When the Cheering Stopped. New York, William Morrow, 1960 (reprinted by Morrow Quill Paperbacks, 1980)

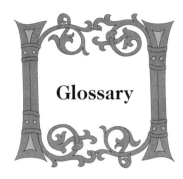

Glossary

absence seizures	Type of seizure in which the patient is briefly unaware of the surroundings, but does not have convulsions.
ACE	*See* angiotensin-converting enzyme.
acetylcholine	A neurotransmitter in the brain, where it helps to regulate memory, and in the peripheral nervous system, where it controls the actions of skeletal and smooth muscle.
activities of daily living (ADL)	Activities, such as dressing, eating, and bathing, that are usually done independently each day by a healthy person.
adenosine	Compound of a sugar called *ribose* and a purine base called *adenine*.
ADL	*See* activities of daily living.
adrenergic	Pertaining to neural activation by catechol-amines such as epinephrine, norepinephrine, and dopamine. Contrast with *cholinergic*.
advance directive	Form of living will whereby patients can direct what medical treatments can be used if they should later become too ill to decide.
afferent	Bringing information toward.

Definitions marked with asterisks are reprinted from Edgerton J, Campbell RJ: *American Psychiatric Glossary,* Seventh Edition. Washington, DC, American Psychiatric Press, 1994. Used with permission.

agnosia	Inability to recognize objects presented by way of one or more sensory modalities that cannot be explained by a defect in elementary sensation or a reduced level of consciousness or alertness.
akinetic mutism	State of apparent alertness with tracking eye movements but no speech or voluntary motor responses.
alexia	Loss of a previously possessed reading facility that cannot be explained by defective visual acuity.
alpha-adrenergic	Type of adrenergic action causing constriction of blood vessels and smooth muscle.
Alzheimer's disease	A progressive, increasing impairment in memory and other intellectual functions/activities beginning with confusion and forgetfulness. The progression, usually after 1–2 years, is shown in disorientation, muscle rigidity, purposeless hyperactivity, and difficulty in speaking. The final stage shows the patient with dementia and in a vegetative state. The dementia is character-ized by continuing and gradual cognitive and functional decline. Early-onset type (sometimes called *presenile dementia*) occurs at age 65 or younger; late-onset type occurs after the age of 65. In the course of deterioration, various syndromes may be superimposed, such as depression, delusions, hallucinations, or other perceptual, behavioral (e.g., violence), commu-nication, or motor skill disturbances.
amygdala	Almond-shaped (amygdaloid) mass of nerve cells near the end of the tail of the caudate nucleus within the temporal lobe of the brain (see Figure A–16).
aneurysm	Abnormal bulging of the wall of an artery.
angiotensin-converting enzyme	Enzyme produced by the kidney that can cause hypertension.

angular gyrus	Area of the cerebral cortex on the lateral surface of the parietal lobe, near the junction with the occipital and temporal lobes (see Figure A–8).
anosognosia	The apparent unawareness of or failure to recognize one's own functional defect (e.g., hemiplegia, hemianopsia).
anterior cerebral artery	Branch of the internal carotid artery supplying the front of the brain (see Figures A–24, A–25, and A–26).
anticholinergic effects or properties	Interference with the action of acetylcholine in the brain and peripheral nervous system by any drug. In psychiatry, the term generally refers to side effects of antipsychotic drugs, tricyclic antidepressants, and antiparkinsonian drugs. Common symptoms of such effects include dry mouth, blurred vision, and constipation.
antioxidant	Substance that slows down metabolism by reducing loss of electrons.
antiphospholipid antibody syndrome (APLAS)	Immunological disorder that can cause multiple strokes in young patients.
aphasia	Loss of a previously possessed facility of language comprehension or production that cannot be explained by sensory or motor defects or by diffuse cerebral dysfunction.
aphonia	Inability to produce normal speech sounds; may be due to either organic or psychological causes.
APLAS	*See* antiphospholipid antibody syndrome.
applied behavior analysis	Analysis of disturbed behavior into component elements, as is done prior to behavior therapy.
apraxia	Loss of a previously possessed ability to perform skilled motor acts that cannot be explained by weakness, abnormal muscle tone, or elementary incoordination.

arcuate nucleus	Nucleus of the thalamus, now called the *ventral posteromedial nucleus,* which receives sensory input from the face.
arrhythmia	Irregular heartbeat.
atherosclerosis	Disease in which plaques of cholesterol build up in the lining of arteries.
atrial fibrillation	Very irregular heartbeat that can cause heart failure or embolisms.
autonomic nervous system	Part of the nervous system that innervates the cardiovascular, digestive, reproductive, and respiratory organs. It operates outside of consciousness and controls basic life-sustaining functions such as heart rate, digestion, and breathing. It includes the sympathetic nervous system and the parasympathetic nervous system.
avoidant personality	Personality disorder characterized by social discomfort and reticence, low self-esteem, and hypersensitivity to negative evaluation. Manifestations may include avoiding activities that involve contact with others because of fears of criticism or disapproval; experiencing inhibited development of relationships with others because of fears of appearing foolish or being shamed; having few friends despite the desire to relate to others; or being unusually reluctant to take personal risks or engage in new activities because they may prove embarrassing.
axon	The fiber-like extension of a neuron through which the cell sends information to target cells.

Babinski

Medical sign, named after a French neurologist, in which the big toe bends upward when the foot is scratched, and which suggests an upper-motor-neuron type of paralysis.

bacterial endocarditis

Infection of the heart valves.

basal ganglia

Clusters of neurons located deep in the brain (see Figures A–3 and A–11); they include the caudate nucleus and the putamen (corpus striatum), the globus pallidus, the subthalamic nucleus, and the substantia nigra. The basal ganglia appear to be involved in higher-order aspects of motor control, such as planning and execution of complex motor activity and the speed of movements. Lesions of the basal ganglia produce various types of involuntary movements such as athetosis, chorea, dystonia, and tremor. The basal ganglia are involved also in the pathophysiology of Parkinson's disease, Huntington's disease, and tardive dyskinesia. The internal capsule, containing all the fibers that ascend to or descend from the cortex, runs through the basal ganglia and separates them from the thalamus.

basal perforating arteries

Central branches of the anterior and middle cerebral arteries that supply the basal nuclei and internal capsule.

basal nuclei

Basal ganglia.

basilar artery

Artery formed by the union of the two vertebral arteries that supply the brain stem and back part of the cerebrum (see Figures A–24, A–25, and A–26).

basis pedunculi	White matter at the front of the midbrain that contains the main tracts of nerve fibers connecting the cerebrum with the spinal cord (see Figure A–18).
behaviorism	An approach to psychology first developed by John B. Watson that rejected the notion of mental states and reduced all psychological phenomena to neural, muscular, and glandular responses. Contemporary behaviorism emphasizes the study of observable responses but is directed toward general behavior rather than discrete acts. It includes private events such as feelings and fantasies to the extent that these can be directly observed and measured.
behaviorist	One advocating or practicing behaviorism.
beta-adrenergic	Type of adrenergic response with increase of heart rate and relaxation of smooth muscle.
beta-blockers	Drugs that block some of the actions of nor-epinephrine, slowing the pulse and reducing blood pressure.
bipolar disorder	In DSM-IV, a group of mood disorders that includes bipolar disorder, single episode; bipolar disorder, recurrent; and cyclothymic disorder. A bipolar disorder includes a manic episode at some time during its course. In any particular patient, the bipolar disorder may take the form of a single manic episode (rare), or it may consist of recurrent episodes that are either manic or depressive in nature (but at least one must have been predominantly manic). Bipolar II disorder is used in some classifications (including DSM-IV) to denote a mood disorder characterized by episodes of major depressive disorder and hypomania (rather than full mania). Other authorities prefer to call such a mood disorder "major depressive disorder with hypomanic episodes."

bipolar illness	Bipolar disorder.
body of Luys	Subthalamic nucleus, corpus luysii.
bradykinesia	Slowness of movement.
brain stem	Part of the brain between the cerebrum and the spinal cord; includes midbrain, pons, medulla, and cerebellum.
calcium blockers	Drugs that block the passage of calcium into and out of nerve and muscle cells.
calcium channel	Part of the wall of a nerve or muscle cell that allows calcium to pass in or out of the cell.
Capgras' syndrome	Delusion that familiar people have been replaced by impostors.
carbamazepine	Drug used in treating epilepsy, especially complex partial seizures, and also used in some psychiatric conditions (trade name is Tegretol).
cardiac monitoring	Continuous recording of the pulse and electrical activity of the heart.
carotid artery	The common carotid artery, which can be felt in the neck, divides into the external carotid artery and internal carotid artery. The latter supplies blood to the brain (see Figures A–24 and A–25).
catecholamines	A group of biogenic amines derived from tyrosine and containing the catechol (3,y-dihydroxyphenyl) moiety. Certain of these amines, such as epinephrine, norepinephrine, and dopamine, are neurotransmitters and exert an important influence on peripheral and central nervous system activity.
caudate nucleus	Mass of nerve cells deep in the brain concerned with regulating the control of movement. The caudate nucleus is one of the basal nuclei (see Figures A–3 and A–11).

central sulcus	Groove on the outer surface of the brain running vertically, and separating the parietal lobe from the frontal lobe. Also called the *fissure of Rolando* (see Figure A–7).
centrum ovale	White matter in the cerebrum above the level of the internal capsule.
cerebellum	Part of the brain, behind the pons and below the cerebrum, concerned with coordination and control of movement and balance.
cerebrum	The largest and uppermost part of the brain with nerve cell bodies (gray matter) on the outside and nerve fibers (white matter) inside.
cholesterol	Fatty substance occurring naturally in the blood and many tissues and giving rise to the plaques in atherosclerosis.
cholinergic	Activated or transmitted by acetylcholine (e.g., parasympathetic nerve fibers). Contrast with *adrenergic*.
choreoathetoid	Describes abnormal movements that are partly twitching (choreic) and partly writhing (athetoid).
cingulate gyrus	Area of the cerebral cortex, on the inner surface, running around the corpus callosum (see Figure A–17).
cingulum	Band of nerve fibers within the cingulate gyrus, running parallel to the surface.
circle of Willis	Set of arteries at the base of the brain connecting the arteries of each side and of the front and back with each other (see Figures A–24 and A–26).
clinical signs	Evidence obtained by examining the patient without the assistance of X rays or blood tests.

cognitive psychology	A reaction to behaviorist psychology; set out to study what went on in the mind *between* the stimulus and the response. These days, it is largely concerned with computerized models of thinking.
complex partial seizure	Form of seizure in which there are complete quasipurposive actions rather than simple muscle jerking; sometimes equated with temporal lobe epilepsy and psychomotor epilepsy.
computed tomography (CT)	Technique for imaging anatomical structures using X ray. Objects are exposed to a series of X-ray beams on a single plane but with origin at different points around a 180-degree arc. A computer algorithm reconstructs the beam absorption data so as to display an image of absorption values at each point in the plane. The process is repeated for each plane to be imaged. Used for anatomical abnormalities such as strokes, tumor, atrophy of the brain.
construct validity	Evidence that the questions in a test all measure the same thing.
contralateral	In the same place on the opposite side.
conversion disorder	One of the somatoform disorders (but in some classifications called a *dissociative* disorder), characterized by a symptom suggestive of a neurological disorder that affects sensation or voluntary motor function. The symptom is not consciously or intentionally produced, it cannot be explained fully by any known general medical condition, and it is severe enough to impair functioning or require medical attention. Commonly seen symptoms are blindness, double vision, deafness, impaired coordination, paralysis, and seizures.
coronal section	Section of the brain made by cutting vertically, parallel to the front and the back of the body.

corpus callosum	Thick band of white matter connecting the right and left halves of the cerebrum (see Figure A–1).
corpus luysii	Subthalamic nucleus; body of Luys.
corpus striatum	The part of the basal ganglia comprising the caudate nucleus together with the lentiform nucleus (see Figure A–11).
cortex	Outer rind of an organ. The cerebral cortex is the layer of nerve cell bodies (gray matter) on the outside of the cerebrum.
cortical	Relating to the cortex.
corticospinal tract	Bundle of nerve fibers (white matter) running down through the spinal cord from the brain, mostly from the opposite side.
countertransference	The therapist's emotional reactions to the patient that are based on the therapist's unconscious needs and conflicts, as distinguished from his or her conscious responses to the patient's behavior. Countertransference may interfere with the therapist's ability to understand the patient and may adversely affect the therapeutic technique. Currently, there is emphasis on the positive aspects of countertransference and its use as a guide to a more empathic understanding of the patient.
cranial nerve	Nerve that arises directly from the brain, instead of from the spinal cord.
CT	*See* computed tomography.
cyclotron	Apparatus for altering atomic structure.
day hospital	Center providing medical and nursing care on a daily basis.

delirium tremens	Alcohol withdrawal delirium occurring within hours of cessation of, or significant reduction in, alcohol use in a person with a pattern of heavy and prolonged drinking. Symptoms may include hand tremor; nausea and vomiting; anxiety; perceptual disturbances such as transient visual, tactile, or auditory hallucinations or illusions with intact reality testing; sweating or increased pulse rate; psychomotor agitation; insomnia; or grand mal seizures.
delusion	A false belief based on an incorrect inference about external reality and firmly sustained despite clear evidence to the contrary. The belief is not part of a cultural tradition such as an article of religious faith.
dementia	A cognitive disorder characterized by defects in memory and executive functioning; aphasia; apraxia; and agnosia. Various forms of dementia are recognized in DSM-IV: 1) dementia due to a general medical condition, including dementia of the Alzheimer type; dementia, vascular; HIV (human immunodeficiency virus) dementia; and dementia due to Pick's disease, Creutzfeldt-Jakob disease, Huntington's disease, and Parkinson's disease; 2) substance-induced persisting dementia (seen with alcohol, inhalants, and sedatives/hypnotics/anxiolytics); 3) dementia due to multiple etiologies; 4) dementia of unknown etiology; and 5) dementia not otherwise specified.

dependent personality disorder	Personality disorder characterized by an excessive need to be taken care of, resulting in submissive and clinging behavior and fears of separation. Manifestations may include excessive need for advice and reassurances about everyday decisions, encouragement of others to assume responsibility for major areas in one's life, inability to express disagreement because of possible anger or lack of support from others, and preoccupation with fears of being left to take care of oneself.
diagnosis-related group (DRG)	Medical-based classification, representing 23 major diagnostic categories, that aggregates patients into case types based on diagnosis. A diagnosis-related group is a subset of a major diagnostic category.
dissecting aneurysm	Bleeding between the layers of the wall of an artery.
distal insufficiency	Insufficient flow of blood in the end branches of an artery.
diuretic	Medication that increases urine output.
do-not-resuscitate (DNR) order	A medical order that extreme measures to prevent death should not be taken.
dopamine	Neurosynaptic transmitter found in the healthy brain, specifically associated with some forms of psychosis and abnormal movement disorders.
Doppler examination	Method of estimating the patency of an artery by the variations in sound waves produced with speed of blood flow.
dorsal longitudinal bundle	Tract of nerve fibers running from the hypothalamus down through the brain stem and probably conveying hypothalamic control to the autonomic nervous system.

dorsomedial nucleus	Part of the thalamus that probably connects with the frontal areas of the cortex. Also known as *mediodorsal thalamic nucleus* (see Figure A–14).
DRG	*See* diagnosis-related group.
DSM-III-R	Revision of the third version of the *Diagnostic and Statistical Manual of Mental Disorders* of the American Psychiatric Association.
DSM-IV	Revision of DSM-III-R.
dysarthria	Difficulty in speech production due to incoordination of speech apparatus.
dystonia (acute, neuroleptic-induced)	Abnormal positioning or spasm of the muscles of the head, neck, limbs, or trunk; develops within a few days of starting or raising the dose of a neuroleptic medication, because of dysfunction of the extrapyramidal system.
edema	Swelling due to pathological increase of fluid in a part of the body.
ego	In psychoanalytic theory, one of three major divisions in the model of the psychic apparatus, the others being the id and the superego. The ego represents the sum of certain mental mechanisms, such as perception and memory, and specific defense mechanisms. It serves to mediate between the demands of primitive instinctual drives (the id), of internalized parental and social prohibitions (the superego), and of reality. The compromises between these forces achieved by the ego tend to resolve intrapsychic conflict and serve an adaptive and executive function. Psychiatric usage of the term should not be confused with common usage, which connotes self-love or selfishness.
embolism	Blockage of an artery by a blood clot or other particles carried from elsewhere in the body.

embolus	Blood clot or other particles causing an embolism.
epileptiform	Resembling epilepsy.
epinephrine	One of the catecholamines secreted by the adrenal gland and by fibers of the sympathetic nervous system. It is responsible for many of the physical manifestations of fear and anxiety. Also known as *adrenaline*.
estrogen	A female sex hormone.
euphoria	An exaggerated feeling of physical and emotional well-being, usually of psychological origin. It is also seen in organic mental disorders and in toxic and drug-induced states.
excitotoxic	Damaging by excess of an excitatory neurotransmitter.
extrapyramidal	A set of nervous mechanisms for control of system movement, supposed to be disordered in conditions such as Parkinson's disease.
factor VIII	One of the substances responsible for blood coagulation.
FDA-approved indication	Purpose for which a drug is officially considered effective by the U.S. Food and Drug Administration.
fibrinolytic	Able to remove blood clots by dissolving fibrin.
first-rank Schneiderian	Belonging to a set of symptoms considered specific to schizophrenia.
folic acid	Water-soluble vitamin of the B group.
fornix	Bundle of nerve fibers deep in the brain, extending from the mammillary bodies to the temporal lobe (see Figures A–9 and A–16).
Framingham study	Large-scale study with long-term follow-up of heart disease and other illness in the population of Framingham, Massachusetts.

frontal lobe	Part of the brain in front of the central sulcus (see Figure A–5).
fusiform gyrus	Part of the cortex of the temporal lobe.
gamma-aminobutyric acid (GABA)	An inhibitory neurotransmitter.
GABA	*See* gamma-aminobutyric acid.
generalized anxiety disorder (GAD)	Anxiety neurosis; characterized by unrealistic or excessive anxiety, apprehensive expectations, and worry about many life circumstances (e.g., occupational, academic, athletic, or social performance). A mother may worry endlessly about her child, who is in no danger. The worry is associated with symptoms such as trembling, muscle tension, restlessness, feelings of being smothered, light-headedness, insomnia, exaggerated startle response, or difficulty in concentrating. The worrying is difficult to control, and, with the associated symptoms, often social or occupational functioning is impaired. When it occurs in childhood or adolescence, GAD is termed *overanxious disorder* by some. Symptoms include multiple, unrealistic anxieties concerning the quality of one's performance in school, at work, or in sports, and of one's health or appearance, accompanied by the need to be reassured.
geniculocalcarine tract	Bundle of nerve fibers carrying visual sensation from the lateral geniculate bodies (see Figure A–20) to the occipital cortex.
Gestalt	German word meaning "the wholeness of a thing"; also applied to a particular school of psychology.
giant cell arteritis	Type of inflammation of the arteries.
globus pallidus	Inner (medial) part of the lentiform nucleus.
glucose intolerance	Tendency to develop abnormally high blood glucose after eating sugar.

glutamic acid

Amino acid involved in many biochemical processes, which also serves as a neurotransmitter.

gray matter

Parts of the brain consisting mainly of nerve cell bodies, as opposed to white matter, which contains the nerve cell processes.

gyrus

Bulge of the cortex.

habenula

Bundle of nerve fibers connecting the pineal body with the back of the thalamus.

half-life

A measure of speed and duration of action of a drug, defined by the length of time it takes for half the dose taken to be used up by the body.

hallucination

A sensory perception in the absence of an actual external stimulus; to be distinguished from an illusion, which is a misperception or misinterpretation of an external stimulus. Hallucinations may involve any of the senses (i.e., auditory, olfactory, somatic, tactile, visual).

Hawthorne effect

Improvement in performance resulting from knowledge that methods to improve performance are being tried.

HDL

See high-density lipoprotein.

health maintenance organization (HMO)

A form of group practice by physicians and supporting personnel to provide comprehensive health services to an enrolled group of subscribers who pay a fixed premium (capitation fee) to belong. Emphasis is on maintaining the health of the enrollees as well as treating their illnesses. HMOs must include psychiatric benefits to receive federal support.

hemianopsia

Loss of vision for one-half of the visual field of one or both eyes.

hemiparesis

Weakness, not amounting to complete paralysis, of one side of the body.

hemiplegia

Paralysis of one side of the body.

Heschl's area (gyrus) — Area of upper surface of the temporal lobe cortex concerned with hearing (see Figure 6–3).

high-density lipoprotein (HDL) — The "good cholesterol."

hippocampus — Set of intermingled layers of nerve cells and fibers within the temporal lobe (see Figures A–2 and A–9).

histological — Relating to the study of tissues under the microscope.

HMO — *See* health maintenance organization.

homonymous hemianopsia — Inability to see objects in half of the field of vision, affecting both eyes.

5-hydroxytryptamine — Serotonin.

hypercholesterolemia — High blood cholesterol.

hyperpathic akinetic mutism — Condition in which the patient is mute and immobile but awake and alert. Coma vigil; vigilant coma.

hypogastric plexus — Part of the sympathetic nervous system in the lower abdomen.

hypothalamus — The complex brain structure composed of many nuclei with various functions. It is the head ganglion of the autonomic nervous system (see Figure A–15) and is involved in the control of heat regulation; heart rate, blood pressure, and respiration; sexual activity; water, fat, and carbohydrate metabolism; digestion, appetite, and body weight; wakefulness; fight-or-flight response; and rage.

hysteria — Mental disorder, no longer in official nomenclatures, consisting of imaginary physical ailments and self-dramatization.

ICD-10 — Tenth revision of the *International Classification of Diseases and Related Health Problems* of the World Health Organization.

idiopathic

Of unknown cause.

inert gas

Gaseous element that cannot combine with other elements.

infarct

Tissue killed by having its blood supply blocked.

infarction

Process of blood-supply blockage whereby tissue is killed.

inferior longitudinal fasciculus

Inferior longitudinal bundle. Tract of nerve fibers running from visual reception centers in the occipital lobe forward to the parietal lobe.

inhibitory amino acid

Amino acid (e.g., GABA, glycine) that acts as an inhibitory neurotransmitter.

insight-oriented therapy

Psychotherapy consisting of talking to get the patient to understand the cause of an emotional problem.

intermittent claudication

Pain in the legs that increases with exercise.

internal capsule

Vertically running nerve fibers (white matter) deep inside the brain (see Figures A–3 and A–10). The lentiform nucleus is medial to the internal capsule. The thalamus and head of the the caudate nucleus are lateral to it. The front part (anterior limb) carries motor impulses downward and the back part (posterior limb) brings sensation upward. The part in between is called the *genu.*

International Classification of Diseases (ICD)

The official list of disease categories issued by the World Health Organization; subscribed to by all member nations, who may assign their own terms to each ICD category. The ICDA (*International Classifications of Diseases,* U.S. Public Health Service adaptation) represents the official list of diagnostic terms to be used for each ICD category in the United States.

intralaminar nuclei of the thalamus

Masses of gray matter lying within an area of white matter inside the thalamus.

intracranial

Inside the skull.

ischemia

Lack of blood supply.

ischemic

Suffering from ischemia.

Jacksonian

Relating to a type of epilepsy described by Hughlings Jackson, and also to his teachings about the hierarchal organization of the nervous system.

Joint Commission on Accreditation of Healthcare Organizations (JCAHO)

Formerly Joint Commission on Accreditation of Hospitals (JCAH); the agency that surveys hospitals and other health facilities and programs and certifies that they have met the standards set by the Joint Commission.

kana

Japanese characters that represent sounds, as in European alphabets.

kanji

Japanese characters that represent concepts, as in the Chinese alphabet.

Korsakoff-type amnesia

Memory disorder associated with Korsakoff's syndrome, characteristically accompanied by confabulation and not by dementia.

late paraphrenia

Condition with paranoid delusions occurring late in life. The relationship to schizophrenia and to dementia is controversial.

lateral

Lying to the left if in the left half of the body, or to the right if in the right half of the body.

lateral geniculate bodies

Group of nerve cells in the back of the thalamus that receive visual sensations from the optic tracts and pass them along in the optic radiation to the occipital cortex (see Figures A–14 and A–20).

lateral lemniscus

Bundle of nerve fibers carrying hearing sensation from the cochlear nuclei to the back of the midbrain *(inferior colliculus)* (see Figure 6–4).

lateral medullary syndrome	Type of stroke affecting the cerebellum and lower cranial nerves. Wallenberg's syndrome; posterior inferior cerebellar artery syndrome.
lateral ventricle	Fluid-filled space within the brain (see Figure A–2).
legal guardian	Person appointed by law to supervise someone and act on his or her behalf.
lenticular nucleus	Lentiform nucleus.
lenticulostriate arteries of Charcot	Central perforating arteries arising from the middle cerebral artery and supplying the basal ganglia, thalamus, and internal capsule (see Figure A–10).
lentiform nucleus	Mass of gray matter (nerve cells) deep in the brain, comprising the putamen and globus pallidus, and forming part of the basal ganglia and corpus striatum. Probably concerned with regulating control of motor activity (see Figures A–3, A–10, and A–11).
lesion	Localized tissue disease or damage from any cause, whether tumor, injury, infection, or infarction.
lexical-phonological	Having to do with the sound and appearance of words rather than the understanding of their use and meaning.
libidinal energy	A motivating force for human actions assumed in Freud's early theories.
libido	The psychic drive or energy usually associated with the sexual instinct. (Sexual is used here in the broad sense to include pleasure and love-object seeking.)
limbic system	Visceral brain; a group of brain structures— including the amygdala, hippocampus, septum, cingulate gyrus, and subcallosal gyrus—that work to help regulate emotion, memory, and certain aspects of movement.

lingual gyrus	Part of the occipital cortex.
lipophilic	Able to combine with or dissolve in fat.
living will	Procedure by which competent persons can, under certain circumstances, direct their physicians to treat them in a prescribed way if they become incompetent (e.g., withdraw lifesaving medical care if in a vegetative state).
locus coeruleus	A small area in the brain stem containing norepinephrine neurons that is considered to be a key brain center for anxiety and fear (see Figure A–22).
longitudinal (spin-lattice) relaxation time	Kind of MRI scan, commonly known as T_1, in which fluid and gray matter look dark and white matter looks white.
long-term potentiation	Process whereby practice increases the ease of passage of a nerve impulse across a synapse.
love-object	In psychoanalytic theory, anything outside the body that is invested with strong feelings.
lower motor neuron	Neuron extending outside the central nervous system and connecting with muscle.
magnetic resonance imaging (MRI)	Technique for showing anatomic structures that involves placing subjects in a strong magnetic field and then, by use of magnetic gradients and brief radio frequency pulses, determining the resonance characteristics at each point in the area to be studied. Used to detect structural or anatomic abnormalities; it is better able to differentiate between gray and white matter than is computed tomography.
mammillary body	Group of nerve cells in the lower part of the hypothalamus (see Figure A–16).
mammillothalamic tract	Bundle of nerve fibers connecting the mammillary body with the anterior nucleus of the thalamus (see Figure A–16).

mania	Bipolar disorder; a mood disorder characterized by excessive elation, inflated self-esteem and grandiosity, hyperactivity, agitation, and accelerated thinking and speaking. Flight of ideas may be present. A manic syndrome may also occur in organic mental disorders.
medial	Toward the midline; that is, left of anything on the right side of the body or right of anything on the left side of the body.
medial forebrain bundle	Bundle of nerve fibers connecting the hypo-thalamus with several other parts of the brain (see Figure A–17).
medial lemniscus	Vertically running bundle of nerve fibers (white matter) bringing sensation up from the spinal cord to the thalamus.
Medicaid	Government program for paying for medical care for the poor.
mesial	Looking at the inner surface of the sagittally split brain; in the middle.
middle cerebral artery	Branch of the internal carotid artery (see Figures A–10, A–24, and A–25).
minimum data set	Records on each nursing-home patient required by the government under the Omnibus Budget Reconciliation Act of 1987 (OBRA '87).
mitral valve prolapse	Abnormal condition of a heart valve that may be asymptomatic.
monoamine oxidase inhibitor (MAOI)	A group of antidepressant drugs that inhibit the enzyme monoamine oxidase (MAO) in the brain and raise the levels of biogenic amines.
MRI	*See* magnetic resonance imaging.
myelin	Fatty sheath surrounding nerve fiber.
myocardial infarction	Death of heart muscle due to obstruction of blood supply.

N-methyl-D-aspartate (NMDA)	An agonist for one type of receptor on nerve cells.
narcissism	Self-love as opposed to object-love (love of another person). In classical psychoanalytic theory, cathexis (investment) of the psychic representation of the self with libido (sexual interest and energy). An excess of narcissism interferes with relations with others. To be distinguished from egotism, which carries the connotation of self-centeredness, selfishness, and conceit. Egotism is but one expression of narcissism. Recent revisions in psychoanalytic theory (self psychology) have viewed the concept of narcissism in less pathological terms.
nerve cell	Cell with ability to receive and emit nerve impulses. Identical with *neuron,* except that it is sometimes used for the nerve cell body rather than its processes.
nerve fiber	Long process of a nerve cell. Usually an axon.
nervi erigentes	Autonomic nerves in the lower abdomen.
neuropsychiatry	Medical specialty that combines neurology and psychiatry, emphasizing the somatic substructure on which emotions are based and the organic disturbances of the central nervous system that give rise to mental disorders.
neuropsychology	Branch of psychology concerned with the structure of the brain and with testing brain function.
NMDA receptor	A type of receptor in the nerve cell wall.
nondominant	Used neurologically for the right hand and left cerebral hemisphere of a left-handed person and the left hand and right cerebral hemisphere of a right-handed one.
nonsignificant trend	Difference between two values that might be attributable to chance.

noradrenergic

Influenced by the neurotransmitter norepi-nephrine.

norepinephrine

A catecholamine neurotransmitter related to epinephrine found in both the peripheral and the central nervous systems. Functional ex-cesses in the brain have been implicated in the pathogenesis of manic states; and functional deficits, in certain depressive states. Also called *noradrenaline*.

nucleus basalis

Mass of gray matter lateral to the front of the hypothalamus (see Figure A–4).

nucleus of Meynert

Nucleus basalis.

nurse's aide

Person with on-the-job training providing patient care.

nursing home

Nursing facility providing long-term or convales-cent care.

OBRA '87

See Omnibus Budget Reconciliation Act of 1987.

obsessive-compulsive neurosis

Persistent intrusion of unwanted and un-controllable ego-dystonic thoughts, urges, or actions. The thoughts may consist of single words, ruminations, or trains of thought that are seen as nonsensical. The actions may vary from simple movements to complex rituals such as repeated hand washing. Referred to as *obsessive-compulsive disorder* in DSM-III-R and DSM-IV.

occipital cortex

Cortex of the occipital lobe.

occipital lobe

Back part of the cerebrum (see Figure A–5).

occupational therapist

Therapist qualified to treat by supervised activities in order to restore function.

oculomotor nerve

Cranial nerve controlling movements of the eye and contraction of the pupil. Third nerve (see Figure A–19).

Omnibus Budget Reconciliation Act of 1987 (OBRA '87)	Act that established new government regulations for nursing homes.
opioids	Group of drugs, originally derived from opium, resembling morphine in their effects.
optic radiation	Bundle of nerve fibers leading from the lateral geniculate body to the occipital cortex.
optic tract	Bundle of nerve fibers leading from the optic chiasma to the lateral geniculate body.
orbital area	Undersurface of the frontal lobe, overlying the orbit of the eye.
organic personality syndrome	A DSM-III-R diagnosis for certain changes due to organic brain damage; included in DSM-IV as "personality change due to a general medical condition."
OTC	*See* over the counter.
over the counter (OTC)	Descriptor applied to medication for which no prescription is needed.
paradigm	Typical example.
parahippocampus	Part of the temporal lobe near the hippocampus.
paranoia	A condition characterized by the gradual development of an intricate, complex, and elaborate system of thinking based on (and often proceeding logically from) misinterpretation of an actual event. A person with paranoia often considers himself or herself endowed with unique and superior ability. Despite its chronic course, this condition does not seem to interfere with thinking and personality. To be distinguished from *schizophrenia, paranoid type.*

parasympathetic nervous system	The part of the autonomic nervous system that controls the life-sustaining organs of the body under normal, danger-free conditions and that is mediated by acetylcholine.
parenchymal	Within the substance of the brain.
parietal lobe	Part of the cerebrum behind the frontal lobe, in front of the occipital lobe, and above the temporal lobe (see Figure A–5).
parkinsonism (Parkinson's disease, *paralysis agitans*)	One of the medication-induced movement disorders, characterized by rapid, coarse tremor; muscular rigidity; or akinesia, developing within a few weeks of starting or raising the dose of neuroleptic medication or of reducing medication used to treat extrapyramidal symptoms.
passive-aggressive personality disorder	Personality disorder cited in older literature and characterized by unassertive resistance and general obstructiveness in response to the expectations of others. Manifestations include procrastination; postponement of completion of routine tasks; sulkiness, irritability, or argumentativeness if asked to do something one does not want to do, and then working unreasonably slowly and inefficiently; or avoidance of obligations by claiming to have forgotten them.
Patient Self-Determination Act of 1991	An act legalizing living wills and advance directives.
pelvic floor	The muscles and ligaments supporting the bladder.
perimeter	Instrument for measuring visual fields.
peripheral sense organ	Organ of sight, hearing, touch, or smell.
peripheral vascular disease	Disease blocking flow of blood to the limbs.

periventricular	Around the fluid-filled central cavities of the brain.
phantom boarder	Delusional belief that uninvited guests have taken up residence in one's home.
phenothiazine derivatives	Neuroleptic subgroup of psychotropic drugs that, chemically, have in common a phenothiazine configuration (i.e., phenyl rings and a heterocyclic ring containing nitrogen and sulfur) but differ from one another through variations in side chains.
photon	Smallest possible quantity of light or other electromagnetic radiation.
physical therapist	Person qualified to treat disease of muscles, nerves, and bones by methods other than medication or surgery.
placebo effect	The production or enhancement of psychological or physical effects using pharmacologically inactive substances administered under circumstances in which suggestion leads the subject to believe that a particular effect will occur.
plain X ray	X ray taken without use of dye injected into the patient.
planum temporale	An area on the upper surface of the temporal lobe.
polycythemia	Abnormally increased number of red blood cells.
pontine	Having to do with the pons, the part of the brain stem above the medulla, below the midbrain, and in front of the cerebellum.
postcentral gyrus	Part of the cortex behind the central sulcus (see Figure A–6).

posterior cerebral artery	Branch of the basilar artery supplying the back of the cerebrum (see Figures A–24, A–25, and A–26).
posterior communicating artery	Artery connecting the carotid artery with the posterior cerebral artery and forming part of the circle of Willis (see Figure A–26).
posterior inferior cerebellar artery	Branch of the vertebral artery supplying the lower part of the brain (see Figure A–26).
posttraumatic stress disorder	Anxiety symptoms resulting from severe emotional stress.
power of attorney	Ability to act legally on someone's behalf.
power requirements	Number of experimental subjects needed to avoid a type II error.
PPO	*See* preferred provider organization.
preferred provider organization (PPO)	Type of HMO with a loose affiliation between providers rather than a central controlling authority.
prefrontal areas	Parts of the frontal lobe in front of the precentral gyrus.
present	Verb, in a medical context, that refers to the signs and symptoms that the patient brings to first medical exam.
progesterone	A female sex hormone.
prognosis	Probable outcome of an illness.
projection	A defense mechanism, operating unconsciously, in which what is emotionally unacceptable in the self is unconsciously rejected and attributed (projected) to others.
prosopagnosia	Inability to recognize familiar faces that is not explained by defective visual acuity or reduced consciousness or alertness.

proton   Subatomic particle.

provincial hospital   Canadian equivalent of an American state hospital.

psychodynamics   The systematized knowledge and theory of human behavior and its motivation, the study of which depends largely on the functional significance of emotion. Psychodynamics recognizes the role of unconscious motivation in human behavior. The science of psychodynamics assumes that one's behavior is determined by past experience, genetic endowment, and current reality.

psychomotor epilepsy   Complex partial seizures. Sometimes equated with temporal lobe epilepsy.

psychosis   A severe mental disorder characterized by gross impairment in reality testing, typically manifested by delusions, hallucinations, disorganized speech, or disorganized or catatonic behavior. Persons with these disorders are termed *psychotic*. Among these illnesses are schizophrenia, delusional disorders, some secondary or symptomatic disorders ("organic psychoses"), and some mood disorders.

pulmonary embolism   Blockage of the pulmonary artery by a blood clot dislodged from a vein.

pupillary reflexes   Contraction of the pupil of the eye in response to light or to see nearby objects.

quality assurance   Activities and programs intended to ensure the standard of care in a defined medical setting or program; such programs must include educational components intended to remedy identified deficiencies in quality.

random	A statistical term that denotes accuracy by chance or without attention to selection or planning. For example, a random sample is a group of subjects selected in such a way that each member of the population from which the sample is derived has an equal or known chance (i.e., probability) of being chosen for the sample.
randomize	Ensure that there is no bias in selection.
rarefaction	Term used in neuroradiology to denote a brain area in which the amount of solid tissue is diminished.
receptor	Specialized area on a nerve membrane, a blood vessel, or a muscle that receives the chemical stimulation that activates or inhibits the nerve, blood vessel, or muscle.
recreational therapist	Person qualified to treat patients by training and encouragement in recreations.
reflex	Involuntary action produced automatically by a stimulus.
renin	Enzyme produced by the kidney causing hypertension.
representative payee	Person allowed to receive Social Security payments on behalf of a patient.
reticular formation	Areas of intermixed gray and white matter in the brain stem; probably concerned with maintenance of consciousness (see Figure A–12).
reversible ischemic neurological defect (RIND)	An interruption of the blood supply to the brain, causing clinical effects lasting longer than those of a TIA, but not resulting in a brain infarct.
rhizotomy	Surgical cutting of the dorsal nerve roots bring sensation to the spinal cord.
RIND	*See* reversible ischemic neurological defect.

sagittal section	Section made by a vertical cut from front to back.
schizophrenia	A group of idiopathic psychotic disorders characterized by both positive and negative symptoms associated with disturbance in one or more major areas of functioning, such as work, academic development or achievement, interpersonal relations, and self-care. Positive symptoms include delusions, which may be bizarre in nature; hallucinations, especially auditory; disorganized speech; inappropriate affect; and disorganized behavior. Negative symptoms include flat affect, avolition, alogia, and anhedonia. Duration is variable: ICD-10 requires that continuous signs of the disturbance persist for at least 1 month; DSM-IV requires a minimum of 6 months.
scotoma	Blind spot.
secondary gain	Advantage produced by an illness.
selectivity	Specificity.
semantic	Concerned with the meaning of words and sentences.
sensitivity	Ability to pick out cases of a condition without excluding true positives; specificity.
serotonin	A neurotransmitter with an indole structure found in both peripheral ganglia and the central nervous system. Its transmitter functions in the central nervous system are less clearly demonstrable than in the gastrointestinal tract. It is implicated indirectly in the psychobiology of depression. Also called *5-hydroxytryptamine*.
serum osmolality	Concentration of dissolved substance in the blood.
sickle cell anemia	Inherited blood disease.
sign	Objective evidence of a disease or disorder.

significant	Unlikely to be due to chance.
Social Security	Federal government pension given to people who are elderly or permanently disabled.
somnolent akinetic mutism	Condition in which the patient is mute and immobile and is not fully alert; also called *apathetic mutism.*
special investigations	Medical tests, such as X rays or blood tests, needing special equipment and not readily performed at the bedside.
specificity	Ability to pick out cases of a condition without including false positives.
spinothalamic tract	Bundle of nerve fibers conveying sensation from the spine to the brain.
spongiform encephalopathy	Brain disease causing microscopically evident spaces between the nerve and glial cells.
state hospital	Large mental hospital run by a state government.
status epilepticus	Continuous epileptic seizures.
straitjacket	Robe used for restraining violent mental patients.
stria terminalis	Bundle of white matter in the floor of the lateral ventricle (see Figure A–17).
subarachnoid	Between the surface of the brain and its covering membranes.
subcortical	Below the cerebral cortex.
substantia nigra	Group of dark nerve cells in the midbrain (see Figures A–18 and A–21).
subthalamic nucleus	Group of nerve cells below the thalamus. Corpus luysii; body of Luys.
supramarginal gyrus	Part of the parietal cortex, near the junction of the frontal, parietal, and temporal lobes and in front of the angular gyrus (see Figure A–8).

supratentorial	In the upper part of the skull.
Sylvian fissure	Fissure separating the temporal lobe from the frontal lobe. Also called *lateral sulcus* and *fissure of Sylvius* (see Figure A–7).
sympathetic nervous system	The part of the autonomic nervous system that responds to dangerous or threatening situations by preparing a person physiologically for "fight or flight."
sympatholytic	Antagonizing the actions of norepinephrine and epinephrine.
sympathomimetic	Producing actions similar to those of the sympathetic nervous system.
synaptic	Relating to the junctions between nerve cells.
syncope	Short sudden spell of unconsciousness.
syndrome	A configuration of symptoms that occur together and that constitute a recognizable condition.
synergy	Increased effectiveness produced by the combining of actions.
systemic lupus erythematosus	Collagen disease affecting the heart, lungs, skin, and kidneys.
systolic blood pressure	The highest blood pressure reached during a heartbeat.
Tarasoff rule	Based on the 1976 California decision *Tarasoff v. Regents of the University of California,* this landmark opinion held that when a patient presents a serious danger of violence to a foreseeable victim, the psychotherapist of that patient has a duty to use reasonable care to protect the intended victim against such danger. No fewer than 30 jurisdictions have issued a ruling or statute involving some variation of the *Tarasoff* "duty to protect" doctrine.

tardive dyskinesia, neuroleptic-induced	A medication-induced movement disorder consisting of involuntary choreiform, athetoid, or rhythmic movements of the tongue, jaw, or extremities developing with long-term use (usually a few months or more) of neuroleptic medication.
Tax Equity and Fiscal Responsibility Act (TEFRA)	Act limiting Medicare payments by establishing diagnosis-related groups.
temporal lobe	Part of the cerebrum below the parietal and frontal lobes and in front of the occipital lobe (see Figure A–5).
temporal lobe epilepsy	Seizure disorder originating in the temporal lobe. The seizures may take the form of complex partial seizures or psychomotor epilepsy.
testamentary capacity	Pertains to the state of mind of an individual at the time he or she writes or executes his or her will. Generally, to have sufficient testamentary capacity, testators must possess a certain level of understanding of the nature and extent of their property, of the persons who are the natural objects of their bounty, and of the disposition that they are making of their property, and must appreciate these elements in relation to each other and form an orderly desire as to the disposition of their property.
thalamus	Area of gray matter deep in the brain, behind the head of the caudate nucleus, that receives sensation from all parts of the body (see Figures A–13 and A–14).
third nerve	Oculomotor nerve (q.v.).
third-party payer	Payer of medical expenses other than the patient, usually an insurance company.
thrombus	Mass of coagulated blood.
transduce	Transform from one kind of action to another.

transverse section	Section cut horizontally.
transverse spin-spin relaxation time	Kind of MRI scan commonly known as T_2, where fluid and gray matter look light and white matter looks dark.
trazodone	Antidepressant drug; trade name is Desyrel.
tricyclic antidepressant	Class of antidepressant drugs that includes imipramine (Tofranil) and amitriptyline (Elavil).
two-point discrimination	Ability to tell whether one is being touched in only one place or in two places close together.
upper motor neuron	Neuron or chain of neurons originating in the brain and connecting with the lower motor neuron.
validity	Ability to truly measure or predict.
vascular	Concerned with the arteries or veins.
vasculitis	Inflammation of arteries or veins.
vasculogenic	Due to the condition of the arteries or veins.
vasogenic	Due to artery dilation.
vasovagal	Due to action of the parasympathetic nervous system on the cardiovascular system.
ventral lateral nucleus	Part of the thalamus that probably receives impulses from the basal ganglia and cerebellum and passes them to the motor cortex. Also called *ventrolateral nucleus of the thalamus* (see Figure A–14).
ventricular hypertrophy	Enlargement of the heart.
ventrolateral nucleus of the thalamus	Ventral lateral nucleus.
vertebral artery	Artery that enters the skull from the neck and then joins with the vertebral artery of the opposite side to form the basilar artery (see Figures A–24 and A–26).

vertebrobasilar	Referring to the vertebral and basilar arteries and their branches.
vertigo	Sensation that the external world is spinning around; a symptom of vestibular dysfunction.
vigilant coma	Condition in which the patient seems alert but does not move or speak. Hyperpathic akinetic mutism; coma vigil.
visual field	Area that can be seen without moving the eyes.
visual field defect	Restriction of the visual field.
Wallenberg's syndrome	Posterior inferior cerebellar artery syndrome; lateral medullary syndrome.
Wernicke's aphasia	Loss of the ability to comprehend language coupled with production of inappropriate language.
Wernicke-Korsakoff syndrome	A disease of central nervous system metabolism due to a lack of vitamin B_1 (thiamine) seen in chronic alcoholism. Wernicke's disease features irregularities of eye movements, incoordination, impaired thinking, and often sensorimotor deficits. Korsakoff's syndrome is characterized by confabulation and, more importantly, by a short-term, but not immediate, disturbance that leads to gross impairment in memory and learning. Wernicke's disease and Korsakoff's psychosis begin suddenly and are often found in the same person simultaneously.
white matter	Parts of the brain composed of nerve cell fibers, as opposed to nerve cell bodies.

Index

*Page numbers in **boldface** type refer to figures or tables.*